D1593746

# Women's Health after Abortion

## The Medical and Psychological Evidence

Second Edition

### Elizabeth Ring-Cassidy
### Ian Gentles

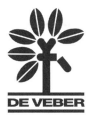

DE VEBER

The deVeber Institute for Bioethics and Social Research

Copyright © 2003 by Elizabeth Ring-Cassidy and Ian Gentles

All rights reserved. No part of this book may be reproduced, transmitted in any form or by any means, electronic, mechanical, photocopying, recording, or otherwise, or stored in a retrieval system, without written permission from the publisher, except by a reviewer who may quote brief passages in a review.

First published in 2002 by
The deVeber Institute for Bioethics and Social Research
3089 Bathurst Street, Suite 316
Toronto, Ontario, Canada
M6A 2A4

www.deveber.org

National Library of Canada Cataloguing in Publication Data


Ring-Cassidy, Elizabeth, 1948-
        Women's health after abortion : the medical and psychological
        evidence / Elizabeth Ring-Cassidy, Ian Gentles. -- 2nd ed.


Includes bibliographical references and index.
ISBN 0-920453-24-4


1. Abortion—Complications.  2. Abortion—Psychological aspects.
3. Women—Health and hygiene.  I. Gentles, Ian  II. deVeber Institute for
Bioethics and Social Research  III. Title.

RG734.R55 2003              618.8'8              C2003-904531-5

Printed in Canada

# Contents

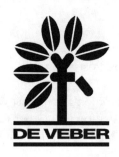

# Preface to the Second Edition

The response to the first edition of this book has been gratifying. We have taken the opportunity of a new edition to make corrections, and update the material in Chapters Two and Four in the light of new research. We owe a great debt of gratitude to many individuals, especially Dr Deborah Zeni for her expert advice and assistance.

September 2003

# Preface to the First Edition

In 1985 the de Veber Institute's predecessor, the Human Life Research Institute, published *Abortion's Aftermath*, an examination of the physical complications and psychological sequelae of induced abortion. Heavy demand resulted in a second edition two years later, which was also well received. In the intervening years there have been many hundreds of studies published, so that our knowledge of the after-effects of abortion is much more extensive than it was in the 1980s. At the same time abortion research has become politicized as never before, and barriers have been raised against the full disclosure to the public – women in particular – of the negative sequelae of abortion.

This book has been written to make available to women and medical personnel new information about the complications of a medical procedure that is undergone by many hundreds of thousands of women in North America each year. Our aim is also to assist all those who are struggling to clarify for themselves the numerous health issues surrounding abortion.

*i*

Much of the material in this book is necessarily scientific and technical. To enhance the book's accessibility to non-medical people we have included a Glossary at the end. In each chapter, the first appearance of a term listed in the Glossary is signalled by the use of italics. For the same reason our referencing style is modified from the practice found in most scientific journals. Full titles of journals, rather than abbreviations, are used, for example, and page numbers are given for quotations.

The boxed quotations that appear in various places throughout the book are taken from the de Veber Institute's questionnaire to physicians across Canada. Entitled the *Survey of Canadian Physicians on Women's Health after Induced Abortion*, it reports the results of questions to doctors about abortion sequelae that they have treated in their practices.

The book falls into two parts. Chapters 1 to 10 deal with the physical or medical consequences, or sequelae, of abortion. Chapters 11 to 16 deal with the psychological consequences. Chapter 17 is an outline of the methodological problems that plague much of the research on induced abortion. Chapter 18 discusses the ethical and legal obligations of medical professionals to provide up-to-date information to patients seeking abortion about the documented risks associated with the procedure.

*Women's Health after Abortion: The Medical and Psychological Evidence* could not have been completed without the active assistance of Dr Will Johnston, Dr Heather Morris, Professors Keith Cassidy and Barrie deVeber, Dr Bridget Campion, Lori Cavanagh, Martha Crean, Bob Fowler, Alan Fujiwara, Barry Jamieson, Jane Hodgins, Denyse O'Leary, Brent Rooney, and Bambi Rutledge. We also owe an immense debt of gratitude to the many friends of the Institute who have contributed generously to the research and publication costs of this study.

# Introduction

It is widely thought that induced abortion is safe and almost risk free. Yet recent research indicates that the procedure carries with it clear hazards to women's physical and psychological health. The findings presented in this study raise the thorny issues of women's right to informed consent – something that is not realizable if all the potential risks of the medical procedure in question are not made known to the patient.

We also alert readers to areas of controversy so that they can make up their own minds in the light of the best current knowledge. Unfortunately there exist elements within the research and medical establishments for whom the paramount consideration appears to be to preserve the image of abortion as simple, safe and easily available to women. Consequently they have been strongly critical of recent studies which make it unmistakably clear that after an abortion a woman is at a much greater risk of breast cancer and a host of other medical complications, as well as ongoing emotional distress. Ironically, research from countries with liberal abortion laws, such as Sweden, Finland and Denmark, offers candid acknowledgement of risks that induced abortion poses to women's physical and psychological health.

Our goals in this book are twofold: first, to inform women who may be contemplating an abortion and the medical professionals who care for them; second, to encourage the North-American medical research establishments to re-examine their existing assumptions about the effects of abortion on women's health, keeping uppermost in their

1

minds the present and future health and well-being of all women dealing with pregnancy.

*Women's Health after Abortion* is based on over 500 articles that have appeared in medical and other journals, chiefly during the past twenty years. Much of the information has been extracted from papers whose primary focus was not abortion. Some of the consequences of abortion do not surface until long after the procedure, or, as in the case of infertility, remain undetected until the woman wishes to bear a child. Yet at present many studies rely on short-term findings; furthermore, researchers often minimize the significance of their findings, and sometimes even arrive at conclusions that flatly contradict their data. The difficulties surrounding the study of abortion have only increased with the dramatic rise over the past decade in the number of procedures performed in clinics, where follow-up of patients is minimal or non- existent. Nonetheless, what research there is, shows that abortion is the source of serious physical and psychological problems for a significant number of women.

The medical risks include ectopic pregnancy, which has risen disturbingly during the period since abortion was legalized. Other risks include uterine perforation, uterine adhesions, and pelvic inflammatory disease (PID). The latter condition is now epidemic in North America, and commonly results in infertility. There is also valid reason for thinking that maternal mortality from abortion is generally underreported in Canada and the U.S. There is increasing evidence too, of a link between abortion and subsequent cancers of the reproductive system, as well as colorectal cancer. Over the past 40 years, there has been overwhelming evidence of a strong link between abortion and the incidence of breast cancer among women. Despite the fact that the evidence has been virtually ignored by much of the research establishment in North America, it has been recognized in Europe, where the Royal College of Obstetricians and Gynaecologists in Britain has recently acknowledged that induced abortion increases the risk of breast cancer.

Among abortion's psychological effects are depression, guilt and low self-esteem. Many women feel pressured into abortion by men. Women who undergo abortions – adolescents in particular – experience a much higher rate of suicide than those who don't. Abortion can also have a devastating impact on existing children in a family whose parents decide to abort a pregnancy. For some men abortion can also be an experience of grief and powerlessness. Finally, it is well established that abortion results in the deterioration of relationships between women and those who are close to them.

Information that we have discovered, and which we present in this book, has frequently been downplayed or even omitted from the discussion or conclusion sections of the papers written by those who came up with the data in the first place. The subject is also bedeviled by the way hospitals report patients' diseases or disorders (coding), and also because the diagnosis is not always correct at the time of discharge. Accordingly, the actual incidence of ill effects, while significant, is still not fully known. Evidence, however, continues to flow in confirming the substantial risks attached to abortion.

In a recent study sponsored by the College of Physicians and Surgeons of Ontario, a comparison was made between 41,039 women who had induced abortions and a similar number who did not undergo induced abortions. The study only concerned itself with short-term consequences, but in the three-month period after the abortion, the hospital patients had a more than four-times higher rate of hospitalizations for infections (6.3 vs. 1.4 per 1000), a five-times higher rate of "surgical events" (8.2 vs 1.6 per 1000), and a nearly five times higher rate of hospitalization for psychiatric problems (5.2 vs. 1.1 per 1000), than the matching group of women who had not had abortions. The community clinic patients fared somewhat better, but the authors cautioned that the clinics "cannot easily follow the medium-term outcomes subsequent to the services they provide".[1]

As the second edition was being prepared for the press, one more study by Reardon and colleagues appeared in the

*Canadian Medical Association Journal,* showing a significantly higher risk of psychiatric admissions among low-income women who have an induced abortion than among those who carry a pregnancy to term. In the face of the number of letters criticizing this study, the *CMAJ* editors penned a strongly worded editorial defending the integrity of the research and stressing the importance of publishing controversial papers whose conclusions may challenge the preconceptions of some of its readers.[2]

A key question raised by our book is, do women have the right to be informed about the physical and psychological risks of abortion? Will doctors be liable to prosecution if they fail to alert their patients to the documented risks associated with induced abortion? We are convinced that the increased risks associated with induced abortion are serious enough to merit dissemination beyond the pages of professional journals. If there is a right to choose, there is also a right to know. Without accurate, up-to-date knowledge, how can informed consent be given in any meaningful sense?

**Notes**

1    Ostbye T, Wenghofer EF, Woodward CA, Gold G, Craighead J. Health services utilization after induced abortions in Ontario: A comparison between community clinics and hospitals. American Journal of Medical Quality 2001 May;6(3):99-106. See Table 3, p. 103, and p. 105.

2(a) Reardon DC, Cougle JR, Rue, VM, Shupping MW, Coleman PK, Ney PG. Psychiatric admissions of low-income women following abortion and childbirth. Canadian Medical Association Journal 2003 May 13;168(10):1253-1256.

2(b)  Editorial. Unwanted results: the ethics of controversial research. CMAJ 2003 July 22;169(2):93.

Chapter 1

# Research on Post-Abortion Complications: An Overview

Induced abortion has been widely used and accepted in North America since the 1970s. In the U.S. the number of abortions rose steadily from 1967 to reach a peak of over 1.5 million in the early 1990s. Since that time the numbers have declined to about 1.3 million annually. In Canada the induced abortion rate has remained steady at about 120,000 per year for the past decade. All together this means that tens of millions of women in North America have now experienced induced abortion. Nevertheless, the reporting of the effects of this widespread procedure on women's health is either neglected or tends to be limited to short-term complications. By contrast, studies from other countries reveal many of the problems women may experience after an abortion, such as *pelvic inflammatory disease (PID), ectopic pregnancies, endometritis*, and other infections. The question arises: Are abortion services more efficient in Canada and the United States or does North-American research methodology miss many complications by relying only on short-term follow up and incomplete coding?

The lifelong risks of repeat, induced, and late-term abortions on women's health are not being addressed in the research literature, and further studies need to be done on the long-term effects of abortion, including a probable link to breast cancer. It seems clear that if women are going to give "informed consent" to an abortion, they should be made aware of the possible consequences of the procedure to their present and future health. It is likely that women are not being made aware of these risks in most abortion facilities in North America.

# Research on Post-Abortion Complications

With about 120,000 induced abortions a year in Canada and 1.3 million in the United States, the health of a significant number of women is affected. What is the impact of this procedure and of the numerous complications that can occur?

## Limitations in the Available Literature

It must be recognized at the outset that there are serious problems with the validity of much research on the physical after-effects of abortion on women:

### 1. Short-term Follow Up

In the first place, the reporting of medical sequelae tends to be based on very short-term findings. Longer-term follow up uncovers issues that would not be discovered immediately, such as infertility, which might not surface until the woman wishes to carry a pregnancy to term, perhaps as long as a decade after the abortion.

However, both Canada and the United States have seen a dramatic increase in the number of abortions occurring in clinics where follow up is negligible. For example, in studies such as one by Ferris and colleagues, which looked at post-abortion complications in Canadian abortion clinics and hospitals, 98.9 per cent of the women had day surgery.[1] The follow up was limited to the few hours after the procedure. Yet it is generally accepted that even short-term complications may appear up to several days or weeks after the procedure.

### 2. Lack of Reporting Policy

To the question, "Do hospitals or clinics in your area notify you if one of your patients has had an induced abortion?" Of 179 respondents, 107 said no, 48 said yes, and 24 were unsure.*

*This and all subsequent boxed quotations are taken from the *Survey of Canadian Physicians on Women's Health after Induced Abortion* conducted in 1997 by the de Veber Institute.

Because no reporting policy exists in Canada or the United States, it is unclear precisely what happens when complications emerge several days or weeks later. For the most part it appears that the diagnosis and treatment of follow-up issues are left to community hospitals or family physicians. These diagnoses and treatments may never be linked statistically to the original abortion procedure, and therefore they will seldom appear in the North-American literature as the sequelae of an induced abortion.

Until this bias is corrected, it is best to assume that data originating from day patient abortion facilities are a minimum baseline that typically ignores complications that did not prevent the patient from leaving the clinic. The data or studies cannot be interpreted as a close look at actual outcomes.

Because there is no standard reporting procedure, the Institute surveyed family physicians across Canada about sequelae reported in their practices. While their reports are anecdotal, they are all that are available at present concerning many longer-term issues. In the chapters that follow we outline some of the methodological difficulties. It is hoped that this will assist in targeting future research in neglected areas.

### 3.  Possible Political Bias in Some Medical Literature
Because abortion is very much a political issue in North America, all research results need to be interpreted with care, bearing in mind the problem cited above – that North-American clinics typically do no follow up and identify only very short-term complications. The authors of many studies are, themselves, abortion providers who have a vested interest in minimizing negative findings.

An additional, highly significant discrepancy has emerged between what North-American journals consider worthy of publication and what European and Oceanic journals publish. For example, Sykes, a New Zealand researcher at Christchurch Women's Hospital, publishing in the *New Zealand Journal of Medicine*, reports that his results are consistent with European and British findings.[3] But Sykes then compares his results with results published in North-American journals: He notes that "Hakim-Elahi et al. report very low abortion complication rates and other American authors suggest complication rates should be lower than reported from Christchurch."[4]

To demonstrate why his own complication rates "should be" lower, Sykes reports research data from Grimes and Cates, and Castadot.[5]

This discrepancy raises the question about where the bias or faulty science originates – in New Zealand or in North America? Indeed, MacLean, another medical researcher from New Zealand, responded to Sykes' findings by suggesting that the cited complication rate was an underestimate because of a) the reluctance of women to attend for treatment and b) the fact that a number of serious complication cases are readmitted to other hospitals.[6]

It is, of course, possible that a real difference between North-American women and women in New Zealand – perhaps based on culture, food, health, or religion – affects abortion complication rates. But no such difference has been documented.

In addition, there are often glaring inconsistencies between the actual research results and the summaries and conclusions of articles. (A number of these will be identified in the following pages, but see in particular, Chapter 17.) Attempts to minimize negative results and to explain away findings that are not consistent with accepted opinion exist throughout the literature on abortion sequelae. A medical practitioner or family counselor is then left to wonder: Whose findings should be accepted? Could researchers such as Sykes, who report a higher complication rate, be published in a North-American journal?

In Chapter 2, we will discuss the case of Dr. Joel Brind, who conducted a *meta-analysis* of all epidemiological studies that showed a positive relationship between abortion and breast cancer.[7] His results were published in *The Journal of Epidemiology and Community Health*, a prestigious international journal that is not known for any extreme political position on the abortion issue. The handling of Brind's research results in North America raises serious questions as to how open North-American medicine is to genuine bad news about abortion sequelae.

## Changes Since the 1970s

### Repeat Abortion

Over the past decade, the trend towards the use of abortion as a primary method of fertility regulation has grown exponentially. For example, the repeat abortion rate now stands at more than 29 per cent in Canada. Among teenagers the repeat rate in 1993 was *four times the rate of first abortions* (81 per 1000 vs. 19 per 1000).[8] Given that almost one in three women attending for abortion is now a repeater, we must consider the effects that a habitual recourse to abortion will have on the medical – and ultimately also the psychological – health of women. This report addresses the issue of repeat abortions and attempts to synthesize and analyze the research data available.

### Chemical Abortion

Abortion induced by drugs as an alternative to surgical intervention is increasingly used for both first- and second-trimester abortions (see Chapter 8). Since this type of abortion has been available for less than ten years, research tends to be short-term and comparative. The main thrust is to justify its use over against the surgical approach. But, generally speaking, long-term complications, such as infertility or psychological issues, are not addressed in the literature.

### Late-term Abortions

Wadhera and Millar from Statistics Canada note that the actual reported numbers of second-trimester abortions decreased from around 10,000 in 1974 to approximately 7000 in 1991.[9] A 1995 Statistics Canada report indicates that complications in late-term abortions are higher than in earlier abortions for women of all ages but that among the oldest group of women (30-39 years) the complication rate is almost 22 per cent for abortions between seventeen and 24 weeks gestation. Similarly, Koonin and colleagues of the Centers for Disease Control (CDC) report that the percentage of abortions occurring after the thirteenth week of pregnancy was twelve per cent in 1991 and thirteen per cent in 1992.[10] The growing use of genetic testing for an increasing variety of conditions or traits will undoubtedly lead to many more second-trimester abortions.

**Pelvic Inflammatory Disease (PID)**
A further concern is the increasing incidence of pelvic inflammatory disease (PID) triggered by an induced abortion. One episode of PID can lead to *secondary infertility* or increase a woman's risk for future ectopic pregnancies. British and Scandinavian researchers have concluded that women who have an untreated *sexually transmitted disease (STD)* at the time of their abortion, have a cumulative 63 to 72 per cent risk of developing early or late PID by observing patients for two years following the abortion.[11]

**Abortion Complications – General Statistics**
The growing number of women who abort, particularly those who are having a second abortion, changes the complication numbers considerably. In Canada, the number of known abortions performed in 1969, the first year that abortion was partially decriminalized, was approximately 8000. By 1994, that number had risen to over 100,000. This is an increase of 1200 per cent, while the total population of Canada in this period grew by only approximately ten per cent. There was a sharp rise in the number of women of child-bearing years, but this rise would not account for the massive increase in abortion.

The UK's Royal College of Obstetricians and Gynaecologists has recently established that the immediate physical complication rate of induced abortion is at least eleven per cent.[12] In 1969 this complication rate affected only 400 Canadian women. But in the 1990s and 2000s, it would mean that over 13,000 Canadian women currently suffer each year from a medical condition related to their abortion. Among the 30 per cent who are undergoing a repeat abortion, the risk of complications is sharply higher. The rise in non hospital abortion facilities (26 per cent from 1989 to 1998 alone) can only have accentuated the problem, since abortion clinics are not well equipped to handle complications. In the 32 years since induced abortion was legalized in Canada, then, somewhere in the neighborhood of 300,000 Canadian women may have required medical services owing to complications after their abortion. In the United States, the current abortion rate of 1.3 million per year means that over 140,000 women a year have an immediate medical complication arising from their elective abortion. Some of these complications have grave consequences for women's health and the health of their future children.

Different complication rates have been reported from different countries. For example, Sykes studied 2879 cases of abortion performed at Christchurch Women's Hospital in New Zealand and found a complication readmission rate of 5.8 per cent, including two patients who presented with immediately life-threatening conditions: a uterine *hemorrhage* due to perforation and a severe sepsis.

Sykes' findings provide a non-political framework in which to evaluate complication rates. If two of every 2879 abortion patients in North America have life-threatening complications, then, of the more than 1.5 million women who abort yearly, 1042 would suffer such complications.

Sykes also reports 167 readmissions for various complications. Of these, fewer than one per cent were immediate complications such as perforations, hemorrhage, endometritis, and retained fetal or placental tissue while 84 per cent required a second *dilation and curettage (D&C)*.

Forty per cent of the admissions were in the first week but some patients still presented more than six weeks later, according to Sykes' report. Although Sykes had all admissions for complications registered, he recognized that the actual complication rate may be much higher than their data showed because some complications might be presented to hospitals other than Christchurch, while other patients could also be lost to follow up as a consequence of being treated privately. One statistic that points to this conclusion is that women who lived outside the region accounted for about nine per cent of the abortions but only six per cent of the complications. It is unlikely that women who happened to live outside Christchurch experienced a lower rate of complication. More likely, these women sought treatment in their home communities.

In a small UK study of *post-abortion morbidity*, Duthie and colleagues found a twelve per cent rate of morbidity due to complications including retained tissue, pelvic inflammatory disease (PID), and infections. Seventy-one per cent of those with PID also tested positive for *chlamydia trachomatis*, while only eight per cent of chlamydia-positive women had "uneventful recoveries". The women displaying these sequelae are described by Duthie as "clinically ill". Like Sykes, Duthie also found that a number of patients (ten per cent) did not return for follow up. Whereas Sykes concludes that such women would also experience complications but seek treatment elsewhere, Duthie's team asserts "we assumed that they remained asymptomatic". No reasons are given for this assumption.[13]

The studies by Sykes and Duthie are confirmed in a recent publication of the Royal College of Obstetricians and Gynaecologists in the UK, which acknowledges an immediate physical complication rate of over eleven per cent. This percentage takes no account of long-term complications such as infertility and cancers of the breast and reproductive tract.

Most recently, an important American study of the psychological responses of women after abortion also discovered that seventeen per cent of these women reported physical complications such as bleeding or pelvic infection after their first-trimester abortion.[14]

When compared with the complication rates reported in other Western countries with advanced medical systems, North-American statistics are strikingly lower. Is this because abortion services in Canada and the United States are safer and more efficient? Or is it because the North-American research methodology misses many complications owing to short-term follow up, incomplete coding, and political bias? The most recent American study, by Major and colleagues, shows that *when women themselves are asked whether they suffered physical complications, at least one in six (seventeen per cent) report that they did.*

## Overview of This Study

It is likely in North America that the complications of induced abortion are under-reported. This report examines the available findings and attempts to map out the areas and degree of risk.

The report also looks at long-term effects of induced abortion. Epidemiological research, particularly on cancer and infertility, has uncovered several long-term consequences of induced abortion. We will focus primarily on three areas: cancers of the breast and reproductive system, future fertility, and difficulties with future pregnancies. We also touch on repeat abortion, pain during the procedure, and maternal mortality in abortion. Finally, in Chapter 17, we provide an account of the limitations of methodology in this field.

To sum up, we believe that women are not usually made aware of the most statistically significant risks of induced abortion. Though it may be difficult to convey to a distressed individual that a given course of action may lead to a different distress some years down the road, everyone who believes in a woman's right to "informed consent" must agree that accurate information should be made available to her when she is about to make a significant and irreversible decision in her life.

**Key Points Chapter 1**

• Limitations exist in the available literature on physical after-effects of abortion.

• There are no standard reporting procedures of complications after abortions in Canada, the United States, or by WHO (the World Health Organization), and those complications which are reported, are only short term.

• The abortion question in North America is very politicized, which may explain why reported negative sequelae are significantly fewer than in medical reports from other countries.

• Since the 1970s, there has been a marked increase in North America in the number of abortions and repeat abortions, which may explain the significant increases in pelvic inflammatory disease (PID), uterine hemorrhage, sepsis, pain due to endometritis, retained fetal or placental tissue, and the increasing evidence of an abortion-breast cancer link.

• What accounts for the significantly lower reporting of negative sequelae after abortion in North America? Are its abortion services more efficient, or are they missing complications as a result of relying on short-term follow up and incomplete coding?

• This study will examine long-term effects of abortion on women's health and the importance of "informed consent" for women considering abortion.

## Notes

1  Ferris LE, McMain-Klein M, Colodny N, Fellows GF, Lamont J. Factors associated with immediate abortion complications. Canadian Medical Association Journal 1996 June 1;154(11):1677-85.

2  Osser S, Persson K. Postabortal pelvic infection associated with Chlamydia trachomatis and the influence of humoral immunity. American Journal of Obstetrics and Gynecology 1984 November 15;150(6):699-703.

3  Sykes P. Complications of termination of pregnancy: a retrospective study of admissions to Christchurch Women's Hospital 1989 and 1990. New Zealand Medical Journal 1993 March 10;106(951):83-5.

4  Hakim-Elahi E, Tovell HM, Burnhill MS. Complications of first-trimester abortion; a report of 170,000 cases. Obsetrics & Gynecology 1990 July;76(1):129-35.

5  Grimes DA, Cates W Jr. Complications from legally-induced abortion: a review. Obstetrical and Gynecological Survey 1979 Mar;34(3):177-91.

Castadot RG. Pregnancy termination: techniques, risks, and complications and their management. Fertility and Sterility 1986 January;45(1): 5-17.

6  MacLean N. Complications of legal abortion [Letter]. New Zealand Medical Journal 1993 May 12;106(955):186.

7  Brind J. Abortion, breast cancer, and ideology. ed. Koterski JW. *Life and Learning VII.* University Faculty for Life; 1997 June; Loyola College, Baltimore, Maryland:139-44.

8  Millar WJ, Wadhera S, Henshaw SK. Repeat abortions in Canada, 1975-1993. Family Planning Perspectives 1997 January-February;29(1):20-4.

9  Wadhera S, Millar WJ. Second trimester abortions: trends and medical complications. Health Reports 1994;6(4):441-54.

10  Koonin LM, Smith JC, Ramick M, Green CA. Abortion surveillance-United States, 1992. Morbidity and Mortality Weekly Report, Centers for Disease Control, Surveillance Summaries 1996 May 3;45(3):1-36.

11  Blackwell AL, Thomas PD, Wareham K, Emery SJ. Health gains from screening for infection of the lower genital tract in women attending for termination of pregnancy. The Lancet 1993 July 24;342(8865):206-10.

Sorensen J, Thranov I, Hoff G, Dirach J. Early- and late-onset pelvic inflammatory disease among women with cervical chlamydia trachomatis infection at the time of induced abortion - a follow-up study. Infection 1994;22(4):242-6.

12  Royal College of Obstetricians and Gynaecologists (UK). The care of women requesting induced abortion: 4. Information for women.2000. www.rcog.org.uk/guidelines/induced_abortion.html.

13  Duthie SJ, Hobson D, Tait IA, Pratt B, Lowe N, Sequeira P, et al. Morbidity after termination of pregnancy in first trimester. Genitourinary Medicine 1987;63:183-7.

14  Major B, Cozzarelli C, Cooper ML, Zubek J, Richards C, Wilhite M, Gramzow RH. Psychological responses of women after first-trimester abortion. Archives of General Psychiatry 2000 August 57(8):777-84, p. 780.

Chapter 2

# Induced Abortion and Breast Cancer

Breast cancer poses a significant threat to the health and survival of women in the Western world. Excess estrogen exposure has emerged as a major risk factor, raising concern about the way in which induced abortion exposes women to the unprotected cancer-inducing effects of the high estrogen environment of early pregnancy. Since 1957, evidence linking induced abortion to the later development of breast cancer has been observed in 23 of 37 studies worldwide, including ten of fifteen U.S. studies. Although the poor quality and confusing presentation of many studies has hidden the significance of the breast cancer risk posed by induced abortion, a recent clarifying meta-analysis has established abortion as a significant independent risk factor, averaging a 30 per cent increased risk. The medical establishment has exhibited some reluctance to accept and respond to this emerging evidence, presumably because of the political controversy over abortion.

# Induced Abortion and Breast Cancer

At the dawn of the 21st century, breast cancer poses a life-time risk to women of greater than one in ten. It now strikes over 170,000 American women and over 5,000 Canadian women every year.[1] Intense interest in the search for possible genetic, dietary, and environmental risk factors is shared by the medical research community and the public at large.

## Possible Abortion and Breast Cancer Link

### Pathophysiology

The observed association between induced abortion and an increased risk of the later development of breast cancer is congruent with our understanding of the hormonal effects of pregnancy on a woman's breast tissue. Prior to her first pregnancy, a woman's breast is composed largely of connective tissue linking ducts which contain few milk-producing cells. Upon conception, a surge of *oestradiol* reaches twentyfold in the first trimester, triggering an explosive growth of breast tissue, a period when breast cells are most likely to be affected by carcinogens. When a woman completes her first full pregnancy, further hormonal changes propel these newly produced breast cells through a state of differentiation, a natural maturing process which greatly reduces the risk of future breast cancer.[2]

An abrupt, premature termination of a first pregnancy by abortion arrests this process before the cancer-reducing evolution of hormone release later in pregnancy can occur, leaving a large population of dangerously-stimulated breast tissue cells in place, greatly raising future cancer risk. On the other hand, "...an early first full-term pregnancy would provide the greatest protection against breast cancer by drastically reducing, early on, the presence of undifferentiated and hence vulnerable breast cells, thereby decreasing the risk of subsequent transformation."[3]

Animal studies support this model. Russo and Russo exposed two groups of rats to a chemical carcinogen. One group, who mated and carried a first pregnancy to term, developed mammary tumors at a rate of six per cent. The other group, who mated, became pregnant, then were aborted (via hysterectomy), developed mammary tumors at an incidence of 78 per cent; virgin rats also developed tumors at a high rate, but not as high as those that were aborted."

**Evidence of Risk in Humans**

In 1994, Dr. Janet Daling, a research epidemiologist at the Fred Hutchison Cancer Institute in Seattle, published a study in the *Journal of the National Cancer Institute* revealing that women who underwent an induced abortion had a 50 per cent greater chance of developing breast cancer than matched control women who had not previously aborted. Importantly, Daling separated out women who had suffered a spontaneous abortion (miscarriage), and found they had no increased risk of breast cancer.[5]

Her findings were not unique. In fact, of fifteen U.S. studies to date, looking specifically at the risk of breast cancer in women with a history of induced abortion, eleven of these studies have shown an increased risk. The first of these, by Pike and colleagues, initially funded by the U.S. National Cancer Institute (NCI) and published in the *British Journal of Cancer*, uncovered a 137 per cent increased risk of breast cancer. They concluded that "a first-trimester abortion...before first full-term pregnancy appears to cause a substantial increase in risk of subsequent breast cancer. Our finding makes biological sense if one considers breast tissue as merely proliferating in early pregnancy; the protective effect of a first full-term pregnancy is then brought about by a combination of cell differentiation and possibly permanently altered hormone levels."[6]

These studies of American women reinforce earlier and subsequent international investigations that now total 37 epidemiological studies worldwide, of which 23 show a higher risk of breast cancer in women who have chosen abortion. The original report of Segi in 1957 based on Japanese women diagnosed with breast cancer between 1948 and 1952 found a 163 per cent increased risk. A later Japanese investigation of women with breast cancer in Tokushima prefecture found a nearly identical 152 per cent increased risk. Along with two other positive Japanese studies, women who have undergone abortion were found to have an

19

increased risk of breast cancer in Russia (71 per cent increase), France (32 per cent increase), Greece (51 per cent increase), and the Netherlands (90 per cent increase).[7]

**Exposure**
Some in the scientific community have maintained that even a 30 per cent increased risk of breast cancer from abortion is quite small compared to, for example, the tenfold increase in lung cancer with smoking. On the other hand, the typical smoker with lung cancer has acquired this risk by smoking a pack of cigarettes a day for anywhere from ten to 40 years, which represents 73,000 to 292,000 cigarettes. And even after thousands of cigarettes, the risk can be partly reversed if a person quits early enough. But a measurable increased risk of breast cancer comes after just one "exposure" to abortion, and abortion is not reversible.

The overall exposure of women to abortion is enormous. Of roughly 1,300,000 abortions in the U.S. each year, over half are performed on women with their first pregnancy. At a baseline rate of development of breast cancer of ten per cent, a 30 per cent increased risk above this could result in 20,000 extra cases of breast cancer per year as these women age through the next few decades. In Eastern Europe, the phenomenon may underlie the recent alarming increase in the incidence of breast cancer in younger women. While the typical breast cancer patient in Western Europe presents in her forties and fifties, a marked increase in breast cancer onset in the late twenties and early thirties has been observed in Lithuanian women, many of whom may have had five or six abortions by their mid-twenties.[8]

**Response in North America**
Despite intense interest among the public and the medical research community in the possible genetic, dietary, and environmental risk factors for breast cancer, the findings of both North American and international studies linking abortion with breast cancer have generally been ignored by North-American cancer research authorities. The official Web site of the U.S. National Cancer Institute (cancernet.nci.nih.gov) minimizes the abortion-breast cancer link, as do other national cancer institutes, for example in Canada (cancer.ca), and among public health information groups (healthlinkusa.com).

Until recently, authoritative medical reviews of breast cancer risks have not even mentioned induced abortion.[9] However, the emancipation of medical information on the internet has led to the development of a "fifth estate" of alternative analyses of medical data (abortioncancer.com).

Where a connection between abortion and an increased risk of breast cancer has been discovered, researchers have often seen their findings either minimized or questioned by the medical and research establishments. Before the 1994 publication in the United States of the Daling research, the *Journal of the National Cancer Institute (JNCI)*, stated about earlier studies: "...recently, foes of abortion and some scientists have been pointing to a few studies that suggest that an aborted pregnancy increases the risk for the disease." When the Daling study was published in the *JNCI*, the journal ran an accompanying editorial that played down Daling's finding of a 50 per cent increased risk of breast cancer attributable to induced abortion among American women.[10] Since Daling's and other research scientists' publication of data linking abortion and breast cancer, the controversy over their findings has been discussed in the mass media, including a newspaper article in *The Wall Street Journal* entitled "The Politics of Breast Cancer". In this article, John McGinnis noted that "Recently...several respected, supposedly impartial scientific researchers have been brushing aside...evidence of a link between abortion and breast cancer, thus allowing the politics of abortion to discourage at least one area of breast cancer research."[11] In the spring of 2003, the U.S. National Cancer Institute convened a workshop to address the growing controversy, but according to reports, the more than four decades of evidence documenting an abortion-breast cancer link did not lead to a significant revision of NCI's published "fact sheet".

**A Clarifying Meta-analysis**
One of the researchers whose work has been most questioned by the cancer establishment is Dr. Joel Brind, a professor of endocrinology at Baruch College, City University of New York. At the same time that Daling was publishing her results, Dr. Brind and his team were sifting through decades of published data on the epidemiology of breast cancer. Using the technique of meta-analysis to look at data from

previous studies, Brind found a significant connection between induced abortion and the later development of breast cancer.

Brind and biostatistician Vern Chinchilli pooled together patients and control subjects from 28 original published reports, establishing stringent and conservative criteria to select data in which exposure to induced abortion could be separated clearly from spontaneous abortion. The overall odds ratio, for any abortion exposure, of the risk of breast cancer was found to be 1.3, a 30 per cent increased risk (where 1.0 represents no increased risk). The study is so statistically powerful that the 95 per cent confidence interval was a tight 1.2 to 1.4 (twenty per cent to 40 per cent increased risk), meaning there is less than a one in twenty likelihood that the increased risk of breast cancer could be anything less than twenty per cent. Statistically, Brind's study is virtually unassailable, yet its publication ignited a storm of controversy.[12] The validity of his finding is gradually being recognized. Dr. Thomas Stuttaford, an eminent medical columnist in Britain, has recently announced a change of mind. Writing in *The Times* (London) he stated, "Breast cancer is diagnosed in 33,000 women in the UK each year; of these, an unusually high proportion had an abortion before eventually starting a family. *Such women are up to four times more likely to develop breast cancer*" [emphasis added].[13]

**Effect of Delayed Childbirth**

A crucial feature of Brind's study was his careful separation of the independent effects of abortion on a woman's breast cancer risk from the previously-known risk of delaying her first full-term completed pregnancy. Some critics in the medical community assert that this delayed first-birth effect is the only explanation for a claimed increased risk of breast cancer. Brind's study conclusively demonstrates that abortion is an *independent* risk factor in its own right. This conclusion was achieved in two ways: 1) By including studies in which the control group (women without breast cancer) included nulligravid women (women who had never been pregnant); and 2) In studies where some women had given birth, at various ages, a calculation was performed to subtract out the effect of age at first live birth. The result? The independent risk of induced abortion was still significant.

Brind and his colleagues argued that the two effects – delayed childbirth and abortion – are additive. If it is assumed, conservatively, that an average woman's lifetime risk of breast cancer is ten per cent (one in ten), it is known that an early full-term pregnancy reduces this risk, from ten per cent to about seven per cent. If a young pregnant woman opts instead for an abortion, she relinquishes the benefit of an early completed pregnancy and, in addition, adds the independent 30 per cent increased risk from the abortion, raising her risk from ten per cent to thirteen per cent. Thus the decision to abort her first pregnancy will nearly double her lifetime risk of breast cancer, from seven per cent to thirteen per cent. A second abortion will add further risk, both from the abortion itself and by further delaying the protective effects of a first completed pregnancy.

Despite the statistical power of Brind's study (or, perhaps, because of it), many in the medical and scientific community were quick to attack his findings. The *New England Journal of Medicine* published a remarkably flawed Danish study which explained away a 44 per cent increased risk of breast cancer in women with a history of abortion as being based on an otherwise unexplained global increase in breast cancer incidence. The JNCI offered a generic criticism of the technique of meta-analysis, stating that "biased studies entered into a meta-analysis produced biased results."[14]

With time, however, the quality of Brind's study has gradually begun to win grudging acceptance among important sectors of the world medical community. In April 2000, Britain's Royal College of Obstetricians and Gynecologists (RCOG) published Evidence-based Guideline *No. 7: The Care of Women Requesting Induced Abortion*, which said of two of the most thorough reviews of the abortion-breast cancer literature, one being Brind's meta-analysis: "These two meta-analyses were independently assessed for the RCOG Group. The assessor concluded that both were carefully conducted reviews and that the Brind paper had no major methodological shortcomings and could not be disregarded."[15]

Even more significant was the inclusion, for the first time, of abortion as a risk factor for breast cancer in a February 2000 review of the subject by Katrina Armstrong and colleagues in the *New England Journal of Medicine*. Although abortion was downplayed as one of four "risk factors...less consistently associated with breast cancer", its inclusion in such a short list represents a significant acknowledgement.[16] A 1992 review in the same journal did not mention abortion, despite 45 years of evidence at that point.[17]

**Recall Bias**

One way of explaining a clearly emerging worldwide trend linking abortion with an increased risk of breast cancer, is the concept of recall bias, proposed by Harris and colleagues. These authors postulated that "a woman with cancer is perhaps more likely to remember and report a previous abortion than a healthy control".[18] If this was true, a falsely elevated apparent risk in breast cancer patients might result. The only support for this notion rests with a set of Swedish data which shows that, rather than non-cancer patients underreporting abortions, several women with cancer seemed to overreport abortions, that is, apparently they declared abortions they never had (based on discordance between a computerized registry and interview data).[19] Few workers in the field accept this concept, which raises questions about the quality of data reporting in that study. Indeed, the Swedish authors of this study eventually retracted their claim.[20] In any event, there are now four studies whose design has conclusively ruled out any evidence of recall bias.[21]

**The Importance of Identifying Precise Studies**

Over two dozen other studies of the association of abortion and breast cancer since 1960 are betrayed by various confounding factors which prevent an examination of uncontaminated data related to induced abortion. The most common error is the failure to separate data from women who have suffered miscarriages (spontaneous abortion) from those who have undergone induced surgical abortion. Spontaneous abortion has long been recognized to offer no increased risk of subsequent breast cancer, and there are clear biological reasons for this. It appears that miscarried pregnancies are doomed from the earliest days after conception by a failure to develop the expected estrogen hormonal surge, thus these women are never exposed to the powerfully high estrogen levels of a healthy pregnancy that is abruptly terminated by abortion. The low maternal oestradiol surge in spontaneous abortion was first observed by Kunz and Keller in 1976, and has recently been confirmed by Stewart and colleagues. This biological difference between spontaneous and induced abortion underlies the flaw inherent in epidemiological studies that pool data from both groups, and points out the value of a meta-analysis such as the one carried out by Brind, which isolates and studies data from induced abortion alone.[22]

A study that mixes spontaneous abortion cases with induced abortion is imprecise, and results in a falsely low apparent risk of subsequent breast cancer. For example, in a 1996 study by Newcombe and colleagues, which garnered prominent attention, the actual increased breast cancer risk of women exposed to induced abortion was 23 per cent, but by mixing in women who had suffered miscarriages, the risk was watered down to twelve per cent.[23] It was this twelve per cent figure that was most quoted in press reports, misleading the public into believing the study showed only a minimal risk of breast cancer from abortion. It is clear that further human studies are needed which separate miscarriages from induced abortions in order to advance our understanding of this important area of women's health research.

**Age at First Abortion**
Only a few studies have looked at the question of whether a woman who has an abortion at a very young age faces a significantly higher risk of developing breast cancer. In noting that the rate of cell proliferation is likely to be highest in the youngest subjects, Daling and her colleagues have suggested that the greater risk for women younger than eighteen at the time of their first abortion may be real, and should be further investigated.[24] One of the most recent studies reconfirmed this point, demonstrating an increased breast cancer risk in women who abort a first pregnancy under age twenty, whereas nulliparous women who abort above age twenty showed no such risk.[25]

**Family History**
Although data on this subject are limited, the observations are ominous. In the Daling study of 2000 women, twelve women had a combination of a positive family history of

breast cancer and an abortion before age eighteen. All twelve women went on to develop breast cancer before age 45. The risk in this study was, therefore, incalculably high.

**The Medical Establishment**
There are serious grounds for believing that induced abortion creates an increased risk of breast cancer, and that this risk may be more significant for women with a positive family history. Research studies in this field have been hampered by the omission of key information, imprecise gathering of data (mixing miscarriages with induced abortions), and the politicized nature of the subject, all of which conspire to create significant barriers to a true understanding of the risk. Many North American researchers who study breast cancer are unwilling to accept induced abortion as a factor worthy of study.

For women considering abortion to have the benefit of a truly informed choice, a major shift in the medical paradigm is required. It has long been observed that the medical establishment is slow to respond to emerging data. The smoking-lung cancer link and the relationship between diet and health are but two examples of concepts which have taken years, even decades, to become accepted. Today they form part of conventional medical wisdom.

**Table 2-1**
**World epidemiological studies on the association of breast cancer with induced abortion.**[26]
To date, twenty-three of thirty-seven studies worldwide have shown an increased risk of breast cancer in women with a history of induced abortion, including twelve of fourteen studies in which statistical significance was reached.

Risk of abortion presented in terms of Odds Ratios (OR), i.e., OR=1.3 represents a 30 per cent increased risk of breast cancer; OR=0.9 represents a ten per cent reduced risk; OR=1.0 represents no particular risk. Variability of the data is represented by the 95 per cent Confidence Intervals (95 per cent CI), means that the true result has a 95 per cent chance of falling within the described range.

Studies whose results are statistically significant are indicated by an asterisk.

par=parous; null=nulliparous; appr=approximate

| Study | Year | OR | 95 per cent CI |
|---|---|---|---|
| **United States** | | | |
| Pike MC, Henderson BE et al. | 1981 | **2.37** | 0.85 - 6.93 |
| Brinton LA, Hoover R et al. | 1983 | **1.2** | 0.6 - 2.3 |
| Rosenberg L, Palmer JR et al. | 1988 | **1.2*** | 1.0 - 1-6 |
| Howe HL, Senie RT et al. | 1989 | **1.9*** | 1.2 - 3.0 |
| Moseson M, Koenig KL et al | 1993 | **1.0** | 0.7 - 1.4 |
| Laing AE, Demenais FM et al. | 1993 | **3.1*** | 2.0 - 4.8 |
| Laing AE, Bonney GE et al. | 1994 | **2.44*** | 1.0 - 6.0 |
| Daling JR, Malone KE et al. | 1994 | **1.36*** | 1.11 -1.67 |
| White E, Malone KE et al. | 1994 | - | - |
| Brinton LA, Daling JR et al. | 1995 | **0.99** | 0.81 - 1.21 |
| Newcomb PA, Storer BE et al. | 1996 | **1.23*** | 1.00 - 1.51 |
| Palmer J, Rosenberg L et al | 1997 | **1.20*** | |
| Lazovich D, Thompson JA et al. | 2000 | **1.10** | 0.8 - 1.21 |
| Newcomb PA, Mandelson MT | 2000 | **0.9** | 0.5 - 1.6 |
| Mahue-Giangreco M, Ursin G et al | 2003 | **1.05 par** | 0.75 - 1.48 |
| | | **0.69 null** | 0.46 - 1.04 |
| **Japan** | | | |
| Segi M, Fukushima I et al. | 1957 | **2.63*** | 1.85 - 3.75 |
| Watanabe H and Hirayama T et al. | 1968 | **1.51** | 0.91 - 2.53 |
| Nishiyama F | 1982 | **2.52*** | 1.99 - 3.20 |
| Hirohata T, Shigematsu T et al. | 1985 | **1.51** | 0.93 - 2.48 |
| **France** | | | |
| Le M-G, Bachelot A et al. | 1984 | **1.32** | 0.97 - 1.77 |
| Andrieu M, Clavel F et al. | 1994 | **1.1** | 0.7 - 1.8 |
| **China** | | | |
| Sanderson M, Shu X-O et al. | 2001 | **0.9** | 0.7 - 1.2 |
| Ye Z, Gao DL et al. | 2003 | **1.06** | 0.91 - 1.25 |
| **Russia** | | | |
| Dvoirin VV and Medvedev AB | 1978 | **1.71** | 0.80 - 3.64 |
| **Yugoslavia** | | | |
| Burany B | 1979 | **0.50** | 0.33 - 0.74 |
| **Slovenia** | | | |
| Robertson C, Van Den Donk et al. | 2001 | **1.1 appr** | - |
| **Denmark** | | | |
| Ewertz M and Duffy SW | 1988 | **2.91** | 0.77 - 16.2 |
| **England** | | | |
| Goldacre MJ, Kurina LM et al. | 2001 | **0.83*** | 0.74 - 0.93 |
| **Sweden/Norway** | | | |
| Harris B-M L, Eklund G et al. | 1989 | **0.9** | 0.5 - 1.3 |
| Adami H-O, Bergstrom R et al. | 1990 | - | - |
| Erlandsson G, Montgomery SM et al. | 2000 | **0.84*** | 0.72 - 0.99 |
| **Italy** | | | |
| Parazzini F, La Vecchia C et al. | 1991 | **0.92** | 0.80 - 1.06 |
| La Vecchia C, Negri E et al. | 1993 | - | - |
| Tavani A., La Vecchia C et al. | 1996 | **1.3** | 1.0 - 1.6 |
| Talamini R, Franceschi S et al. | 1996 | - | - |
| **Greece** | | | |
| Lipworth L, Katsouyammi K et al. | 1995 | **1.51*** | 1.24 - 1.84 |
| **Netherlands** | | | |
| Rookus MA and van Leeuwen FE | 1995 | **1.9*** | 1.2 - 3.1 |
| **Meta-Analysis** | | | |
| Brind J, Chinchilli VM et al. | 1996 | **1.3*** | 1.2 - 1.4 |

**Key Points Chapter 2**

• Abortion increases a woman's overall risk of breast cancer by 30 per cent.

• The risk is likely much higher in women who have a first abortion at a young age, or who have a family history of breast cancer.

• Since 1957, 23 of 37 worldwide studies show an increased breast cancer risk with abortion, a risk as high as 310 per cent.

• Ten of fifteen U.S. studies confirm the abortion-breast cancer link.

• The biological rationale for breast cancer development is related to the woman's unprotected internal exposure to estrogen when a pregnancy is abruptly terminated early in gestation.

• The magnitude of the risk has, until recently, been hidden by studies of poor quality, many of which have failed to separate induced abortion from low-risk spontaneous miscarriage.

• The medical establishment is often slow to accept and respond to emerging data, slowed further, in this case, by the conflicting politics of abortion.

## Notes

1  Ries LAG, Kosary CL, Hankey BF, Miller BA, Clegg L, Edwards BK, eds. SEER Cancer Statistics Review, 1973-1996: Bethesda, Maryland: National Cancer Institute; 1999.

Hamilton Regional Cancer Centre. Early Stage Breast Cancer. Cancer Centre Update 1997;5(1):1-8.

2  Kelsey JL. A review of the epidemiology of human breast cancer. Epidemiologic Reviews 1979;1:74-109.

Kelsey JL, Fischer DB, Holford TR, LiVoisi VA, Mostow ED, Goldenberg IS et. al. Exogenous estrogens and other factors in the epidemiology of breast cancer. Journal of the National Cancer Institute 1981 Aug;67(2):237-233.

Ewertz M, Duffy SW. Risk of breast cancer in relation to reproductive factors in Denmark. British Journal of Cancer 1988 Jul;58(1):99-104.

3  Krieger N. Exposure, susceptibility, and breast cancer risk: a hypothesis regarding exogenous carcinogens, breast tissue development, and docial gradients, including black/white differences, in breast cancer incidence. Breast Cancer Research and Treatment 1989 Jul;13(3):205-223.

4  Russo J, Russo IH. Susceptibility of the mammary gland to carcinogenesis. II. Pregnancy interruption as a risk factor in tumor incidence. American Journal of Pathology 1980 Aug;100(2):497-512.

5  Daling JR, Malone KE, Voigt LF, White E, Weiss NS. Risk of breast cancer among young women: relationship to induced abortion. Journal of the National Cancer Institute 1994 Nov(2);86(21):1584-92.

6  Pike MC, Henderson BE, Casagrande JT, Rosario I, Gray GE. Oral contraceptive use and early abortion as risk factors for breast cancer in young women. British Journal of Cancer 1981 Jan;43(1):72-6.

7  Segi M, Fukushima I, Fujisaku S, Kurihara M. Saito S, Asano K, et al. An epidemiological study of cancer in Japan. GANN 48, Supplement (April 1957):1-43.

Nishiyama F. The epidemiology of breast cancer in Tokushima prefecture. Shikou Ichi 1982;38:333-43.

Dvoirin V, Medvedev AB. Role of women's reproductive status in the development of breast cancer. In: *Methods and Progress in Breast Cancer Epidemiology Research*, Tallin, 1978. Moscow: Oncology Science Centre of the USSR Academy of Sciences, 1978. pp. 53-63.

Le M, Bachelot A, Doyon F, Kramar A, Hill C. Oral contraceptive use and breast or cervical cancer: preliminary results of a French case-control study. In *Hormones and Sexual Factors in Human Cancer Aetiology*, eds. Wolff J-P and Scott JS, 139-47. Amsterdam: Elsevier, 1984.

Lipworth L, Katsouyanni K, Ekbom A, Michels KB and Trichopoulos D. Abortion and the risk of breast cancer: a case-control study in Greece. International Journal of Cancer 61, 1995 Apr;61(2):181-184.

Rookus MA, van Leeuwen FE. Induced abortion and risk of breast cancer: reporting (recall) bias in a Dutch case-control study. Journal of the National Cancer Institute 1996 Dec 4;88(23):1759-1764.

8   Rich V. Breast cancer in Lithuania. The Lancet 1994;344:947.

9   Armstrong K, Eisen A, Weber B. Assessing the risk of breast cancer. New England Journal of Medicine 2000 Feb 24;342(8):564-571.

10  Parkins T. Does abortion increase breast cancer risk? Journal of the National Cancer Institute 1993 Dec 15;85(24):1987-88.

Rosenberg L. Induced abortion and breast cancer: more scientific data are needed. Journal of the National Cancer Institute 1994 Nov 2;86(21): 1569-70.

11  McGinnis J. The politics of cancer research. The Wall Street Journal 1997 Feb 28.

12  Brind J, Chinchilli VM, Severs WB, Summy-Long J. Induced abortion as an independent risk factor for breast cancer: a comprehensive review and meta-analysis. Journal of Epidemiology and Community Health 1996 Oct;50(5):481-496.

13  Stuttaford, T. *The Times*, 17 May, 2001. p. 8.

14  Melbye M, Wohlfahrt J, Olsen JH, Frisch M, Westergaard T, Helweg-Larsen K, et al. Induced abortions and the risk of breast cancer. New England Journal of Medicine 1997 Jan 9;336(2):81-85.

Weed DL, Kramer BS. Induced abortion, bias, and breast cancer. Why epidemiology hasn't reached its limit. Journal of the National Cancer Institute 1996 Dec 4; 88(23):1698-1700.

15  Royal College of Obstetricians and Gynaecologists. Evidence-based Guideline No. 7: The Care of Women Requesting Induced Abortion. London; 2000 Apr.

16  Armstrong et al. 2000. See n. 9.

17  Harris JR, Lippman ME, Veronesi U, Willett W. Breast cancer (1). New England Journal of Medicine 1992 Jul 30; 327(5):319-28.

18 Harris BM, Eklund G, Meirik O, Rutqvist LE, Wiklund K. Risk of cancer of the breast after legal abortion during first trimester: a Swedish register study. British Medical Journal 1989 Dec 9;299(6713):1430-1432.

19 Harris et al. 1989. See n. 18.

Meirik O, Lund E, Adami HO, Bergstrom R, Christoffersen T, Bergsjo P. Oral contraceptive use and breast cancer in young women. A joint national case-control study in Sweden and Norway. The Lancet 1986 Sep 20; 2(8508):650-654.

20 Meirik O, Adami HO, Eklund G. Letter on: Relation between induced abortion and breast cancer. Journal of Epidemiology and Community Health 1998 Mar;52(3):209-211.

21 Watanabe H, Hirayama T. Epidemiology and clinical aspects of breast cancer [translation of Japanese title]. Nippon Rinsho 1968 Aug;26(8): 1843-1849.

Howe HL, Senie RT, Bzduch H, Herzfeld P. Early abortion and breast cancer risk among women under age 40. International Journal of Epidemiology 1989 Jun;18(2):300-304.

Daling et al. 1994. See n. 5.

Lipworth et al. 1995. See n. 7.

22 Kunz J and Keller PJ. HCG, HPL, oestradiol, progesterone and AFP in serum in patients with threatened abortion. British Journal of Obstetrics and Gynaecology 1976 Aug;83(8):640-6.

Stewart DR, Overstreet JW, Nakajima ST, Lasley BL. Enhanced ovarian steroid secretion before implantation in early human pregnancy. Journal of Clinical Endocrinology and Metabolism 1993 Jun;76(6):1470-1476.

Brind et al. See n. 12.

23 Newcomb PA, Storer BE, Longnecker MP, Mittendorf R, Greenberg ER and Willett WC. Pregnancy termination in relation to risk of breast cancer. Journal of the American Medical Association 1996 Jan;275(4):283-7.

24 Howe 1989. See n. 21.
Daling et al. 1994. See n. 5.

25 Mahue-Giangreco M, Ursin G, Sullivan-Halley J, Bernstein L. Induced abortion, miscarriage, and breast cancer risk of young women. Cancer Epidemiology Biomark Prevention 2003;12:209-14.

26 Table 2-1

**United States**

Pike 1981. See n. 6.

Brinton LA, Hoover R, Fraumeni JF Jr. Reproductive factors in the aetiology of breast cancer. British Journal of Cancer 1983 Jun;47(6):757-762.

Rosenberg L, Palmer JR, Kaufman DW, Strom BL, Schottenfeld D, Shapiro S. Breast cancer in relation to the occurrence and time of induced and spontaneous abortion. American Journal of Epidemiology 1988 May;127(5):981-989

Howe et al. 1989. See n. 21.

Moseson M, Koenig KL, Shore RE, Pasternack BS. The influence of medical conditions associated with hormones on the risk of breast cancer. International Journal of Epidemiology 1993 Dec;22(6):1000-1009.

Laing AE, Demenais FM, Williams R, Kissling G, Chen VW, Bonney GE. Breast cancer risk factors in African-American women: the Howard University Tumor Registry experience. Journal of the National Medical Association 1993 Dec;85(12):931-939.

Laing AE, Bonney GE, Adams-Campbell L, et al. Reproductive and lifestyle factors for breast cancer in African-American women. Genetic Epidemiology 1994;11:285-310, p. 300.

Daling et al. 1994. See n. 5.

White E, Malone KE, Weiss NS, Daling JR. Breast cancer among young U.S. women in relation to oral contraceptive use. Journal of the National Cancer Institute 1994 Apr 6;86(7):505-514.

Brinton LA, Daling JR, Liff JM, Schoenberg JB, Malone KE, Stanford JL. Oral contraceptives and breast cancer risk among younger women. Journal of the National Cancer Institute 1995 Jun 7;87(11):827-835.

Newcomb et al. 1996. See n. 23.

Palmer J, Rosenberg L, Rao R, Zauber A, Strom B, Warshauser M, et al. Induced and spontaneous abortion in relation to risk of breast cancer (United States). Cancer Causes and Control 1997;8:841-849.

Lazovich D, Thompson J, Mink P, Sellars T, Anderson K. Induced abortion and breast cancer risk. Epidemiology 2000;11:76-80.

Newcomb PA, Mandelson MT. A record-based evaluation of induced abortion and breast cancer risk (United States). Cancer Causes Control 2000;11(9):777-811.

Mahue-Giangreco M, Ursin G, Sullivan-Halley J, Bernstein L. Induced abortion, miscarriage, and breast cancer risk of young women. Cancer Epidemiology Biomark Prevention 2003;12;209-14.

**Japan**
Segi et al. 1957. See n. 7.

Watanable et al. 1968. See n. 21

Nishiyama 1982. See n. 7.

Hirohata T, Shigematsu T, Nomura AM, Nomura Y, Horie A, Hirohata I. Occurrence of breast cancer in relation to diet and reproductive history: a case-control study in Fukuoka, Japan. National Cancer Institute Monograph 1985 Dec:187-190.

**France**
Le M et al. 1984. See n. 7.

Andrieu N, Clavel F, Gairard B, Piana L, Bremond A, Lansac J, Flamant R et al. Familial risk of breast cancer and abortion. Cancer Detection and Prevention 1994;18(1):51-55.

**China**
Sanderson M, Shu X-O, Jin F, Dai Q, Wen WQ, Hui Y, Gao YT, Zheng W. Abortion history and breast cancer risk: results from the Shanghai breast cancer study. American Journal of Epidemiology 2000;151(abstract only).

Ye Z, Gao DL, Qin Q, Ray RM, Thomas DB. Breast cancer in relation to induced abortions in a cohort of Chinese women. British Journal of Cancer 2002; 87(9):977-81.

**Russia**
Dvoirin and Medvedev 1978. See n. 7

**Yugoslavia**
Burany B. [Gestational characteristics in women with breast cancer]. Article in Serbo-Croatian (Roman). Jugosl Ginekol Opstet 1979 Sep-Dec;19(5-6):237-247.

**Slovenia**
Robertson C, Van Den Donk M, Primic-Zakelj, Macfarlane T, Boyle P. The association between induced and spontaneous abortion and risk of breast cancer in Slovenian women aged 25-54. Breast 2001;10:291-8.

**Denmark**
Ewertz and Duffy 1988. See n. 2.

**England**
Goldacre MJ, Kurina LM, Seagroatt V, Yeates. Abortion and breast cancer: a case-control record linkage study. Journal of Epidemiology and Community Health 2001;55:336-7.

**Sweden/Norway**
Harris 1989. See n. 18.

Adami HO, Bergstrom R, Lund E, Meirik O. Absence of association between reproductive variables and the risk of breast cancer in young women in Sweden and Norway. British Journal of Cancer 1990 Jul;62(1):122-126.

Erlandsson G, Montgomery SM, Cnattingius S, Ekbom A. Abortions and breast cancer: a record-based case-control study. International Journal of Cancer 2003;103:676-9.

**Italy**
Parazzini F, LaVecchia C and Negri E. Spontaneous and induced abortion and risk of breast cancer. International Journal of Cancer 1991 Jul30;48(6):816-20.

LaVecchia C, Negri E, Franceschi S and Parazzini F. Long-term impact of reproductive factors on Cancer risk. International Journal of Cancer 1993 Jan 21;53(2):215-219.

Tavani A, La Vecchia C, Franceschi S, Negri E, D'Avanzo B, Decarli A, et al. Abortion and breast cancer risk. International Journal of Cancer 1996;65:401-405.

Talamini R, Franceschi S, La Vecchia C, Negri E, Borsa L, Montella M, et al. The role of reproductive and menstrual factors in cancer of the breast before and after menopause. European Journal of Cancer 1996;32A(2):303-310.

**Greece**
Lipworth et al. 1995. See n. 7.

**Netherlands**
Rookus and van Leeuwen 1995. See n. 7.

**Meta-Analysis**
Brind et al. 1996. See n. 12.

# Chapter 3

# Induced Abortion and Other Cancers

It is difficult to draw definitive conclusions regarding possible links between induced abortion and a higher risk of cancer because spontaneous and induced abortions are frequently not separated in the literature. In addition, inconsistencies exist between studies and from country to country. There have been a number of studies done in the past twenty years, however, that indicate an increased risk of cervical and ovarian cancer when there has been a history of previous abortion(s). Women who have had more than one previous abortion seem particularly to be at a higher risk of ovarian cancer, while research indicates that childbirth provides women with protection from cancers of the reproductive system. A higher incidence of rectal cancer also seems to be related to induced abortion, though further research is needed to study this connection.

The link between induced abortion and breast cancer is particularly important, and is explored in Chapter 2.

# Induced Abortion and Other Cancers

Spontaneous and induced abortion are often not separated in the literature which makes it difficult to draw conclusions. Inconsistency between studies and from country to country compounds the problem. But a history of previous induced abortion may play a role in cancers such as uterine, cervical, colorectal, endometrial, and breast. (The relationship of abortion to breast cancer is discussed in Chapter 2.)

**Cancers of the Reproductive System**
Cancer of the cervix (the entrance of a woman's uterus) was found to be increased in Australian women with a history of previous induced abortion.[1] After researchers adjusted for other possible causes, no statistically significant link was found, although there was a trend towards an increased cancer risk in women who had undergone two or more abortions. La Vecchia and colleagues isolated a cervical cancer risk following one induced abortion and reported that "...cervical cancer was directly associated with induced abortions".[2] In another study, Schwartz and colleagues found a significant relationship between *leiomyosarcoma* and a history of induced abortion.[3]

Studies of cancer of the ovary have presented conflicting evidence regarding a possible association with induced abortion. As late as 1990 Larissa Remennick commented in the *Journal of Epidemiology and Community Health* that the possible influence of abortion on ovarian cancer had hardly ever been examined.[4] Yet in 1995 Bernal and colleagues reported that "ovarian cancer cases show important fetal loss".[5] With four abortions, the *relative risk* rose to 3.66 – meaning a 266 per cent increased risk. Regrettably, the study made no distinction between spontaneous and induced abortions. A year later Chen and colleagues determined that incomplete pregnancies, including abortions, do not provide women with the protective effect of full-term pregnancies against the onset of ovarian cancer.[6] This is significant, because the risk of developing ovarian cancer has been shown to decrease with the number of full-term pregnancies.[7] Finally, Albrektsen and colleagues have determined that childbirth furnishes protection against cancers of the reproductive system, thanks to "a mechanical shed of malignant or pre-malignant cells at each delivery".[8] Such protection is not found in pregnancies ended by induced abortion.

McPherson and colleagues found that for ovarian cancer "a history of ever (versus never) having had an induced abortion was a factor that remained statistically significant." The increase in risk is 150 per cent (relative risk = 2.5). They also determined that the time of a spontaneous abortion in a woman's life was also significant – "a miscarriage late in reproductive life followed by lack of a subsequent full-term pregnancy" is a risk factor for ovarian cancer. It is unfortunate that they provide no discussion of the sequence of pregnancy interruptions because induced abortion is known to contribute to later spontaneous abortions. If a consistent pattern turned out to be, for instance: 1) induced abortion of first pregnancy; 2) subsequent spontaneous abortions; 3) ovarian cancer, the finding would be significant.

**Colorectal Cancer**
Kvale and Heuch report that "having had many abortions was associated with high risk of colorectal cancer of all subsites. However, the association was statistically significant for rectal cancer only",[10] where the relative odds were found to be 1.72, in other words 72 per cent higher than among women who had had no abortions.

These researchers go on to suggest that "international correlational studies have demonstrated a positive relationship between the incidence of colorectal cancer and that of breast cancer and women with breast cancer are at increased risk of developing a second primary cancer of the colon...this suggests that colon and breast cancer have, at least in part, a common etiology".[11] Given the established link between abortion and breast cancer discussed in Chapter 2, and given that colorectal cancer and breast cancer share some common causes or triggers, then induced abortion may prove to be a common risk factor for both cancers even though Kvale and Heuch assert that "the results have not been consistent" with regard to reproductive factors in the etiology of colorectal cancer.[12]

**Conclusion**

At present, research indicates that after an induced abortion (and especially after more than one abortion), there is an apparent higher risk of contracting cervical, ovarian, or rectal cancer, though the exact links are inconclusive. Researchers have found that a full-term pregnancy resulting in childbirth seems to provide a protective effect for women against cancers of the reproductive system. It is remarkable that with the increase in cancers of the reproductive system in women – and the very serious threat these cancers pose to their health and longevity – there is so little agreement on whether or not induced abortion(s) increase women's risk of cancer. As in other areas of the effects of abortion on women's health, more objective studies are needed.

**Key Points Chapter 3**

•   A history of previous induced abortion(s) may play a role in cancers of the reproductive system and rectal cancers.

•   Inconsistencies between studies and countries where the studies are done, in addition to the fact that in the literature, spontaneous and induced abortions are often not separated, make it difficult to draw definitive conclusions.

•   Recent studies have connected a higher risk of cervical and ovarian cancers to previous abortions, though the degree of risk varies from study to study.

•   A consistent finding has been the protective effect of full-term pregnancies against the onset of cancers of the reproductive system.

•   Researchers have found a connection between abortion and rectal cancer.

•   With reproductive and rectal cancers on the increase in women, more studies are needed, specifically to examine the connection between abortion and cancer.

## Notes

1   Brock KE, Berry G, Brinton LA, Kerr C, MacLennan R, Mock PA, et al. Sexual, reproductive and contraceptive risk factors for carcinoma-in-situ of the uterine cervix in Sydney. Medical Journal of Australia 1989 February 6;150(3):125-30.

2   La Vecchia C, Negri E, Franceschi S, Parazzini F. Long-term impact of reproductive factors on cancer risk. International Journal of Cancer 1993 January 21;53(2):215-9, p. 217.

3   Schwartz SM, Weiss NS, Daling JR, Newcomb PA, Liff JM, Gammon MD, et al. Incidence of histologic types of uterine sarcoma in relation to menstrual and reproductive history. International Journal of Cancer 1991 September 30;49(3):362-7.

4   Remennick LI. Induced abortion as cancer risk factor: a review of epidemiological evidence. Journal of Epidemiology and Community Health 1990 December;44(4):259-64, p. 262.

5   Bernal A, Mendez-Moran L, Fajardo-Gutierrez A, Gonzalez-Lira G, Escudero P, Ortiz H. Univariate and multivariate analysis of risk factors for ovarian cancer: case-control study, Mexico City. Archives of Medical Research 1995, Autumn;26(3):245-9.

6   Chen MT, Cook LS, Daling JR, Weiss NS. Incomplete pregnancies and risk of ovarian cancer (Washington, United States). Cancer Causes and Control 1996 July 7;7(4):415-20.

7   Whittemore AS, Harris R, Itnyre J. Characteristics relating to ovarian cancer risk: collaborative analysis of 12 US case-control studies. II. Invasive epithelial ovarian cancers in white women. Collaborative Ovarian Cancer Group. American Journal of Epidemiology 1992 November 15;136(10):1184-203.

8   Albrektsen G, Heuch I, Tretli S, Kvale G. Is the risk of cancer of the corpus uteri reduced by a recent pregnancy? A prospective study of 765,756 Norwegian women. International Journal of Cancer 1995 May 16;61(4):485-90, p.485.

9   McPherson CP, Sellers TA, Potter JD, Bostick RM, Folsom AR. Reproductive factors and risk of endometrical cancer. The Iowa Women's Health Study. American Journal of Epidemiology 1996 June 5;143(12):1195-202, p. 1195.

10  Kvale G, Heuch I. Is the incidence of colorectal cancer related to reproduction? A prospective study of 63,000 women. International Journal of Cancer 1991 February 1;47(3):390-5, p. 392.

11  Kvale 1991. See n. 10, p. 390.

12  Kvale 1991. See n. 10, p. 390.

Chapter 4

# Impact on Subsequent Pregnancies

Induced abortion creates future reproductive complications for women. These complications include: cervical damage leading to future problems in carrying a pregnancy to term; uterine damage resulting in *placenta previa* which increases the morbidity and mortality risks for both mother and infant; and ectopic pregnancy. Data indicate that in the past twenty years the incidence of these complications has risen sharply. Studies reveal that induced abortion can put a woman at a seven-fold increased risk of placenta previa and a 30 to 510 per cent increased risk of delivering a premature infant. Children born prematurely are at an enormously increased risk of developing cerebral palsy. Ectopic pregnancies are reaching epidemic proportions, the rates having doubled or tripled in many parts of the world in direct proportion to the increase in induced abortions. Yet North American researchers continue to minimize the seriousness of the risk of induced abortion to women's health and its effects on future pregnancies, with their statistical data often being at odds with their conclusions.

# Impact on Subsequent Pregnancies

Induced abortions complicate subsequent pregnancies by increasing the risk of cervical incompetence that causes late spontaneous abortions (miscarriages at eighteen to 22 weeks of age); placenta previa; premature labour and the delivery of premature infants as well as ectopic pregnancies.

Some issues dealt with in this chapter, such as ectopic pregnancy, also affect future fertility. If the primary effect of an induced abortion presents during a subsequent pregnancy we discuss it here. The medical conditions which cause infertility or sterility are found in Chapter 5.

### Uterine or Cervical Damage and Subsequent Pregnancies
One point of agreement among researchers working in the field of post-abortion research is that cervical or uterine damage caused by induced abortions continues to lead to major ongoing complications that affect subsequent pregnancies.

### Cervical Dilation
During the course of a normal pregnancy the cervix needs to resist the tendency to dilate under the downward pressure of the infant in the uterus. A decrease in cervical resistance leads to the premature dilation of the cervix with a subsequent late second trimester spontaneous abortion as the cervix becomes incompetent. Molin examines this problem of decreased cervical resistance following induced first trimester abortions. His study suggests that cervical resistance is correlated with the ability to continue subsequent pregnancies to term and a "fall in resistance to dilatation corresponds to a tear in the cervical tissue of more than two millimeters".[1] He demonstrates that if the cervix is dilated to nine millimeters during an induced abortion prior to the evacuation of the fetus, this can lead to a fall in cervical resistance in 12.5 per cent of patients, while dilating the cervix to eleven millimeters leads to decreased cervical resistance in two thirds (66.7 per cent) of the women. This finding did not change according to whether or not the woman had borne a child.

To reduce such injuries Molin suggests that *prostaglandins* and *laminaria tents* be used for all induced abortions. In many public and university hospitals, such precautions are part of the standard abortion preparation but the practices of private facilities may vary widely.

Injury to the cervix can be a possible cause of later spontaneous abortions. Zlatnik and colleagues determined that such cervical incompetence was associated with a wide cervical canal.[2]

Slater and colleagues reported lower birth weights in subsequent pregnancies when in a previous abortion the dilatation of the cervix was greater than twelve mm. It was also found that the subsequent pregnancies were shorter in duration, although the difference was not statistically significant.[3]

Although the *D&C* method described by Slater and colleagues is no longer used, dilation remains part of present-day *dilation and evacuation (D&E)* procedures. Also, the women who were aborted by D&C may well experience the longer-term effects of the abortion as long as they remain in the childbearing years. Thus a young woman having an abortion in 1985 at the age of seventeen is in her mid-thirties today. This maternal age is now common for a first planned pregnancy.

**Uterine Perforation**

A more recent American study found that *"most traumatic uterine perforations during first-trimester abortions are unreported or even unsuspected"* [emphasis added]. Data from the 1970s showed that tears to the wall of the uterus occurred up to 6.4 times per 1000 abortions. However, they conclude that this was a significant underestimate because such injuries are only detected during later gynecological surgeries. Accordingly, they now report "the true incidence of uterine perforations in the laparoscopic group was... 19.8/1000 procedures."[4] Although few serious consequences result, the women at high risk for such injuries are those who have had children before, who abort under general anesthetic, and are over the age of 35.

Another recent report cautions about the maternal *morbidity* following second-trimester D&E abortions. American

43

practitioners note that "dilation and evacuations between twelve and sixteen weeks...have the potential to cause significant morbidity and mortality." Because of the possible uterine complications, the researchers conclude that such procedures should only be used where intensive emergency treatment can be initiated immediately.[5]

**Placenta Previa**

*Placenta previa* (when the placenta implants in the lower part of the uterus near or over the cervix) may be diagnosed if the placenta is located in the lower uterine segment and extends to the *cervical os* or covers the cervix. The reason for this has been identified by Barrett and colleagues[6] and Rose and Chapman who found an association between uterine scarring and curettage.[7] Where there is scarring of the upper uterus, future pregnancies cannot implant properly and so the new pregnancy becomes attached to the lower uterine segment near or over the cervix. This is known as faulty placentation. This condition is a complication in five of every 1000 deliveries annually in Canada and the United States and can result in serious injury to the mother and death to the baby during delivery, owing to severe *hemorrhage* before or during birth and severe *neonatal hypotension*.

Taylor and colleagues undertook a case-controlled, retrospective, and comparative study of all white women in the state of Washington from 1984 to 1987 whose pregnancies were complicated by placenta previa. They used birth records for this group as well as records of miscarriages and induced abortions. They found that women with a previous history of induced abortion were 28 per cent more likely to have a later pregnancy complicated by placenta previa. They labeled this risk as "minor" and downplayed the finding of Barrett and colleagues who in their 1981 study reported a seven-to fifteen-fold (i.e., 600 to 1400 per cent) excess risk among women who had undergone a legal abortion. They alleged that the Barrett study had failed to account for the dramatic increase in cesarean rates, which had occurred during the same period.

Taylor's study excluded 250 nulliparous women with placenta

previa. Thus the analysis was restricted to women who reported one or more previous live births. The 250 excluded placenta previa cases would have increased the sample by 50 per cent. The possible effect of including women with previous abortions but no live births was not considered in Taylor's discussion.

Taylor concludes that if induced abortion were shown to increase placenta previa, "...it would be of considerable import. However, we found only a small increased risk in association with induced abortion so its clinical or public health significance seems minor."[8] Taylor's conclusion provides a useful illustration of a fact noted elsewhere in this study: That the conclusions of research studies on abortion after-effects often minimize the significance of the data gathered (see Chapter 17 on methodological problems). Others might question this dismissal of a 28 per cent increased risk, as well as the casual disregard of Barrett and colleagues' finding of a *sevenfold* increased risk. Furthermore, while Taylor's study involved fewer than 2200 women, Barrett and colleagues surveyed over 5000.

# Premature or Preterm Births

### Prematurity

A direct consequence of both cervical incompetence and infection is premature or preterm birth (meaning birth at less than 37 weeks gestation). Prematurity is the leading cause of infant death before the age of one. Premature infants who do not die are at a much higher risk for physical and mental handicaps. Indeed pre-term birth is "the leading cause of infant morbidity and mortality."[9] Writing in the *Eugenics Review* about the East-European experience of legalized abortion, Malcolm Potts expressed "little doubt that there is a true relationship between the high incidence of therapeutic abortion and prematurity".[10] Prematurity is therefore a very serious consequence of induced abortion.

What is the magnitude of this risk? Forty-nine studies between 1963 and 2001 in ten countries (The United States, Britain, Germany, Japan, France, Australia, Denmark, Hungary, Greece, and Singapore) point to a statistically significant increased risk of preterm births after abortion.[11] The classic book on the subject is Dr Barbara Luke's *Every Pregnant Woman's Guide to Preventing Premature Birth*, in which she writes "If you have had one or more induced abortions, your risk of prematurity with this pregnancy increases by about 30 per cent."[12]

The leading authority on prematurity is Dr Emile Papiernik. In a recent article he and his colleagues reported:

1. an 86 per cent increased risk of very preterm birth (meaning less than 33 weeks gestation) for women with previous first-trimester abortions.

2. a 267 per cent increased risk of very preterm birth for women with previous second-trimester abotions.[13]

In the same year (1999), Zhou and colleagues in Denmark surveyed 15,727 women whose pregnancies were ended by first-trimester abortions and compared them with 46,026 women whose pregnancies were not interrupted by induced abortions. They discovered the following increased risk of preterm births:

1. after one abortion:          89 per cent
2. after two abortions:         166 per cent
3. after three or more abortions:  103 per cent

They concluded, "The study showed an increase in preterm and post-term pregnancies after induced abortions."[14]

A large German study of 106,345 births showed that previous induced abortions pushed up the likelihood of a subsequent premature delivery by percentages that increased strikingly with the number of previous abortions.

**Increased risk by number of previous abortions**[15]

|                                            | 1   | 2   | 3   |
|--------------------------------------------|-----|-----|-----|
| Delivery at less than 32 weeks (per cent)  | 150 | 460 | 510 |
| Delivery at less than 37 weeks (per cent)  | 50  | 110 | 260 |

Finally, a French study of 12,432 women found an overall increased risk of pre-term birth associated with previous induced abortions to be 40 per cent.[16]

Papiernick's, Zhou's, Martius', and Henriet's are only the most recent of 49 studies from around the world that have found varying degrees of risk of prematurity after abortion. All of these studies' findings were statistically significant. Not surprisingly they demonstrate that the more the abortions the greater the risk. More unexpected is the revelation that the linkage between abortion and prematurity is strongest with extremely premature deliveries (meaning under 32 weeks' gestation).

Why does abortion increase the likelihood of prematurity? According to Dr Luke:

> The procedures for first-trimester abortion involve dilating the cervix slightly and suctioning the contents of the uterus...The procedures for second-trimester abortion are more involved, including dilating the cervix wider and for longer periods, and scraping the inside of the uterus. Women who had had several second-trimester abortions may have a higher incidence of incompetent cervix, a premature spontaneous dilation of the cervix, because the cervix has been artificially dilated several times before this pregnancy.[17]

A second major cause of prematurity mentioned by experts in the field is infection. Dr Janet Daling and colleagues report that if the previous pregnancy ended in induced abortion the risk of intraamniotic infection increased by 140 per cent.[18] As Dr Judith Lumley explains, "One possible mechanism is that cervical instrumentation can facilitate the passage of organisms into the upper part of the uterus, increasing the probability of inapparent infection and subsequent preterm birth."[19]

In short, the greater the number of previous induced abortions the higher the risk of prematurity as a consequence of either cervical incompetence or infection.

**Cerebral Palsy and Other Disabilities Resulting from Prematurity**
The implications of this finding are enormous. In a sweeping survey of 111 studies of prematurity led by Dr Gabriel Escobar of the Kaiser Permanente Medical Center in California, it was determined that *the rate of disability among very low birthweight infants (less than 1500 grams) was 25 per cent. The rate of cerebral palsy was 7.7 per cent.* Given that the rate of cerebral palsy is about 0.2 per cent (or two in a thousand) among the general population, this means that *prematurity at below 1500 grams birth multiplies the risk of the baby's contracting this serious condition over 38 times.*[20]

Further research is needed on the statistical relationship between the rise of induced abortion and the rising incidence of cerebral palsy. There is no doubt however, that more induced abortion means more subsequent preterm births, and more preterm births mean a greatly increased incidence of cerebral palsy. It comes as no surprise to discover that since abortion was legalized in the late 1960s and early 1970s, the incidence of premature births has also risen. Between 1981 and 2001, the rate of premature births rose from 9.4 to 11.9 per cent - a net increase of 27 per cent during these two decades.[21]

The clear link between induced abortion, preterm births and cerebral palsy have implications for informed consent by women who undergo abortion. The point has already been made that the liability costs for cerebral palsy are exceptionally high. Induced abortion, therefore, unless it is accompanied by very detailed informed consent, "may carry an unsupportable legal liability." A consent form that "does not inform women of the elevated future risk of a preterm delivery, and that the latter constitutes a risk factor for devastating complications such as cerebral palsy, may not satisfy courts."[22]

At least three European governments have responded to the greatly increased risk of prematurity and other threats to women's health posed by induced abortion, by sharply curtailing the availability of the procedure. In the early 1970s the Hungarian government, alarmed by the striking increase in premature births to women with a record of induced abortion, and worried also by the striking increase in physically and mentally handicapped babies born to such women, rewrote its abortion law. By restricting access to the procedure it reduced the abortions by 40 percent between 1973 and 1974. This reduction has remained permanent, as Hungary's abortions in 2000 remained below the 1974 total.[23]

Poland is the second country to have cut back the availability of abortion, making it legally permissible only for rape, threat to the mother's life, or serious illness. Since the new law was passed in 1993 the recorded incidence of induced abortion has tumbled from almost 60,000 in 1990 to under a thousand per year.[24]

Finally, in the summer of 2003, as this book goes to press, we learn that the government of Russia has introduced sweeping legislation to enforce stringent criteria before a woman can be approved for an induced abortion. The health impact of abortion on women and their subsequent children are a major thrust behind this legislation.[25]

**Ectopic Pregnancy**
An ectopic pregnancy occurs when an embryo implants outside of the uterine cavity, generally in the fallopian tubes. Rupture of an ectopic pregnancy accounts for ten to fifteen per cent of maternal deaths. The occurrence of ectopic pregnancies has increased significantly in recent years. Goldner used the United States Centers for Disease Control Surveillance Summaries to determine that between 1970 and 1989 "the rate increased almost fourfold from 4.5 to 16.0 ectopic pregnancies per 1000 reported pregnancies."[26]

There are two separate issues regarding the relationship of induced abortion to ectopic pregnancies: 1) The increased risk of ectopic pregnancy occurring subsequently as a result of an induced abortion; 2) The increased health risk incurred when an abortion is performed for an unrecognized ectopic pregnancy.

**Ectopic Pregnancies Subsequent to Induced Abortions**

There is a documented relationship between induced abortion and the occurrence of a subsequent ectopic pregnancy. Michalas and colleagues note "a worldwide epidemic of ectopic pregnancy," and have found that "induced abortions were positively related to ectopic pregnancy."[27]

Even a single abortion increases a woman's risk of having an ectopic pregnancy in the future with the relative risk of a subsequent ectopic pregnancy for a woman who has had an abortion double that experienced by women who have not had induced abortions. They referred to a small study from Boston that reported a 2.6-fold increase in the risk of ectopic pregnancy after two of more induced abortions. Levin in a retrospective study found that the "possible association of multiple prior induced abortions with subsequent ectopic pregnancy persists."[28] In addition, Yugoslav and Japanese studies reported crude relative risks at least double those of women with no history of induced abortion. Parazzini and colleagues in Italy found that the risk of ectopic pregnancy after induced abortion continued to escalate with each subsequent induced abortion a woman underwent.[29] They determined that the ectopic pregnancy risk in women having multiple abortions was thirteen times higher than for women who carried to term. Combined, these five studies all reveal that induced abortion results in a two to thirteen-fold increase in the risk of a subsequent ectopic pregnancy.

Why do induced abortions lead to ectopic pregnancies? Chung and colleagues "showed a highly significant association" between both retained products of conception and pelvic infection following induced abortion and the later occurrence of ectopic pregnancies. They conclude that these two medical complications of abortion lead to a five-fold increase in the rate of ectopic pregnancies.[30] The most common cause of an ectopic pregnancy is pelvic infection.[31] Induced abortions increase the incidence of pelvic infections which cause scarring within the fallopian tubes. The scar tissue interferes with normal tubal motility or flexibility. As a consequence the fertilized ovum is entrapped and then implants in the tube. The presence of post-abortion pelvic inflammatory disease is predictive of a greater likelihood of an ectopic pregnancy in the future.

### Undiagnosed Ectopic Pregnancies at the Time of an Induced Abortion

Ectopic pregnancies can be difficult and costly to identify.[32] A woman with an ectopic pregnancy generally presents six to eight weeks after her last menstrual period with a history of abdominal pain and vaginal bleeding. Twenty per cent of women with an ectopic pregnancy will not experience abdominal pain [33] Therefore a woman with an ectopic pregnancy could have an abortion and, assuming that she is not longer pregnant, dismiss her symptoms of pain and bleeding as normal post-abortion side-effects. This is of special concern because most abortion clinics advise women to expect cramping and bleeding for up to three weeks and no period for six to eight weeks. For two vital reasons a woman with an undiagnosed ectopic pregnancy is placed in a vulnerable position by this advice: 1) It may not only cause a significant delay in making the correct diagnosis; 2) it may also increase her risk of serious medical complications and death.

Concerns regarding abortion and missed ectopic pregnancies are underscored by recent publication in Archives of Pathology which note that certain jurisdictions have not yet adopted the recommendation that all tissue removed at the time of an induced abortion be examined for fetal parts. Studies have found that medical follow-up was required in 28 per cent of cases where the pathology was abnormal. Obviously the absence of fetal tissue would alert medical personnel to the possible presence of an ectopic pregnancy and potentially avert a life-threatening event.

Because ectopic pregnancies are a significant cause of maternal deaths request have been made to the Centers for Disease Control to investigate all deaths from ectopic pregnancies to determine if a woman has had a recent abortion. Any identified deaths would then be attributed to induced abortions, not pregnancy. (see Chapter 6 for a further discussion of maternal mortality).

**Limitations in the North-American Data**

Daling and colleagues found that women who had two or more induced abortions increased their risk of ectopic pregnancy 2.6 times. While admitting that this finding is "worrisome", they nonetheless concluded that "it remains unresolved whether having a legal induced abortion in the United States imparts an excess risk of EP [ectopic pregnancy]." The abstract to the study states that the research shows that abortion "does not carry a large excess risk." Here again, the conclusion is at odds with the data.[34]

Many observers would consider a risk of a 2.6 times increase in a potentially life-threatening condition to be "excess[ive]." As we have noted above in the section on *Placenta Previa*, there is a marked tendency in the North-American literature on abortion for researchers to minimize their own findings. Those interested in the subject are well advised to read the numerical data and compare them carefully with the abstract and conclusions, rather than relying on either the abstract or conclusions alone. Comparisons are also recommended with literature from European countries, particularly Great Britain and the Scandinavian countries, where population size and sophisticated medical linkage data bases make data collection more accurate and comprehensive.

Another compromising factor is that North-American statistics do not always break down the risks by population group. This is a limitation because some ethnocultural groups in North America are at significantly greater risk than the aggregate data show. African-American women, for example, are more likely to die from an ectopic pregnancy present at the time of an induced abortion.[35] Goldner notes that "...deaths from complications were consistently higher for blacks and other racial minorities than for whites throughout the period."[36]

**Conclusion**

A survey of the literature makes it clear that "an underreporting of information particularly with respect to an induced abortion" is a major flaw in all retrospective research.[37] Underreporting is clearly a problem in the North-American case data as well. There are many procedures which aborting women are subject to, whose consequences put them at higher risk for future health problems: Cervical dilation, still used in D&E, can lead to cervical incompetence which often results in miscarriage; uterine perforations may be three times higher than previously believed; abortion produces an increase of up to sevenfold in the risk of placenta previa; and there is a disturbing rise in ectopic pregnancies which are significant contributors to maternal deaths and which are very likely associated with the increase in induced abortions over the past 30 years. Indeed, the five studies we surveyed reported *an increased risk, anywhere from twofold to thirteenfold, that induced abortion will lead to an ectopic pregnancy.*

The gravest consequence of induced abortion for future pregnancy is a rise in the rate of premature births ranging from 30 to 700 per cent. Preterm babies weighing less than 1500 grams suffer an incidence of cerebral palsy over 38 times greater than full-term babies. Thus induced abortion tremendously increases a woman's risk of later bearing a child with cerebral palsy.

Too many North-American studies minimize these findings with serious implications for the present and future health of North-American women, especially those who are African-American.

**Key Points Chapter 4**

• Subsequent pregnancies are negatively affected by induced abortion.

• The main complications are: cervical incompetence leading to future miscarriages; uterine perforations and placenta previa with serious implications to the health of the woman and her child(ren) in later pregnancies; and ectopic pregnancies which, if undiagnosed and not treated, can lead to a woman's death.

• Forty-nine studies of preterm or premature births from Europe and North America found increased risks ranging from 30 per cent to 510 per cent.

• The consequence of this significantly increased risk of prematurity after abortion is that the rate of cerebral palsy among premature infants weighing less than 1500 grams at birth is 38 times greater than among the general population. Induced abortion, in other words, is directly responsible for many thousands of cases of cerebral palsy – in North America alone – that otherwise would not have occurred.

• Despite the data which point to the link between induced abortion and future serious health risks, many North-American research studies fail to point these out.

• Numerical data should be carefully compared to research abstracts and conclusions because they often do not correlate; in other words, where data clearly indicate increased health risks, they are often minimized in the abstracts and conclusions of medical articles.

• In light of the growing knowledge of the impact of abortion on the rate of prematurity, abortion providers may soon incur greatly increased liability for obtaining informed consent from women contemplating induced abortion.

## Notes

1  Molin A. Risk of damage to the cervix by dilatation for first-trimester-induced abortion by suction aspiration. Gynecologic and Obstetric Investigation 1993;35(3):152-4.

2  Zlatnik FJ, Burmeister LF, Feddersen DA, Brown RC. Radiological appearance of the upper cervical canal in women with a history of premature delivery II. Relationship to clinical presentation and to tests of cervical compliance. Journal of Reproductive Medicine 1989 August;34(8):525-30.

3  Slater PE, Davies AM, Harlap S. The effect of abortion method on the outcome of subsequent pregnancy. Journal of Reproductive Medicine 1981 March;26(3):123-8.

4  Kaali SG, Szigetvari IA, Bartfai GS. The frequency and management of uterine perforations during first-trimester abortions. American Journal of Obstetrics and Gynecology 1989 August;161(2):406-8; p. 407.

5  Trott E, Ziegler W, Levey J. Major complications associated with termination of a second trimester pregnancy: a case report. Delaware Medical Journal 1995 May;67(5):294-6.

6  Barrett JM, Boehm FH, Killam AP. Induced abortion: a risk factor for placenta previa. American Journal of Obstetrics and Gynecology 1981 December 1;141(7):769-72.

7  Rose GL, Chapman MG. Aetiological factors in placenta praevia--a case controlled study. British Journal of Obstetrics and Gynaecology 1986 June;93(6):586-8.

8  Taylor VM, Kramer MD, Vaughan TL, Peacock S. Placenta previa in relation to induced and spontaneous abortion: a population-based study. Obstetrics and Gynecology 1993 July;82(1):88-91; p. 91.

9  Thorp JM, Hartmann KE, Shadigian E. Long-term physical and psychological health consequences of induced abortion: review of the evidence. Obstetrical and Gynecological Survey 2003;58(1):67-79; p.75.

10 Potts M. Legal abortion in Eastern Europe. Eugenics Review 1966-1967; 58-59:232-250, p. 235.

11 Zhou W, Sorensen HT, Olsen J. Induced abortion and subsequent pregnancy duration. Obstetrics & Gynecology 1999 Dec;94(6):948-53.

Pickering RM, Forbes J. Risk of preterm delivery and small-for-gestational age infants following abortion: A population study. British Journal of Obstetrics and Gynaecology 1985;92:1106-1112.

Michielutte R, Ernest JM, Moore ML, Meis PJ, Shrp PC, Wells HB, Buescher PA. A comparison of risk assessment models for term and preterm low birthweight. Preventive Medicine 1992;21:98-109.

Berkowitz GS. An epidemiologic study of preterm delivery. American Journal of Epidemiology 1981;113;81-92.

Lieberman E, Ryan KJ, Monson RR, Schoenbaum SC. Risk factors accounting for racial differences in the rate of premature birth. New England Journal of Medicine 1987;317:743-748.

Lang JM, Lieberman E, Cohen A. A comparison of risk factors for preterm labor and term small-for-gestational-age birth. Epidemiology 1996;7:369-376.

Mueller-Heubach E, Guzick DS. Evaluation of risk scoring in a preterm birth prevention study of indigent patients. American Journal of Obstetrics and Gynecology 1989;160:829-837.

Shiono PH, Lebanoff MA. Ethnic differences in preterm and very preterm delivery. American Journal of Public Health 1986;76:1317-1321.

Pantelakis SN, Papadimitrious GC, Doxiadis SA. Influence of induced and spontaneous abortions on the outcome of subsequent pregnancies. American Journal of Obstetrics and Gynecology. 1973;116:799-805.

Lumley J. The association between prior spontaneous abortion, prior induced abortion and preterm birth in first singleton births. Prenatal and Neonatal Medicine 1998;3:21-24.

Van Der Slikke JW, Treffers PE. Influence of induced abortion on gestational duration in subsequent pregnancies. British Medical Journal 1978;1:270-272.

Richardson JA, Dixon G. Effect of legal termination on subsequent pregnancy. British Medical Journal 1976;1:1303-1304.

Pickering RM, Deeks JJ. Risks of delivery during 20th to the 36th week of gestation. International Journal of Epidemiology 1991;20:456-466.

Koller O, Eikhom SN. Late sequelae of induced abortion in primigravidae. Acta Obstetricia et Gynecologica Scandanavica 1977;56:311-317.

Papaevangelou G. Vrettos AS, Papadatos D, Alexious C. The effect of spontaneous and induced abortion on prematurity and birthweight. Journal of Obstetrics and Gynaecology of the British Commonwealth May 1973;80:418-422.

Bognar Z, Czeizel A. Mortality and morbidity associated with legal abortions in Hungary, 1960-1973. American Journal of Public Health 1976;66:568-575.

Martius JA, Steck T. Oehler MK, Wulf K-H. Risk factors associated with preterm (<37+0 weeks) and early preterm (<32+0 weeks): univariate and multi-variate analysis of 106 345 singleton births from 1994 statewide perinatal survey of Bavaria. European Journal of Obstetrics & Gynecology and Reproductive Biology 1998;80:183-189.

Lekea-Karanika V, Tzoumaka-Bakoula C and Golding J. Previous obstetric history and subsequent preterm delivery in Greece. European Journal of Obstetrics & Gynecology and Reproductive Biology 1990 November;37:99-109.

Ancel PV, Saurel-Cubizolles MJ, Renzo GCD, Papiernik E, Breait G. Very and moderate preterm births: are the risk factors different? British Journal of Obstetrics and Gynaecology 1999; 106:1162-1170.

Lumley J. Very low birth-weight (<1500g) and previous induced abortion: Victoria 1982-1983. Australian and New Zealand Journal of Obstetrics and Gynecology 1986;26:268-272.

Twenty-nine additional studies are listed in Rooney B, Calhoun BC. Induced abortion and the Risk of later premature births. Journal of American Physicians and Surgeons 2003 (Summer) [See footnote 22].

12  Luke B. *Every Pregnant Woman's Guide to Preventing Premature Birth*. 1995 [foreword by Emile Papiernik], New York: Times Books; p. 32.

13  Ancel P-Y, Saurel-Cubizolles M-J, Renzo GCD, Papiernik E, Breart G. Very and moderate preterm births: Are the risk factors different? British Journal of Obstetrics and Gynaecology 1999; 106:1162-1170.

14  Zhou et al. 1999. See n. 11, p. 948.

15  Martius et al. 1998. See n. 11.

16  Henriet L, Kaminski M. Impact of induced abortions on subsequent pregnancy outcome: The 1995 French national perinatal survey. British Journal of Obstetrics and Gynaecology 2001; 108: 1036-1042; p.1036

17  Luke 1995. See n. 12, pp. 32-33.

18  Krohn MA, Daling JR, , Miscarriage or termination in the immediately preceding pregnancy increases the risk of intraamniotic infection in the following pregnancy. American Journal of Epidemiology 1992;136:1013

19  Lumley 1998. See n. 11.

20  Escobar GJ, Littenberg B, Petitti DB. Outcome among surviving very low birthweight infants: a meta-analysis. Archives of Disease in Childhood 1991;66:204-211.

21  Martin JA, Hamilton BE, Ventura SJ, Menacker F, Park MM, Sutton PD. Births: Final Data for 2001. National Vital Statistics Reports 2002 December 18;51(2). http://www.cdc.gov/nchs/releases/02news/precare.htm

22  Rooney, B, Calhoun, BC. Induced abortion and the risk of later premature births. Journal of American Physicians and Surgeons 2003 (summer); 8 (2): 46-49, p. 47.

23  Hungary, 2001, in Demographic Yearbook, 2001 ed., on line, Council of Europe. Available at http://www.coe.int/t/e/social%5fcohesion/population/demographic%5fyear%5fbook/2001%_Edition/Hungary%202001.asp. http://www.johnstonsarchive.net/policy/abortion/ab-hungary.html

24  Gentles, I. In the matter of child care, Canada could learn from Poland. The Report 2000 (9 October 2000), p. 46]

25  Russia prepares to end its embrace of abortion: tighter laws reverse tradition of tolerance. Globe and Mail [Toronto] 2003 (2 July), p. A1;

25  Russians Feel Abortion's Complications; used as birth control in Soviet times, practice has led to widespread infertility. Washington Post 2003 (22 February), A16, Final Edition.

26  Goldner TE, Lawson HW, Xia Z, Atrash HK. Surveillance for ectopic pregnancy--United States, 1970-1989. Morbidity and Mortality Weekly Report, Centers for Disease Control Surveillance Summary 1993 December;42((SS-6)):73-85.

27  Michalas S, Minaretzis D, Tsionou C, Maos G, Kioses E, Aravantinos D. Pelvic surgery, reproductive factors and risk of ectopic pregnancy: A case controlled study. International Journal of Gynecology and Obstetrics 1992 June;38(2):101-5, pp. 101, 103.

28  Levin AA, Schoenbaum SC, Stubblefield PG, Zimicki S, Monson RR, Ryan KJ. Ectopic pregnancy and prior induced abortion. American Journal of Public Health 1982 March;72(3):253-6.

29  Parazzini F, Ferraroni M, Tozzi L, Ricci E, Mezzopane R, La Vecchia C. Induced abortions and risk of ectopic pregnancy. Human Reproduction 1995 July;10(7):1841-4.

30  Chung CS, Smith RG, Steinhoff PG, Mi MP. Induced abortion and ectopic pregnancy in subsequent pregnancies. American Journal of Epidemiology 1982 June;115(6):879-87; p. 884.

31  Tenore J. Ectopic Pregnancy. American Family Physician 2000 (Feb.15): 1080-1088.

32  Wong TW, Lau CC, Yeung A, Lo L, Tai CM. Efficacy of transabdominal ultrasound examination in the diagnosis of early pregnancy complications in an emergency department. Journal of Accidental and Emergency Medicine 1998 May;15(3),155-8

33  Abbott J, Emmans LS, Lowenstein SR. Ectopic pregnancy: ten common pitfalls in diagnosis. American Journal of Emergency Medicine 1990;8:515-522.

34  Daling JR, Chow WH, Weiss NS, Metch BJ, Soderstrom R. Ectopic pregnancy in relation to previous induced abortion. Journal of the American Medical Association 1985 February;253(7):1005-8.

35  Atrash HK, Koonin LM, Lawson HW, Franks AL, Smith JC. Maternal mortality in the United States, 1979-1986. Obstetrics & Gynecology 1990 December;76(6):1055-60.

Atrash HK, MacKay HT, Hogue CJ. Ectopic pregnancy concurrent with induced abortion: incidence and mortality. American Journal of Obstetrics and Gynecology 1990 March;162(3):726-30.

36  Goldner et al. 1993. See n. 26.

37  Taylor et al. 1993. See n. 8.

Chapter 5

# Future Fertility

Infertility research clearly shows that abortion can lead to problems for women who later wish to conceive and carry a pregnancy to full term. This is especially true for women who had no successful pregnancy prior to one or more abortions. Lax coding systems in hospitals and lack of follow up by abortion clinics have delayed our recognition of the magnitude of the link between induced abortion and hysterectomy, pelvic inflammatory disease (PID), ectopic pregnancy, miscarriage, and premature birth of a non-surviving baby. Many years may elapse between an induced abortion and the woman's later difficulty in having a child. This long interval may obscure the link between the two experiences.

# Future Fertility

Some post-abortive *sequelae* that affect future fertility are not apparent until the woman attempts to conceive a child and seeks a medical explanation of her inability to do so. These may include *pelvic inflammatory disease; Chlamydia trachomatis*; uterine perforation; *Asherman's Syndrome*; *endometrial ossification; endometrial adhesions*; and *ectopic pregnancy*.

By the term "infertility" we mean problems with conceiving naturally and giving birth to at least one full-term, live infant. Infertility problems do not rule out the possibility that repeated attempts using fertility drugs or high-tech fertility treatment, such as *in vitro fertilization*, might succeed.

It should be noted, however, that the women who can afford the costs of infertility treatment do not make up the total population of infertile women who want to conceive. Some women who wish to have a child cannot afford in vitro fertilization as it is not covered by government or private health plans; others view technological approaches to conception as incompatible with their present belief or value system.

It is also important to separate infertility as a medical condition from the desire to conceive children. Most subjects for infertility studies are recruited from infertility clinic populations. Women who do not seek to have further children after having an abortion may never know about their infertility. They may believe that a method of contraception they are using is effective. As a result, they will not be included in research studies on infertility following abortion. (They may, however, appear in studies citing effective contraception following abortion.) Given these limitations, the figures in the post-abortion literature should be understood as representing the minimum of women who are infertile following abortion rather than the total percentage.

The term "sterility" refers to occurrences that seem to rule out future pregnancies altogether, for example, a complete *hysterectomy*. Complications of abortion can produce sterility if they require the removal of reproductive organs.

**Immediate Complications Producing Sterility**

The immediate medical complications of induced abortion may on rare occasions necessitate a hysterectomy.[1] Castadot notes that pelvic infection with at least three days fever at 38°C, bleeding requiring transfusion, and a second surgery due to problems from the first represent 88 per cent of all major complications. He says, "Sometimes a hysterectomy is the only alternative."[2] Without this surgery the patient will die from hemorrhage or peritonitis. With this surgery the patient is rendered sterile.

It is not clear from the present research how often outcomes that produce sterility occur. Numerous occurrences are reported from patient records identified in a 1996 survey of official medical and legal files.[3] But Ferris and colleagues removed hysterectomy from their study because there was only one case.[4] If the removal of such cases is common research practice it is difficult to pinpoint the actual numbers of women who experience this complication.

Likewise, the coding system of hospitals may make it difficult to determine any link between a hysterectomy and a recent induced abortion. Just such a case is identified in Chapter 17, Section A.3.e, where a physician reports that the final code entered in the patient records did not show that the hysterectomy was the complication of an induced abortion performed three weeks earlier.

Hysterectomy may be an immediate consequence of an abortion when lacerations or abrasions to the uterus occur, or when bleeding from a severed uterine artery can be stopped only by removing the entire uterus. Such incidents have also been documented when damage occurs to the bowel or small intestine.

How often does this happen? A major unknown factor in assessing the number of emergency hysterectomies that are required is whether a patient who experienced severe bleeding after discharge from a day patient abortion clinic would return to the clinic. It is the policy of most private day clinics to instruct the patient to go to a hospital if complications arise. In such cases, the problems she experiences may not enter the abortion statistics.

"I have seen post-TA [therapeutic abortion] bleeds in ER [Emergency Room] and they are not readily identified."
*Survey of Canadian Physicians on Women's Health after Induced Abortion*

### General Studies of Post-Abortion Infertility

Abortion of a first pregnancy may have an effect on future fertility according to a large study in the United Kingdom undertaken by Frank and colleagues for the Royal College of Physicians and Surgeons. Using both prospective and retrospective approaches, they studied two groups of women: one group, who form the prospective cohort, were women who had an unplanned pregnancy followed by a planned pregnancy, or an attempt to conceive; the second group, the retrospective cohort, was made up of women with a planned pregnancy. These women were interviewed regarding their reproductive histories.[5]

This Royal College paper is widely regarded as the seminal study of fertility following abortion. Using the "Planning Time" construct as the basis for between group comparisons, it found that the abortion group experienced six per cent lower fertility than the non-abortion group, but concluded that induced abortion does not have "an important effect" on future fertility. "Similarly there was no significant relationship between a history of previous induced abortion and the planning time of women attending ante-natal clinics." Yet its conclusions continued, "one potentially important association was found which has not been reported previously. *Primigravid* women [women who are pregnant for the first time] who had an abortion had a lowered fertility when compared with primigravid whose first pregnancy had a natural conclusion."

This finding is confirmed by European research which concludes, "When a woman has not previously given birth, her risk of contracting post-abortal complication is found to be significantly greater than in women with one or more births...post-abortal PID (*pelvic inflammatory disease*) significantly increased rates of subsequent infertility and spontaneous abortion."[6] Women whose first pregnancies end in abortion are susceptible to uterine perforations, to uterine adhesions or to retained fetal fragments, and infections that lead to PID, all of which can negatively affect their ability to conceive and bear children in the future. Likewise, these women are not going to benefit from the protective effect that a first full-term pregnancy imparts. Recent *epidemiological* studies have also identified childbirth as protective against later onset cancers[7] (see Chapter 3 on induced abortion and other cancers).

**Pelvic Inflammatory Disease and Chlamydia Trachomatis**
According to the Canadian Pelvic Inflammatory Disease Society, pelvic inflammatory disease (PID) is epidemic in Canada and much of the world. Almost 100,000 Canadian women contract PID each year. The Society estimated that one in four North-American women would have had PID by the year 2000. They noted that pelvic inflammatory disease can also be caused by "any procedure which dilates a woman's cervix or introduces bacteria into the pelvic organs." They also commented that "Researchers estimate that 30 to 50 per cent of PID is not diagnosed."[8] PID has grave implications for a woman's future fertility. Writing in *The Lancet*, Blackwell and colleagues note that "at least ten per cent of women who have a single episode of pelvic infection will become subfertile."[9]

Pelvic inflammatory disease triggered by the presence of Chlamydia trachomatis, apart from any immediate health consequences, is probably the largest single inhibitor of women's future fertility. It can also be the underlying cause of a later ectopic pregnancy which reduces or ends fertility. Where PID is triggered by an abortion, a chain of events links abortion and later ectopic pregnancy, though it may not be pointed out in the literature as such.[10]

The relationship between induced abortion and episodes of PID is well established. For example, Levallois and colleagues report that "Pelvic infection is the most common complication of curettage abortion. Although the rate of postabortal infections is low, it is of public concern for two reasons: First, abortion is a procedure commonly performed on young women; second, pelvic infection can lead to serious sequelae."[11] Sorensen and colleagues conclude that "Pelvic inflammatory disease is the most frequent complication after induced abortion...." Contradicting Lavallois and colleagues, they refer to "...*the high incidence of postabortal PID*, [emphasis added] with potential long-term risks of chronic pelvic pain, *dyspareunia*, subfertililty and ectopic pregnancy".[12]

The abortion procedure can trigger an episode of PID in any woman, but those post-abortion women who already have Chlamydia are at far higher risk of PID than women who do not carry the organism. Women can be asymptomatic and still harbor Chlamydia trachomatis in the lower genital tract. If the abortion clinic does not test for this and prescribe the appropriate antibiotic regime, the woman may only discover the Chlamydia while being treated for post-abortion PID. By then it may be too late to avoid later fertility problems.

Much of the research on the relationship between abortion and pelvic inflammatory disease has been carried out in Europe, particularly in Scandinavia, and the United Kingdom. The research confirms a prospective incidence rate range of six to 30 per cent for post-abortion infection. Even more worrying, the large Danish study by Nielsen and colleagues found that even administering the antibiotic ofloxacin before the abortion "[did] not significantly decrease the rate of post-abortal PID, neither among women with a history of PID nor among those without previous PID".[13]

These findings contrast with an American study, which found that "the incidence [of postabortal upper genital tract infection] may be as low as 0.5 per cent."[14]

Jonsson and colleagues established a *seroprevalence* rate for Chlamydia of 24.7 per cent among sexually active women in Sweden. They also found that the number of sexual partners, age at first coitus, history of induced abortion, and previous PID were "independently correlated with seropositivity [a positive blood test for an organism causing PID]".[15] Women with a history of induced abortion were an astoundingly *3.15 times more likely to be seropositive than women without a history of induced abortion.* To put it another way, 45.8 per cent of aborting women were later shown to be seropositive.

While claiming that rates of infection following abortion are low, Sawaya and colleagues report, from a *meta-analysis* of articles, that "Long-term sequelae of post-abortal infection include chronic pelvic pain, dyspareunia and infertility."[16]

Delay in the onset of symptoms is a critical factor when considering PID caused by Chlamydia following abortion. Blackwell and colleagues found from their patient records that women continued to develop symptoms at eleven weeks, 24 weeks, and 36 weeks post-abortion.[17] Osser and Persson found it to be variable: If the woman was positive for Chlamydia before the abortion, the time of onset for *salpingitis* (infection of the fallopian tubes) was 14.1 days and for *endometritis* (infection of the uterus) 8.2 days. As they report, "chlamydia-associated infections were diagnosed on the average three to ten days later than cases without chlamydia."[18] Such complications would not be identified by abortion clinics as immediate sequelae, or coded as being related to an abortion at all.

Because most women undergoing curettage abortion in the United States are young, unmarried, and have never had a child, upper genital tract infections and subsequent infertility can be devastating. Moreover, "the financial costs associated with treating pelvic infection and its sequelae are substantial".[19]

Tables 5-1 and 5-2 show that the percentage of women who test positive for Chlamydia trachomatis at the time of abortion has increased steadily over the past fifteen years.

But it should be remembered that these numbers are from well-regulated hospital clinics associated with research facilities. Private abortion clinics might not conduct these tests.

**Table 5-1**
**Percentage of aborting women testing positive for Chlamydia at the time of their abortion**[20]

| author/date | % women positive |
|---|---|
| Westergaard 1982 | 10 |
| Qvigstad 1983 | 12.6 |
| Osser and Persson 1984 | 6.3 |
| Barbacci 1986 | 17.6 |
| Sorensen 1992 | 8 |
| Blackwell 1993 | 8 |
| Jonsson 1995 | 2.7 |

**Table 5-2**
**Percentage of women who develop pelvic inflammatory disease following abortion, by Chlamydia status**[21]

| author/date | % chlamydia negative | % chlamydia positive |
|---|---|---|
| Westergaard 1982 | 10 | 28 |
| Qvigstad 1983 | 1.6 | 20 |
| Osser and Persson 1984 | 6.3 | 37.7 |
| Sorensen 1992 | 13 | 43 |
| Blackwell 1993 | - | 63 |
| Nielsen 1993 | 11.9 | 17 |
| Sorensen 1994 | - | 72 |
| Oakeshott 1994 | 5 | 19 |

The research findings noted above show just how pervasive and international is the problem of PID following abortion. Giertz and colleagues found that Chlamydia is a major cause of post-abortion PID, particularly in young women in Scandinavia.[22] Their research confirmed the early finding of Westergaard and colleagues and Qvigstad and colleagues.[23] Induced abortion is a trigger that can often move the infection into the uterine cavity and produce effects that Chlamydia by itself might not cause.

Barbacci found that 17.6 per cent of patients presenting for abortion at the Johns Hopkins Hospital tested positive for

Chlamydia. The doctors found "A significant correlation between the isolation of C[hlamydia] trachomatis from the endocervical canal of patients undergoing therapeutic abortion and subsequent development of endometritis within two weeks of the [abortion]".[24] Many of these women were asymptomatic before the abortion. Sorensen and colleagues found that *untreated women with Chlamydia infection at the time of abortion had a cumulative risk of 72 per cent of developing early and/or late PID* if observed for 24 months. The risk was reduced to eight per cent if the infection was treated at the time of the abortion. They conclude that these women run the "risk of serious sequelae such as ectopic pregnancy".[25]

In the general population of women in the childbearing years who develop pelvic inflammatory disease, Washington and colleagues report that 30 to 50 per cent of all PID is caused by Chlamydia trachomatis representing 402,200 episodes of Chlamydia PID each year in the United States.[26] If one uses the conservative estimates in Tables 3-1 and 3-2 above, about six to ten per cent of aborting women are positive for Chlamydia. With over 1,300,000 abortions each year in North America, roughly 100,000 of these women probably carry this *sexually transmitted disease (STD)*. If abortion clinics are not pretesting and treating STD with *prophylactic antibiotics*, then seventeen to 63 per cent of these women go on to develop PID. Again, using conservative estimates, somewhere in the range of 15,000–65,000 cases of PID may occur each year to Chlamydia-positive women who undergo induced abortion. Chlamydia often goes undetected. But even if every woman infected with it were treated at the time of her abortion, over 10,000 would still contract PID as a result of the abortion.

**Prevention of Pelvic Inflammatory Disease and Chlamydia**
There has been a growing literature discussing the efficacy of pre-abortion testing and treatment for Chlamydia. Sawaya and colleagues report that, based on their meta-analysis, there is "a substantial protective effect of antibiotics in all subgroups of women undergoing therapeutic abortion, even women in low-risk groups."[27] At the same time, the

European research suggests that a single antibiotic dose before abortion has little protective effect and may not decrease post-abortion PID. Because the onset can occur anywhere from one to 36 weeks (nine months) following the procedure, pretesting and aggressive antibiotic therapy for those infected is necessary to prevent development. Blackwell and colleagues utilize a ten-day regime of antibiotics, but recognize the limitation discussed by Brewer and problems with post-abortion compliance: "...although all were given a five-day course of prophylactic oxytetracycline (antibiotic), many left their tablets behind. Most women feel well after abortion. Others may not want to be reminded of it."[28]

Sorensen and colleagues report that erythromycin given prophylactically is effective against PID. But they found that when post-abortion PID was not associated with Chlamydia, "erythromycin prophylaxis did not have any effect on these women, nor did it have an effect on nulliparous women or in those with no previous pregnancies." Similarly, Nielsen and colleagues found that "A single oral dose of ofloxacin (400 mg) did not reduce the incidence of Postabortive PID...."[29]

**Risk Factors for Abortion-Related PID**
Heisterberg and colleagues provided evidence for an increased rate of complications in women who had never borne a child. Nielsen has identified the risk factors for PID as: previous PID incident, no previously borne children, a previous induced abortion. Levallois and colleagues found that in a sample of Quebec women attending for abortion at Laval University Hospital those patients who were repeat abortion seekers and who "...were nulliparous with multiple sex partners developed pelvic infection nearly three times more frequently than others not having these characteristics".[30]

The evidence suggests that single, sexually active, never-previously-pregnant young women are the most likely to suffer from PID following an induced abortion. An incident of PID in adolescence may mean that the woman will never achieve a successful pregnancy.

**Uterine Perforation**

Leibner notes that "Although uterine perforation with intra-abdominal injury is a well-described complication of vacuum aspiration termination of pregnancy, most post-abortion perforations go undetected".[31] Women may remain asymptomatic or may develop abdominal discomfort many weeks after the abortion, which may signal damage to surrounding organs such as the small bowel.

Kaali and colleagues discovered this to be true during a study of 6408 first-trimester abortions.[32] They found that the resulting true uterine perforation rate was actually about seven times higher than the practitioner typically suspected. Practitioners suspected a rate of 2.8 per 1000 procedures when "the instrument was passed beyond the expected distance." However, Kaali also checked the number of perforations found in patients whose abortions were performed along with *laparoscopic sterilization*. The total showed a detected perforation rate of 19.6 per 1000 procedures, "*sevenfold higher* than the perforation rate recognized with traditional methods" (i.e., surgeon's suspicion) [emphasis added]. They also note that "...most traumatic uterine perforations during first-trimester abortions are unreported or even unsuspected".[33] The presence of such injuries is only detected later when scarring prevents implantation of a subsequent pregnancy or when women have difficulty conceiving or carrying a pregnancy to term.

This raises the question of what happens to women who have an abortion without sterilization by laparoscopy? It may be assumed that their rate of undetected perforation is also seven times higher. But, insofar as they were not also sterilized, they would not likely know about it and would not know that this event could affect their future fertility. Untreated uterine perforations may produce scar tissue that can affect the implantation of an embryo in a future pregnancy.

**Asherman's Syndrome**

The diagnosis of Asherman's Syndrome (intrauterine adhesions or IUA, also known as *synechia uteri*), typically occurs in the context of menstrual difficulties or infertility. Schenker looked for the causes of this disorder and concluded that all evidence suggests that it is the result of trauma to the pregnant uterus, mostly through abortions: "Gestational changes bring about the softening of the uterus; consequently, the traumatizing effect of eventual curettage is more intense". Therefore it is possible that the depth of curettage may cause "denudation of the basal layer, the regenerative reservoir of the endometrium."[34] Of the IUA cases reported as connected to pregnancy, 66.7 per cent, occurred after curettage for abortion while 21.5 per cent happened after post-partum curettage and two per cent followed cesarian section. Abortion was by far the leading factor. Schenker suggests that because Asherman's will not necessarily occur immediately but may do so after a delay, physicians should be suspicious when *amenorrhea* or *hypomenorrhea* (absent or scanty menstrual periods), habitual spontaneous abortion, and infertility develop in a patient following mechanical trauma to a pregnant uterus.

Schenker goes on to graph the outcome for untreated intrauterine adhesions: Of the 133 patients, 78 conceived a total of 165 times, but only 50 of these pregnancies progressed to term delivery while 38 had premature deliveries and 66 miscarried. The remaining pregnancies experienced other obstetrical complications which resulted in loss. Even if treated, the success rate varied with the severity of the adhesions. In cases of mild adhesions, 95 per cent pregnancy was achieved with a fifteen per cent spontaneous abortion (miscarriage) rate, while with severe adhesions the pregnancy rate was only 60 per cent with a spontaneous abortion rate of 50 per cent.

A recent French study headed by Sylvie Capella-Allouc confirms that "The most common cause [of Asherman's Syndrome] is dilatation and curettage (D&C) of a recently pregnant uterus", whether the pregnancy was ended by spontaneous or induced abortion, or by live birth. The incidence of intrauterine adhesions after one D&C was found to be sixteen per cent; after two and three procedures the incidences were fourteen and 32 per cent respectively, of which more than 50 per cent were severe adhesions.[35]

At present we do not know how common Asherman's Syndrome is following induced abortion, but uterine adhesions are present in "68 per cent of women with secondary infertility who have a past history of two or more uterine curettages [D&C]."[36] What is most pernicious about Asherman's Syndrome is that women may appear asymptomatic while at the same time reporting a variety of ill-defined disorders such as menstrual irregularity or ongoing infertility.[37]

**Endometrial Ossification (Retained Fetal Bones)**
Documentation of future infertility as a result of endometrial ossification (retained fetal bones) is seldom found in the abortion literature.[38] But it often occurs in clinical studies in gynecology or emergency medicine. Chan discusses the circumstances around this type of infertility and reports other presenting symptoms such as *dysmenorrhoea* (pain or discomfort before a menstrual period) or *menorrhagia* (heavy menstrual flow). Chan concludes that "Some bony fragments may be embedded in the endometrium or myometrium [the muscular wall of the uterus] and may not be identified at curettage." For this reason he suggests, "Retained fetal bones should be considered in all patients with infertility, dysfunctional uterine bleeding, dysmenorrhoea or other symptoms dating from a pregnancy or pregnancy termination."[39]

Ruiz-Velasco and colleagues found that the presence of bone fragments in the endometrium, brought on by ossification around fetal remains, can cause infertility over a number of years, and comment that these problems "are not very rare, that is to say that they are more frequent than thought"[40] Torne and colleagues conclude that in endometrial ossification "the common feature in most reported cases is a previous history of abortion, and the result can be secondary infertility."[41]

Moon and colleagues describes eleven cases of uterine calcification and infertility after *all eleven* had undergone "operative termination of mid-trimester pregnancy. Dilation and curettage or *hysteroscopy* confirmed residual fetal bony fragments." These cases came to light as the women were treated for secondary infertility.[42]

Marcus and colleagues identified secondary infertility and endometrial ossification in two women who had undergone induced mid-trimester abortions four and twelve years earlier and they conclude that this condition should always be considered in any infertility patients, particularly those who have undergone previous induced abortions. They state flatly that "a history of previous abortion is usually present" in cases of endometrial ossification.[43]

Zoricic and colleagues found a 22 mm long fetal bone lodged in the uterine cavity of an infertile patient who had had an induced abortion nineteen years earlier. The authors report that these findings *"strengthen once again the association between abortion and infertility"* [emphasis added].[44] Once again, non-North-American researchers more readily acknowledge the negative consequences of abortion.

Sometimes the outcome of sterility and infertility occur together in the literature. For example, an Italian study, Coccia and colleagues report that cases of *"osseous metaplasia of the endometrium,"* were often the result of the presence of bone within the uterus.[45] The bone prevents the implantation of any fertilized ova while also producing *endometritis* in the patient.

Shimizu and Nakayama diagnosed endometrial ossification in a woman following histological examination of endometrial tissue following curettage. The pathological sample contained a "mature bone." The authors urge caution in diagnosis to avoid a "misdiagnosis of malignant mixed *mullerian tumor."* It is their contention that the symptoms of retained foreign [fetal] bone, particularly vaginal discharge, may present as a tumor and may be difficult to identify if an accurate reproductive history is not available and careful diagnosis not undertaken.[46]

So far these problems are rare, but how many more go simply unreported? It is hard to know because, as we have seen, some cases of infertility, including those mentioned here, were only detected when the patients went to a clinic for fertility treatment or in vitro fertilization. Fertility treatments are quite expensive and are not covered by most health plans. The patients are typically those able to afford private clinics. They are not a random sample of all those who may suffer from the condition.

There are various theories as to how endometrial ossification leads to infertility. They include the following possibilities: retained bone prevents implantation; retained bone causes early abortion; changes in the uterine cavity and an increase in the production of prostaglandins act as a natural contraceptive or abortifacient. What is interesting, however, is the length of time that is reported to have elapsed between the abortion and the identification of the condition: four and twelve years as reported by Marcus and colleagues, and nineteen years as reported by Zoricic and colleagues.

**Table 5-3**
**Length of time between abortion and identification of endometrial ossification**[47]

| | | |
|---|---|---|
| Marcus | 1993 | 4, 12 years |
| Zoricic | 1994 | 19 years |
| Ruiz-Velasco | 1997 | 4-18 years |
| Torne | 1996 | 1-4 months |
| Shimizu and colleagues | 1997 | No time given but patient was 62 years old. |

**Ectopic Pregnancy**

Although we have dealt with the increased risk of ectopic pregnancy following abortion, primarily in terms of its threat to life (see Chapter 4), ectopic pregnancy also impairs fertility. Tuomivaara used a prospective rather than retrospective approach and determined that "the present study confirmed that an ectopic pregnancy dramatically increases the risk of secondary infertility." The study also found that patients with ectopic pregnancy "had more legal abortions" than the control group.[48] Contrast this with the claim by Holt and colleagues that abortion "has little or no influence on a woman's risk of ectopic pregnancy." These researchers dismiss their own finding of twenty per cent greater likelihood of ectopic pregnany (i.e., 1.2 relative risk) after two induced abortions, as possibly occurring by chance.[49] They make this conclusion even though several other studies point in the same direction of increased risk:

Daling and colleagues:
- 40 per cent after one induced abortion and 80 per cent after two or more;

Levin and colleagues:
- 30 per cent after one induced abortion and 160 per cent two or more;

Chung:
- 20 per cent after abortion(s) in general.[50]

When all these studies are considered together, a clear inter-connection emerges between abortion, ectopic pregnancy, and infertility.

**Conclusion**

It is apparent from the research cited here that women who have abortions, especially single young women who have never carried a baby to term, risk experiencing greater difficulty in conceiving and carrying future pregnancies to term. Because very little follow up is done in abortion clinics concerning the negative sequelae of an abortion (such as Chlamydia trachomatis, PID, perforations of the uterus, ectopic pregnancy, endometrial ossification), many women do not even know that they are at risk or should be seeking medical treatment. Long-term effects of these medical problems are complications in future pregnancies and in the most serious cases, inability to have children.

**Key Points Chapter 5**

• No previous births and an earlier abortion put a woman at significant risk of post-abortion complications leading to possible infertility.

• Coding systems at hospitals often make it difficult to link abortion with medical sequelae.

• Much larger numbers of women than previously suspected are negatively affected by induced abortion with PID and ectopic pregnancies at much higher levels than ever before in North America and Europe.

• Other serious sequelae also on the rise are uterine perforations, endometriosis, Chlamydia trachomatis, endometrial ossification (bone fragments left in the uterus), all of which compromise future fertility.

• Many of these medical problems go undetected at the time of abortion and are only discovered years later when women are treated for infertility.

## Notes

1 Trott E, Ziegler W, Levey J. Major complications associated with termination of a second trimester pregnancy: A case report. Delaware Medical Journal 1995 May;67(5):294-6.

Mittal S, Misra SL. Uterine perforation following medical termination of pregnancy by vacuum aspiration. International Journal of Gynaecology and Obstetrics 1985 February;23(1):45-50

2 Castadot RG. Pregnancy termination: techniques, risks, and complications and their management. Fertility and Sterility 1986 January;45(1):5-17.

3 Crutcher M. *Lime 5*. Denton, Texas: Life Dynamics, 1996.

4 Ferris LE, McMain-Klein M, Colodny N, Fellows GF, Lamont J. Factors associated with immediate abortion complications. Canadian Medical Association Journal 1996 June 1;154(11):1677-85.

5 Frank P, McNamee R, Hannaford PC, Kay CR, Hirsch S. The effect of induced abortion on subsequent fertility. British Journal of Obstetrics and Gynaecology 1993 June;100(6):575-80.

6 Heisterberg L, Kringelbach M. Early complications after induced first-trimester abortion. Acta Obstetricia et Gynecologica Scandanavica 1987;66(3):201-4, p. 204.

7 Newcomb PA, Storer BE, Longnecker MP, Mittendorf R, Greenberg ER, Willett WC. Pregnancy termination in relation to risk of breast cancer. Journal of the American Medical Association 1996 January;275(4):283-7.

Andrieu N, Duffy SW, Rohan TE, Le MG, Luporsi E, Gerber M, et al. Familial risk, abortion and their interactive effect on the risk of breast cancer--a combined analysis of six case-control studies. British Journal of Cancer 1995 September;72(3):744-51.

8 Canadian Pelvic Inflammatory Disease Society. Submission to the Royal Commission on Health Care and Costs. Vancouver, British Columbia: 1990 October.

9 Blackwell AL, Thomas PD, Wareham K, Emery SJ. Health gains from screening for infection of the lower genital tract in women attending for termination of pregnancy. The Lancet 1993 July 24;342(8865):206-10, p.209.

10 Westrom L. Clinical manifestations and diagnosis of pelvic inflammatory disease. Journal of Reproductive Medicine 1983 October;28(10 Supplement):703-8, p.703.

11  Levallois P, Rioux JE. Prophylactic antibiotics for suction curettage abortion: results of a clinical controlled trial. American Journal of Obstetrics and Gynecology 1988 January;158(1):100-5, p. 100.

12  Sorensen JL, Thranov I, Hoff G, Dirach J, Damsgaard MT. A double-blind randomized study of the effect of erythromycin in preventing pelvic inflammatory disease after first-trimester abortion. British Journal of Obstetrics and Gynaecology 1992 May;99(5):434-8, p.436.

13  Nielsen IK, Engdahl E, Larsen T. No effect of single dose ofloxacin on postoperative infection rate after first-trimester abortion. A clinical, controlled trial. Acta Obstetricia et Gynecologica Scandanavica 1993 October;72(7):556-9, p. 558.

Westergaard L, Philipsen T, Scheibel J. Significance of cervical Chlamydia trachomatis infection in postabortal pelvic inflammatory disease. Obstetrics & Gynecology 1982 September;60(3):322-5.

Osser S, Persson K. Postabortal pelvic infection associated with chlamydia trachomatis and the influence of humoral immunity. American Journal of Obstetrics and Gynecology 1984 November 15;150(6):699-703.

14  Sawaya GF, Grady D, Kerlikowske K, Grimes DA. Antibiotics at the time of induced abortion: the case for universal prophylaxis based on a meta-analysis. Obstetrics & Gynecology 1996 May;87(5 pt 2):884-90, p. 884.

15  Jonsson M, Karlsson R, Persson K, Juto P, Edlund K, Evander M, et al. The influence of sexual and social factors on the risk of Chlamydia trachomatis infections: a population-based serologic study. Sexually Transmitted Diseases 1995 November-December;22(6):355-63, p. 355.

16  Sawaya et al. 1996. See n.14.

17  Blackwell et al. 1993 See n. 9.

18  Osser S, Persson K 1984. See n. 13, p. 703.

19  Sawaya et al. 1996. See n. 14, p. 884.

20  Table 5-1

Westergaard et al. 1982. See n. 13.

Osser and Persson 1984. See n. 13.

Barbacci MB, Spence MR, Kappus EW, Burkman RC, Rao L, Quinn TC. Postabortal endometritis and isolation of Chlamydia trachomatis. Obstetrics and Gynecology 1986 November;68(5):686-90, p.690.

Sorensen JL, Thranov IR, Hoff GE. Genital Chlamydia trachomatis infection in abortion seekers. Strategy of examination and treatment in order to reduce the sequelae of infection. Ugeskr Laeger 1992 October 26;154(44):3047-53.

Blackwell et al. 1993. See n. 9.

Jonsson et al. 1995. See n. 15.

21  Table 5-2

Westergaard 1982. See n. 13.

Qvigstad E, Skaug K, Jerve F, Fylling P, Ulstrup JC. Pelvic inflammatory disease associated with Chlamydia trachomatis infection after therapeutic abortion. A prospective study. British Journal of Venereal Disease 1983 June;59(3):189-92.

Osser and Persson 1984, See n. 13.

Sorensen 1992. See n. 20.

Blackwell et al. 1993. See n. 9.

Nielsen 1993. See n. 13.

Sorensen, Jl, I Thranov, G Hoff and Dirach J. Early and late-onset pelvic inflammatory disease among women with cervical Chlamydia trachomatis infection at the time of induced abortion - a follow-up study. Infection 22, no. 4 (1994): 242-6.

Oakeshott P, Hilton S, Hay P. Treatment and causes of female infertility. The Lancet 344, no. 8918 (30 July 1994): 334.

22  Giertz G, Kallings I, Nordenvall M, Fuchs T. A prospective study of Chlamydia trachomatis infection following legal abortion. Acta Obstetricia et Gynecologica Scandanavica 1987;66(2):107-9.

23  Qvigstad et al. 1983. See. n. 21.

24  Barbacci et al. 1986. See n. 20, p.690.

25  Sorensen et al. 1994. See n. 21, p. 245.

26  Washington AE, Johnson RE, Sanders LL Jr. Chlamydia trachomatis infections in the United States. What are they costing us? Journal of the American Medical Association 1987 April;257(15):2070-2.

27  Sawaya et al. 1996. See n. 14.

28  Brewer C. Prevention of post-abortion infection. The Lancet 1993 September 25;342(8874):802.

29 Nielsen et al. 1993. See n. 13.

30 Levallois and Rioux 1988. See n. 11, pp. 103-4.

31 Leibner EC. Delayed presentation of uterine perforation. Annals of Emergency Medicine 1995 November;26(5)·643-6, p. 643.

32 Kaali SG, Szigetvari IA, Bartfai GS. The frequency and management of uterine perforations during first-trimester abortions. American Journal of Obstetrics and Gynecology 1989 August;161(2):406-8.

33  Kaali et al. See n. 32, p. 407.

34  Schenker JG. Etiology of and therapeutic approach to synechia uteri. European Journal of Obstetrics and Gynecology and Reproductive Biology 1996 March;65(1):109-13, p. 109.

35  Capella-Allouc S et al. Hysteroscopic treatment of severe Asherman's Syndrome and subsequent fertility. Human Reproduction. 1999 May;14(5)1230-1233, p. 1230.

36  Bacelar AC, Wilcock D, Powell M, Worthington BS. The value of MRI in the assessment of traumatic intra-uterine adhesions (Asherman's Syndrome). Clinical Radiology 1995 February;50(2):80-3.

37 Rock JA, Murphy AA. Anatomic abnormalities. Clinical Obstetrics & Gynecology 1986 December;29(4):886-911.

38  Bellingham FR. Endometrial bone formation. Australian and New Zealand Journal of Obstetrics and Gynecology 1996 February;36(1):109-10.

39 Chan NS. Intrauterine retention of fetal bone. Australian and New Zealand Journal of Obstetrics and Gynecology 1996 August;36(3):368-71.

40  Ruiz-Velasco V, Gonzalez Alfani G, Pliego Sanchez L, Alamillo Vera M. Endometrial pathology and infertility. Fertility and Sterility 1997 April;67(4):687-92, p. 692.

41  Torne A, Jou P, Pagano R, Sanchez I, Ordi J, Vanrell JA. Endometrial ossification successfully treated by hysteroscopic resection. European Journal of Obstetrics and Gynecology and Reproductive Biology 1996 May;66(1):75-7.

42  Moon HS, Park YH, Kwon HY, Hong SH, Kim SK. Iatrogenic secondary infertility caused by residual intrauterine fetal bone after midtrimester abortion. American Journal of Obstetrics and Gynecology 1997 February;176(2):369-70.

43  Marcus SF, Bhattacharya J, Williams G, Brinsden P, Hamou J. Endometrial ossification: a cause of secondary infertility. Report of two cases. American Journal of Obstetrics and Gynecology 1994 May;170 (5 Pt 1):1381-3, p. 1381.

44  Zoricic D, Ambrozic B, Peric D. [A fetal bone as a foreign body in the uterus][Article in Serbo-Croatian (Roman)]. Lijec Vjesn 1994 November-December;116(11-12):298-300.

45  Coccia ME, Becattini C, Bracco GL, Scarselli G. Ultrasound-guided hysteroscopic management of endometrial osseous metaplasia. Ultrasound Obstetrics & Gynecology 1996 August;8(2):134-6.

46  Shimizu M, Nakayama M. Endometrial ossification in a post-menopausal woman. Journal of Clinical Pathology 1997 February;50(2):171-2

47  Table 5-3

Marcus 1993. See n. 43.

Zoricic 1994. See n. 44.

Ruiz-Velasco, 1997. See n. 40.

Torne 1996. See n. 41.

Shimizu et al. 1997. See n. 46.

48  a) Tuomivaara L, Kauppila A. Ectopic pregnancy: a case-control study of aetiological risk factors. Archives of Gynecology and Obstetrics 1988;243(1):511.

   b) Tuomivaara L, Kauppila A. Radical or conservative surgery for ectopic pregnancy? A followup study of fertility of 323 patients. Fertility and Sterility 1988 October;50(4):5803.

49  Holt VL, Daling JR, Voigt LF, McKnight B, Stergachis A, Chu J, et.al. Induced abortion and the risk of subsequent ectopic pregnancy. American Journal of Public Health 1989 September;79(9):1234-8.

50  Daling JR, Chow WH, Weiss NS, Metch BJ, Soderstrom R. Ectopic pregnancy in relation to previous induced abortion. Journal of the American Medical Association 1985 February;253(7):1005-8.

Levin AA, Schoenbaum SC, Stubblefield PG, Zimicki S, Monson RR, Ryan KJ. Ectopic pregnancy and prior induced abortion. American Journal of Public Health 1982 March;72(3):253-6.

Chung CS, Smith RG, Steinhoff PG and Mi MP. Induced abortion and ectopic pregnancy in subsequent pregnancies. American Journal of Epidemiology 1982 June;115(6): 879-87.

Chapter 6

# Maternal Mortality

Although infrequently, women do die as a result of abortion, yet abortion-related maternal mortality is generally underreported. One reason for this is that codes in hospitals report only the presenting cause of death, not the underlying reason which, for example, in the case of abortion-related death, might be hemorrhage, infection, embolism, or ectopic pregnancy. In fact, the reporting systems in Canada, the United States and in the World Health Organization are so imprecise that deaths related to a previous abortion are hard to track: Death certificates are inaccurately completed and, either to protect the privacy of the woman and her family or to avoid a possible lawsuit, hospital staff or doctors may deliberately avoid coding an abortion-related death.

Another reason for underreporting bias is that many of the statistics provided by the Centers for Disease Control (CDC) come from unreliable hospital and clinic records. Statistics from abortion providers in both Canada and the United States tend to underreport negative findings, presumably so that abortion will be seen as a safe procedure. At highest risk of death related to abortion are African-American and other minority women.

A recent authoritative Scandinavian study has established that women who undergo induced abortion experience, over the following twelve months, a death rate nearly four times greater than women who give birth to their children. In addition to this, the suicide rate associated with childbirth was six times lower than the suicide rate associated with abortion. The link between abortion and suicide is of particular note and is examined in detail in Chapter 14 "Behavioral Outcomes, Suicide, Healing".

# Maternal Mortality

### Causes of Maternal Mortality in Abortions

Maternal mortality is a small but persistent aspect of induced abortion. Causes of maternal death that arise specifically from abortions include hemorrhage, infection, *embolism*, and *cardiomyopathy*. These causes of maternal death are generally underreported.

Approximately fourteen per cent of all deaths from *legal abortion* in the United States are due to general anesthesia complications. According to Atrash and colleagues anesthesia-related deaths for legal abortion have not decreased, possibly because "pregnancy increases the sensitivity to the respiratory depressant effects of all these [anesthetic] agents". Furthermore, "an increasing proportion of these [abortion-related deaths] were anesthesia related deaths...resulting from cardiopulmonary arrest".[1]

In six of the countries formerly part of the Soviet Union – Russia, Ukraine, Belarus, Estonia, Latvia and Lithuania – the very high frequency of abortion contributes to the "deleterious" population decline and maternal mortality remains "unacceptably high". "It is particularly worrying," write Mogilevkina and colleagues, "that induced abortions make up twenty per cent to 35 per cent of all maternal mortality".[2]

For an in-depth examination of suicide after abortion, see Chapter 14.

### Underreporting of Maternal Deaths

In the United States and Canada, as well as in the World Health Organization (WHO) there is a general and systematic underreporting of maternal deaths – deaths of women during pregnancy or delivery, or in the six weeks following the termination of a pregnancy.

According to recent analyses of mortality statistics using linkage studies, "more than half of such deaths...are probably still unreported".[3] The death rates identified by these new linkage studies, connecting and cross-referencing various sources of vital statistics data, show that the Centers for Disease Control's Pregnancy-Related Mortality Surveillance System "does not identify all pregnancy-related deaths".[4] In other words, women have died as a result of pregnancy, but their pregnancy was never connected to official death records.

**Underreporting of Abortion-Related Maternal Deaths**
The system used in linkage studies to identify maternal deaths works back from a recorded birth. Because of this, it "cannot identify pregnancy-related deaths that do not generate a record of pregnancy outcome (e.g. ectopic pregnancies...induced or *spontaneous abortions*)".[5] In any event, Centers for Disease Control (CDC) reports combine maternal deaths by miscarriages and induced abortions into a single category and these combined numbers are accepted as accounting for all maternal deaths, even though demographic researchers recognize that there is systematic underreporting. (For instance, many maternal deaths from ectopic pregnancies and other causes are not recorded as related to abortion; see Chapter 4.)

Recently, Bégin, a Canadian health researcher, has found that the problem of underreporting of maternal and abortion-related deaths is not limited to the United States (and Canada), but is also the result of flawed reporting guidelines from the World Health Organization (WHO). WHO's claim that legal abortion (an abortion procedure performed by a licensed practitioner) is safe depends on a voluntary system of death certification which has been shown to be inherently unreliable. WHO's statistics come from physicians who are not told that they must specify the type of abortion that led to maternal death – spontaneous, induced, legal or illegal.[6] Physicians are not even told that they must specify that the terminal illness (e.g. sepsis) followed an abortion.

In addition, the July 1999 CDC Surveillance on Abortion noted that official statistics show twelve per cent fewer abortions than does the Alan Guttmacher Institute, the research arm of Planned Parenthood.[7] Before raising this issue, Surveillance reports maternal death rates as if their own numbers are accurate, with no further explanation.

Of interest here is the fact that institutions such as the American Medical Association (AMA)[8] use the CDC data. Indeed, the AMA (1992) insists that the reporting practices on abortion of the Centers for Disease Control are accurate and complete because "the CDC conducts a thorough investigation of each reported abortion-related death to verify the cause and circumstances surrounding the death".[9] But this statement overlooks the CDC's own admission that it may be missing more than 132,000 actual abortion cases. In any case, the death must first be identified as abortion-related before it can be investigated as such, and this is precisely where information slippage can occur.

**How the Reporting System Works**
The success of the CDC system depends entirely on whether a report is made in the first place. Unless induced abortion is identified as an immediate cause of death, it will not be investigated or recorded by the CDC. Inaccuracies may creep into the reporting process in a number of ways:

> 1. In the United States, 93 per cent of all abortions are performed in free-standing abortion clinics. A woman whose post-abortion condition is life-threatening will be admitted to a general hospital through an emergency department. The attending emergency room doctor will not be the physician who performed the abortion and may not record a subsequent death as resulting from an abortion.

> 2. If the woman dies, it is not usually the abortion provider but a casualty officer or the family doctor who must complete the death certificate, and it is this information upon which the death may or may not be reported to the CDC.[10] In 1995, Statistics Canada noted that "if complications ensue after a patient has been discharged from hospital, the condition is treated as a separate case and does not appear in the original abortion record".[11]

> 3. Inadequate information may be provided on the physician's or coroner's report. For example, the

death may be noted as related to a previous abortion, but insufficient detail may make it impossible to determine whether the abortion was induced or spontaneous. In general, Canadian Medical Certificates of Death have been found to contain major errors 32.9 per cent of the time.[12] At present, given the politicization of the issue, it is not surprising that the records of abortion-related deaths are incomplete.

4. Hospital coding may not reflect the international numbering system. A woman who dies from a hemorrhage may have the event recorded simply as "hemorrhage" but with no code that would connect the bleeding to an earlier induced abortion. Codes such as embolism or cardiomyopathy can stand alone, with no reference to an induced abortion as the cause.

5. Hospital staff may avoid using the full coding in order to protect the privacy of the deceased patient, and/or the family, or to avoid legal or political entanglement.

6. Incomplete, indirect, or subtle coding, if it occurs, may also assist the abortion practitioner who otherwise might run a greater risk of civil liability. Malpractice is a significant issue for all physicians but recent, concerted civil litigation by women injured by abortion has made abortion providers particularly vulnerable.[13]

Bégin has reviewed death statistics and the medical coding methods used to attribute death to maternal causes. She found that the Health Records of four of the seven Canadian provinces and eighteen American states do not permit deaths to be classified as maternal if they occur more than 42 days after the termination of a pregnancy. Bégin goes on to quote Donna Hoyet, the CDC expert on maternal mortality coding: "unless it specifically states that the death was within 42 days we assume it is not a maternal death...If death occurred 43 days or more after a termination of pregnancy...[we] do not [use] code ICD 630-676 [Pregnancy-abortion related]." If the woman has died, then, from abortion-related complications such as ectopic pregnancy, abortion will not be noted; the only cause of death referred to in this case would be "ectopic pregnancy".

If death is immediate, it is not required to specify on the death certificate what kind of an abortion was performed, and if maternal death happens 43 days after an abortion, the death will not be linked to it. As this situation makes clear, accurate reporting on maternal abortion-related deaths is not, at present, a reality in North America.

**Doubtful Data**

Another problem in obtaining accurate information is that data analyses use different comparative categories. For example, Meyer and Buescher, statisticians with the North Carolina Health and Environmental Statistics Bureau, use one type of reporting in which abortion mortality statistics are presented in terms of the number of live births in the state but not in terms of the number of abortions performed.[14] The American Medical Association reported that this approach would exaggerate the danger of pregnancy.

As we have seen, death certificates may not connect the direct cause of death with the preceding abortion event. A death from cardiac arrest may be listed as such, and not as a cardiac arrest due to a reaction to the anesthetic given during an abortion. Jacob found that in the statistics of maternal mortality, the greatest errors in classification occurred for women who had recently undergone an induced abortion.

More to the point, in 1992 the AMA Council on Scientific Affairs reported maternal death rates relying not on the CDC data for post-abortion death rates, but on data from Planned Parenthood.[15] The CDC now concedes that the overall abortion figures of the Alan Guttmacher Institute (the Research Branch of Planned Parenthood) show significantly more abortions each year than the official numbers, but a recent publication does not discuss death rates. As the largest abortion provider in the United States, Planned Parenthood keeps track of the number of abortions, but is clearly in a position of conflict of interest in reporting abortion deaths. In any event, the references found in the CDC report are most often from Planned Parenthood. From a reading of the most recent Surveillance Summary, one might infer that all such deaths are accurately recorded. But it is only from a careful analysis of the literature on the problems of reporting deaths that questions arise.

**Accurate Statistics from Finland**
Further light is shed on the unsatisfactory nature of North-American abortion mortality statistics by the recent experience of Finland. Finland is one of the few countries in the world that has accurate birth, death, and abortion registries. A study of all Finnish women who died between 1987 and 1994 found the following maternal mortality for every 100,000 registered, ended pregnancies.

**Table 6-1**
**Maternal deaths within twelve months of end of pregnancy per 100,000 women**

| | |
|---|---|
| Births | 26.7 |
| Miscarriages or ectopic pregnancies | 47.8 |
| Induced abortions | 100.5 |

*Source:* Gissler (1997)

In other words *the maternal death rate after abortion was nearly four times greater than the maternal death rate after childbirth.*[17] Add to this the finding that the *suicide rate associated with childbirth was six times lower than the suicide rate associated with abortion.*[18] The findings, reported in prestigious British and Scandinavian medical journals, call seriously into question the oft-repeated claim that induced abortion is safer than childbirth. They also illustrate the need for large, record-linkage-based studies to establish the real rate of maternal death from abortion.

**Table 6-2**
**Finland: suicide rate per 100,000 women within twelve months of end of pregnancy**

| | |
|---|---|
| After birth | 5.9 |
| After miscarriage | 18.1 |
| After induced abortion | 34.7 |
| (Mean annual rate) | 11.3 |

*Source:* Gissler and colleagues (1996)

Gissler and colleagues cautiously conclude that "Increased risk for a suicide after an induced abortion can...result from a negative effect of induced abortion on mental wellbeing"[19].

The comparison of death rates from causes other than suicide is almost as striking. *Women who have an induced abortion are more than three times as likely to die within a year as women who give birth:*

**Table 6-3**
**Finland: death rate per 100,000 women within twelve months of end of pregnancy (omitting suicide)**

| | |
|---|---|
| After birth | 20.8 |
| After miscarriage | 29.7 |
| After induced abortion | 65.8 |

*Source:* Gissler and colleagues (1997)

**Reliable Demographic Information?**
What is also known is the greater likelihood that minority women (such as African-Americans) will suffer death while seeking a *legal abortion*. For example, the AMA Council on Scientific Affairs reported, "Death from legal abortion is more common among minority women than white women, women over the age of 35 and those who undergo the procedure during the second trimester."[20]

Berg and colleagues analyzed the U.S. Centers for Disease Control Statistics of overall maternal deaths for the period 1987 to 1990 and reported that the death ratio has increased

from seven per 100,000 births in 1987 to ten per 100,000
in 1990, the majority of this ratio being accounted for by the
dramatic increase in the deaths of African-American
women.[21] In 1990, the rate of death for African-American
women was 26.7 per 100,000 births while in the same period
white women had a rate of only 6.5 per 100,000 births.

There may be some doubt, however, about the true final
figures because some states were missing from the CDC
report. Still, there is no particular reason to believe that if all
the data were available, the alarming trend towards increase
in African-American maternal mortality would disappear.
Berg and colleagues report 1453 maternal deaths from the
CDC statistics in the four years from 1987 to 1990. Of these,
81 are attributed to abortion, but induced and spontaneous
abortions are lumped together. The report did separate the
causes of death of these women (50 per cent from infection,
twenty per cent from hemorrhage, and eleven per cent
"unknown"). At least 70 per cent of the identified causes of
death are known major complications in the post-induced
abortion period. The authors note that the mortality rate due
to infection rose 36 per cent, with the largest increase in the
group of women who died following abortion.

A different study by Ferris and colleagues, which looked at
short-term complications after an abortion, provided some
useful information, suggesting there are few immediate
complications.[22] Studies like this, however, do not report the
many possible complications that could lead to death in the
weeks following abortion. Berg found that among maternal
deaths, at least 43 per cent did not occur until more than
one week following the termination of pregnancy, while
six per cent of the deaths occurred over six weeks after
the abortion, the usual time limit used by statisticians to
categorize deaths as maternal.

When the issue of abortion is not the main topic of an
article, the mortality figures cited are often more straightforward. Lee P. Shulman cites abortion mortality rates in
relation to the type and time of procedure.

**Table 6-4**
**Number of deaths for every 100,000 abortions by procedure**[23]

| Procedure | 1st trimester | 2nd trimester |
|---|---|---|
| Suction Curettage | 0.8 | N/A |
| Dilation and Evacuation | 5.1 | 4.9 |
| Instillation | N/A | 10.1 |
| Saline Injection | N/A | 11.6 |
| Prostaglandin Injection | N/A | 6.4 |
| Hysterectomy/Hysterotomy* | 40.7 | 90.8 |

*These two figures have been re-calculated from the tables on pages 315 and 320 of Shulman.

**General Underreporting Bias**

Despite disclaimers to the contrary, there is a general underreporting bias in abortion and abortion-related maternal deaths. For example, Jones and Forrest of the Alan Guttmacher Institute report that, in using the national survey data in the United States between 1976 and 1988, "...abortions are characteristically underreported...Abortion reporting is found to be highly deficient in all the surveys, although the level varies widely. Whites are more likely to report their abortions than nonwhites."[24] In that case, we must ask, how different would abortion numbers be if they reflected accurately the number of African-American women dying from this procedure? At present, they appear to be underreported.

**Conclusion**

Women continue to die from induced abortion, but this fact is underreported, principally because current methods of gathering and reporting statistics are deficient. Of particular concern is an apparent rise in the death rate of African-American women, combined with the tendency to underreport all abortion deaths. A failure to provide comprehensive and accurate statistics coupled with delays in disseminating available statistics further complicates the problem of reporting abortion-related mortality. It is possible that legal abortion, because of its high prevalence, has now caused more maternal deaths than the previous system of restricted abortion access which was also devoid of accurate documentation. The Finnish method of accurate recording of births, deaths, and abortions shows higher mortality and suicide rates among women who have had abortions compared to those who give birth. It underlines the unreliability of North-American statistics and explodes the myth that abortion is safer for a woman than childbirth.

**Key Points Chapter 6**

• Women die from abortion-related problems but, owing to irregular and biased reporting, it is difficult to know how many.

• Reasons for maternal mortality related to abortion are many, including hemorrhage, infection, embolism, ectopic pregnancy, and cardiomyopathy.

• Coding deaths in hospitals and reasons for death on death certificates frequently record only the presenting problem as the cause of death, which results in many abortion-related deaths going unreported.

• The American Medical Association (AMA) relies on the Centers for Disease Control (CDC) for its statistics concerning abortion-related deaths and, given that the CDC uses hospital and clinic records (which underreport maternal deaths from abortion) for its data, the AMA does not recognize the full extent of abortion-related deaths.

• At most risk of abortion-related deaths are African-American and other minority women.

• A large-scale, authoritative Scandinavian study establishes post-pregnancy death rates within one year that are nearly four times greater among women who abort their pregnancies than among women who bear their babies. The suicide rate is nearly six times greater among aborting women than among women who give birth. These findings refute the oft-heard claim that induced abortion is safer than childbirth.

• There is an urgent need for independent studies of maternal mortality related to abortion, and medical facilities should be required to keep more accurate and informative records so that women may be better served in this area.

## Notes

1   Atrash HK, Cheek TG, Hogue CJ. Legal abortion mortality and general anesthesia, American Journal of Obstetrics and Gynecology 1988 February;158(2):420-4, p. 423, p. 420.

2   Mogilevkina I, Markote S, Avakyan Y, Mrochek L, Liljestrand J, Hellberg D. Induced abortions and childbirths: trends in Estonia, Latvia, Lithuania, Russia, Belarussia and the Ukraine during 1970 to 1994. Acta Obstetricia et Gynecologica Scandanavica 1996 November;75(10):908-11, p. 910.

3   Berg CJ, Atrash HK, Koonin LM, Tucker M. Pregnancy-related mortality in the United States, 1987-1990. Obstetrics & Gynecology 1996 August;88(2):161-7, p. 161.

4   Berg 1996. See n. 3, p. 166.

5   Jacob S, Bloebaum L, Shah G, Varner MW. Maternal mortality in Utah. Obstetrics & Gynecology 1998 February;91(2):187-91, p. 190.

6   Bégin I. Mortalilty and Morbidity Coding in Canada and the World – Pitfalls and Shortcomings. 1999. Ottawa (unpublished paper).

7   Koonin LM, Strauss LT, Chrisman LE, Montalbano MA, Bartlett LA, Smith JG. Abortion Surveillance - United States, 1996. Morbidity and Mortality Weekly Report, Centers for Disease Control, Surveillance Summaries 48(SS04), 1999 July 30:1-42.

8   Council on Scientific Affairs AMA. Induced termination of pregnancy before and after Roe v Wade. Trends in the mortality and morbidity of women. Journal of the American Medical Association 1992 December 9;268(22):3231-9.

9   JAMA 1992. See n. 8, p. 3235.

10  Henshaw SK, Van Vort J. Abortion services in the United States, 1991 and 1992. Family Planning Perspectives 1994 May-June;26(3):100-6, 112.

11  Wadhera S, Millar WJ. Second trimester abortions: trends and medical complications. Health Reports 1994;6(4):441-54

12  Myers KA, Farquhar DR. Improving the accuracy of death certification. Canadian Medical Association Journal 1998 May 19;158(10):1317-23.

13  Collett TS. Abortion malpractice: Exploring the safety of legal abortion. In *Life and Learning; vol. V.* ed. Koterski JW, Fifth University Faculty for Life Conference; 1995 June; Marquette University:243-72.

14  Meyer RE, Buescher PA. Maternal mortality related to induced abortion in North Carolina: a historical study. Family Planning Perspectives 1994 July-August;26(4):179-80, 191.

15  Henshaw SK, Forrest JD, Van Vort J. Abortion services in the United States, 1984 and 1985. Family Planning Perspectives 1987 March-April;19(2):63-70.

16  Gissler M, Kauppila R, Merilainen J, Toukomaa H, Hemminki E. Pregnancy-associated deaths in Finland 1987-199–definition problems and benefits of record linkage. Acta Obstetricia et Gynecologica Scandanavica 1997 Aug;76(7):651-7.

17  Gissler et al. 1997. See n. 16.

18  Gissler M, Hemminki E, Lonnqvist J. Suicides after pregnancy in Finland, 1987-94: register linkage study. British Medical Journal 1996 December 7;313(7070):1431-4.

19  Gissler et al. 1996. See n. 18, p. 1434.

20  Council on Scientific Affairs 1992. See. n. 8.

21  Berg et al. 1996. See n. 3.

22  Ferris LE, McMain-Klein M, Colodny N, Fellows GF, Lamont J. Factors associated with immediate abortion complications. Canadian Medical Association Journal 1996 June 1;154(11):1677-85.

23  Shulman LP, Pregnancy termination procedures. Joe Leigh Simpson and Sherman Elias, eds., *Essentials of Prenatal Diagnosis* (N.Y.: Churchill Livingstone, 1993), pp. 314-15, 320.

24  Jones EF, Forrest JD. Underreporting of abortion in surveys of U.S. women: 1976 to 1988. Demography 1992 February;29(1):113-26, p. 113.

Chapter 7

# Repeat Abortion

There is not a great deal of research on the effects of repeat abortion on women's future ability to conceive and carry a pregnancy to term. What statistics there are concerning this connection are shown in studies dealing with women's reproductive histories as they relate to gynecological problems they are experiencing after abortion(s). These problems include Asherman's Syndrome, pelvic inflammatory disease, and cervical incompetence (caused by surgical instruments widening the cervix), which can significantly limit their ability to conceive and, if conception does take place, to carry their pregnancy to term. Because there are no studies directly dealing with the negative impact of repeat abortion on women's future fertility, the question arises: Before an abortion, are women being informed of its possible negative effects on their future health, especially their ability to have children? If this is not happening, then why not?

# Repeat Abortion

As increasing numbers of women undergo repeated pregnancy terminations, their risk of subsequent pelvic infections may be multiplied with each succeeding abortion. *Asherman's Syndrome* may also occur after *septic* abortion. "The pregnancy rate after treatment of this syndrome is low."[1]

Repeat abortion is not often studied by itself. Rather, the impact of multiple abortions is found in the reproductive histories that are recorded for *epidemiological* studies, mainly in the areas of cancer and fertility treatment. U.S. government statistics note that in 1997, 48 per cent of all reported abortions were classified as repeat abortions.[2] In Ontario a 1996 study of all abortions in that province found that 30 per cent were repeat abortions.[3] Of women with previous pregnancies who participated in a 1996 study of pain during abortion at a Planned Parenthood clinic, 29 per cent having repeat abortions and six per cent had had two or more previous abortions.[4]

In 1980 Levin and colleagues published a large study of the impact of multiple induced abortions on subsequent pregnancy loss.[5] As with so many other research initiatives, this study provides important information that is not central to the study but is part of the reproductive history of the women in the sample. Reported in Table 7-1 below are the effects of abortion on aspects of women's health.

**Table 7-1**
**Occurrence rate (per cent) of gynecological problems following induced abortions**

| women with: | no abortion | 1 abortion | 2+ abortions |
|---|---|---|---|
| Gonorrhea | 3.2 | 5.9 | 17.5 |
| PID* | 4.4 | 7.9 | 9.5 |
| Cervical Incompetence | 1.2 | 1.6 | 3.2 |

\* PID = Pelvic Inflammatory Disease
*Source*: Levin and colleagues (1980), p. 2497.

A history of *sexually transmitted disease* predisposes women to higher levels of complications in other areas, such as *pelvic inflammatory disease (PID)*. Nielsen and colleagues confirmed that women who have previously had a legal abortion are statistically more likely to develop PID.[6]

The 1996 statistical report on induced abortion in the United States, released in 1999, shows that in the state of Maryland the repeat abortion rate was 70 per cent, and that one-third of the women had had three or more abortions. A similar pattern occurred in New York City where 64 per cent were repeat abortions with again one-third having had three or more pregnancy terminations.[7]

**Conclusion**
From the studies dealing with gynecological problems encountered in women who have had multiple abortions, it is clear that repeat abortions have a significant negative impact on their future fertility. Unfortunately, the effect of repeat abortions on a woman's later ability to bear children has not been central to studies of gynecological diseases. It seems clear that if women's better health interests are to be served in the area of fertility, studies are needed that focus directly on the impact of repeat abortion on future pregnancies and women need to be informed of the risk.

**Key Points Chapter 7**

- There have been no attempts to study the effects of repeat abortion on women's future fertility.

- Women's reproductive histories when being treated for gynecological problems such as Asherman's Syndrome, PID, and cervical incompetence, often reveal one or more past abortions.

- A significant number of women who experience pregnancy loss have had multiple induced abortions.

- Many women are not aware of the connection between repeat abortion and their future ability to have children.

- There is a need for studies that focus directly on the connection between multiple abortions and pregnancy loss and that inform women of the risks of repeat abortion to their future health.

## Notes

1  Huggins GR, Cullins VE. Fertility after contraception or abortion. Fertility and Sterility 1990 October;54(4):559-73.

2  Koonin LM, Strauss LT, Chrisman CE, Parker WY. Abortion surveillance--United States, 1997. Morbidity and Mortality Weekly Report, Centers for Disease Control, Surveillance Summaries 2000 December 8;49(SS-11): 1-43, p. 39 (Table 13).

3  Ferris LE, McMain-Klein M, Colodny N, Fellows GF, Lamont J. Factors associated with immediate abortion complications. Canadian Medical Association Journal 1996 June 1;154(11):1677-85.

4  Wiebe ER. Abortion induced with methotrexate and misoprostol. Canadian Medical Association Journal 1996 January 15;154(2):165-70.

5  Levin AA, Schoenbaum SC, Monson RR, Stubblefield PG, Ryan KJ. Association of induced abortion with subsequent pregnancy loss. Journal of the American Medical Association 1980 June 27;243(24):2495-9.

6  Nielsen IK, Engdahl E, Larsen T. [Pelvic inflammation after induced abortion] Danish. Ugeskr Laeger 1992 September 28;154(40):2743-6.

7  Koonin L, Strauss L, Chrisman L, Montalbano M, Bartlett L, Smith J. Abortion Surveillance—United States, 1996: Morbidity and Mortality Weekly Report, Centers for Disease Control, Surveillance Summaries 1999 July 30;48(4):1-42.

Chapter 8

# Drug-Induced or "Medical" Abortion

Since 1985, when the drug *RU-486* was introduced by the
French pharmaceutical company, Roussel-Uclef, women have
had an alternative to surgical abortion. RU-486 and other
similar drugs expel the fetus from the uterus without women
going to a hospital or clinic, but they must have several
follow-up appointments with a doctor in case of complications. In general, *medical abortion* requires more clinic visits
than surgical abortion, and is far from being the simple,
quick procedure that is often portrayed in the media.

At present, there are no long-term, follow-up studies on the
impact of drug-induced abortion, but what studies there are
make it clear that this method is not free of failure, and there
may be a number of unpleasant side effects such as nausea,
diarrhea, vomiting, blood loss, prolonged hemorrhaging, high
temperatures, and infections, especially during second-
trimester abortions. In some cases, if the drug does not
successfully expel the fetus from the womb, a surgical
abortion is then performed. Pain is also an issue, with some
women reporting more pain than with surgical abortion,
but more studies into the actual impact of drug-induced
abortions need to be carried out. As in other questions about
the effects of abortion on women's health, many of these
findings have been understated by North-American
researchers.

# Drug-Induced or "Medical" Abortion

With the introduction in 1985 of RU-486 (misopristone) by the French pharmaceutical company Roussel-Uclef, the use of drugs as a non-surgical alternative to first-trimester abortion became possible. Drug-induced abortion is referred to as "medical" abortion as opposed to "surgical" abortion, based on the traditional division of clinical units by medical or surgical designations. It is not to be confused with abortion performed for medical (maternal health) reasons.[1] Nor is it to be confused with the "morning-after pill", taken within 48 hours of unprotected intercourse.

With drug-induced abortion, the actual expulsion of the fetus occurs outside of a clinic or hospital. Although pronounced "safe and effective", the procedure is presently associated with a higher complication rate, including failure to abort, which subsequently necessitates a surgical abortion. It can also require anywhere from one to several days following the drug injection(s) to complete the fetal delivery.[2]

According to O'Connor, "Initial tests have shown that, when taken within the first seven weeks of pregnancy, RU-486 causes shedding of the fertilized embryo after implantation in the uterine wall 95 percent of the time." Her study also maintains that "The administration of a pill, or two drugs in combination, would allow more physicians to perform or facilitate abortions in their offices, because there would be no need for surgical intervention – thus making abortions available to many more women...."[3]

Two articles by Creinin, however, paint a less glowing picture.[4] There are frequent complications including "prolonged" vaginal bleeding lasting an average of 29 days.[5] A further disadvantage is the average delay of 24 days between treatment and the onset of vaginal bleeding. "...[T]his wait," Creinin dryly observes, "may be unacceptable to some women".[6] Finally, because the use of these chemicals requires several appointments with the administering doctor and numerous laboratory and radiological tests, the method has not become established as the simple alternative to surgery that the quotation by O'Connor suggests.

These problems are acknowledged in a review of the question that appeared recently in the *New England Journal of Medicine*. While endorsing the procedure, the authors of the review concede that "medical abortion is associated with higher rates of prolonged bleeding than in surgical abortion, and the rate of use of analgesic drugs is greater...Moreover, medical abortion has a lower rate of success than surgical abortion." In addition, "medical abortion requires more clinic visits than surgical abortion...and it should be offered only by well-trained clinicians who can provide surgical treatment in the event of a failed abortion or excessive bleeding. Women who choose medical abortion must have access to a specialized center where suction curettage is available, should heavy bleeding occur and blood transfusion be required."[7]

The controversy over the importation of misopristone into Canada and the United States has resulted in other drugs undergoing clinical trials as abortifacients, particularly prostaglandin analogues, such as misoprostol (cytotec) which were developed for use in medical conditions such as gastric ulcers, and methotrexate, a folic acid antagonist used to treat cancer, psoriasis and rheumatoid arthritis. Ferris and Basinski state that some physicians are "counselling women about [the] availability of [misoprostol] as off-label therapy for early termination of intrauterine pregnancy". Yet because of the significant failure rate of drug-induced abortion they declare this practice to be "insupportable".[8] The manufacturer of cytotec has also emphasized the inadvisability of its use in pregnancy.

To date there have been no long-term, follow-up studies of chemical abortion. Many of the studies that do exist are comparative, often analyzing two different drug regimes or patient satisfaction with drugs as they compare to surgery.[9]

**Failed Drug-Induced or "Medical" Abortion**
Drug-induced abortion often fails because the fetus is not fully expelled. Creinin and Vittinghoff studied two different methods of chemical induction and found that there was a 90 per cent effectiveness rate for one of their groups of

patients and a 47 per cent effectiveness rate for another group. In the end ten per cent and 53 per cent, respectively, underwent a surgical abortion in a hospital. As Table 8-1 indicates, this high failure rate remains a major concern of researchers.

**Table 8-1**
**Failure rates in drug-induced or "medical" abortion studies**[10]

| study | date | % failure |
|---|---|---|
| Silvestre and colleagues | 1990 | 4 |
| U.K. Multicentre Trial | 1990 | 6 |
| Bugalho and colleagues | 1993 | 8.3; 14 |
| WHO (Van Look) | 1993 | 4.5 |
| Ferguson and colleagues* | 1993 | 3 |
| Henshaw | 1994 | 5.8 |
| Creinin and Vittinghoff | 1994 | 10; 53 ** |
| Hausknecht | 1995 | 4 |
| El-Refaey and colleagues | 1995 | 3 |
| Wiebe | 1999(a) | 7 |
| Wiebe | 1999(b) | 17.2; 10.9** |

\* Second Trimester
\** Failure percentage depends upon drug administered

**Complications of Drug-Induced or "Medical" Abortion**
The side effects reported in the above studies are also daunting: Ferguson and colleagues found that within their study of 62 women, 38 different symptoms were associated with drug-induced abortion. These symptoms included diarrhea, blood loss, high temperature, and infection. In fact, five women displayed delayed symptoms which did not appear until two weeks following the induction.[11]

Henshaw and colleagues note that there is a "higher rate of unpleasant sequelae during medical abortion...At 50-63 days gestation medical abortion becomes more unpleasant and its efficacy starts to wane...."[12] During the second trimester, according to Guidozzi and colleagues, medical abortion "means a nearly *fivefold increase* in the incidence of complications both major and minor."[13] These complications are summed up by Grimes in his comprehensive review of the literature in the following way: "Disadvantages of medical abortion include the longer process, noxious gastrointestinal side effects, prolonged bleeding, occasional hemorrhage, higher failure rate, the inconvenience of several visits [to the doctor], and lack of immediate confirmation of success for some patients."[14]

In 1996 Ellen Wiebe studied 100 Canadian women who had undergone drug-induced abortions using misoprostol and methotrexate.[15] She found that these women reported 53 side effects, including nausea, diarrhea, fever, headaches, chills, and vomiting, but the number of individuals among whom the effects occurred was not given. Her study reported that eleven women underwent a surgical abortion following the failure of the drugs to complete the abortion.

**Pain in Drug-Induced or "Medical" Abortion**
Pain in surgical abortion (see Chapter 9) is reported to be as intense as the pain associated with non-terminal cancer and phantom limb pain.[16] Researchers inform us that "medical" abortion can also be painful. Women in Wiebe's study of abortion rated their level of pain. It is assumed that the McGill Pain Questionnaire was employed, since Wiebe was also involved in that study.[17]

Pain from drug-induced or "medical" abortions was rated at 5.8,[18] while pain from surgical abortions was only rated at 4.2.[19] These measures are based on a ten-point scale. Drug-induced abortion would seem to be more painful.

Creinin and Vittinghoff note in their study of different drugs for the induction of abortion that only nineteen per cent did not require pain medication, while "Pain was not as well tolerated by women in [the other group using different drugs]." Of the 60 per cent in this second group who required medication, 27 per cent needed narcotics and ten per cent required very high dose narcotics.[20] Henshaw and colleagues found that the unacceptability of "medical" abortion was correlated with the degree of pain that the woman experienced: " ...the more painful the medical abortion, the less acceptable the procedure."[21]

**Psychological Aspects of Drug-Induced or "Medical" Abortion**
Twenty per cent of the women in Henshaw's 1993 study reported that they wished to be assigned to the drug-induced abortion group rather than the surgery group because they viewed the procedure as "less invasive" and more "natural." Similarly, some women in Wiebe's 1996 Canadian sample reported that they were satisfied with the procedure because it "felt more natural" than surgical abortion.

However, induced abortion is not a natural event; nor is it without risk of complications. Further research may be needed to provide an answer to one question that this perception raises: If drug-induced or "medical" abortion is perceived as more "natural" by some, is there a risk that the possibility of pregnancy will be overlooked?

**Conclusion**
No long-term or epidemiological follow up has been carried out on women who have drug-induced or "medical" abortions; however, taking a drug to induce an abortion is not a simple, risk-free alternative to the surgical procedure. Despite Grimes' statement that "Medical abortion with mifepristone or methotrexate in combination with a prostaglandin is safe and effective", he admits that "...the risk of hemorrhage and gastrointestinal side effects is greater with medical abortion [than with surgical abortion]."[22] In one study, women reported up to 53 unpleasant side effects including diarrhea, vomiting, blood loss, hemorrhage, high temperatures, and infection. In addition to these medical complications, frequent visits to the doctor and to medical laboratories for tests are required with no guarantee that the abortion will be successful. In some instances, a surgical abortion is required to expel the fetus fully. As we have pointed out in Chapter 1 and in Chapter 17, "Methodology and Bias", these outcomes are often understated in North-American studies.

**Key Points Chapter 8**

• With the introduction of RU-486 and other similar drugs women can now avoid surgical abortion to terminate a pregnancy.

• There are no long-term, follow-up studies of the consequences of drug-induced or "medical" abortion.

• Studies show that some women choose drug-induced abortion because they consider it "more natural."

• Drugs, however, are not always effective in expelling the fetus. This can lead to a second, surgical, abortion.

• There are a number of unpleasant side effects, including nausea, various gastrointestinal discomforts, prolonged bleeding, and infections sometimes leading to subsequent surgical abortion.

• Pain is an issue for many women and needs further study.

• Many of these unpleasant sequelae are understated in the North-American literature on abortion, leading to the question: Are women in Canada and the United States being fully informed of the medical risks of the procedure?

## Notes

1   O'Connor K. *No Neutral Ground? Abortion Politics in an Age of Absolutes*. Boulder, Colorado: Westview, 1996.

2   Grimes D. Medical abortion in early pregnancy: A review of the evidence [Review]. Obstetrics & Gynecology 1997 May;89(5 Pt 1):790-6.

3   O'Connor 1996. See n. 1; p. 174, p. 178.

4   Creinin MD, Darney PD. Methotrexate and misoprostol for early abortion. Contraception 1993(a) October;48(4):339-48.
Creinin MD. Methotrexate for abortion at <42 days. Contraception 1993(b) December;48(6):519-25.

5   Creinin 1993(a). See n.4, p. 346.

6   Creinin 1993(b). See n. 4, p. 523.

7   Christin-Maitre S, Bouchard P, Spitz IM. Medical termination of pregnancy. New England Journal of Medicine 2000 March 30;342(13):946-956, p. 954.

8   Ferris LE, Basinski AS. Medical abortion: what does the research tell us? Canadian Medical Association Journal 1996 January 15;154(2):185-7, p. 187.

9   Henshaw RC, Naji SA, Russell IT, Templeton AA. A comparison of medical abortion (using mifepristone and gemeprost) with surgical vacuum aspiration: Efficacy and early medical sequelae. Human Reproduction 1994 November;9(11):2167-72.

Creinin MD, Vittinghoff E. Methotrexate and misoprostol vs. misoprostol alone for early abortion: A randomised controlled trial. Journal of the American Medical Association 1994 October 19;272(15):1190-5.

Holmgren K. Women's evaluation of three early abortion methods. Acta Obstetricia et Gynecologica Scandanavica 1992 December;71(8):616-23.

Hausknecht RU. Methetrexate and misoprostol to terminate early pregnancy. New England Journal of Medicine 1995 August 31;333(9):537-40.

10  Table 8-1
Silvestre L, Dubois C, Renault M, Rezvani Y, Baulieu EE and Ulmann A. Voluntary interruption of pregnancy with mifepristone (RU 486) and a prostaglandin analogue. A large-scale French experience. New England Journal of Medicine 1990 March 8;322(10):645-8.

UK Multicentre Trial. The efficacy and tolerance of mifepristone and prostaglandin in first trimester termination of pregnancy. British Journal of Obstetrics and Gynaecology 1990 June;97(6): 480-6.

Bugalho A, Bique C, Almeida L, Bergstrom S. Pregnancy interruption by vaginal misoprostol. Gynecologic and Obstetric Investigation 1993;36(4): 226-9.

World Health Organisation Task Force on Post-ovulatory Methods of Fertility Regulation. Termination of pregnancy with reduced doses of mifepristone. British Medical Journal 1993 August 28;307(6903)·532-7.

Ferguson JE 2d, Burkett BJ, Pinkerton JV, Thiagarajah S, Flather MM, Martel MM, and colleagues. Intraamniotic 15(s)-15-methyl prostaglandin F2 alpha and termination of middle and late second-trimester pregnancy for genetic indications: A contemporary approach. American Journal of Obstetrics and Gynecology 1993 August;169(2 Pt 1):332-9; discussion 339-40.

Henshaw RC, Naji SA, Russell IT, Templeton AA. Comparison of medical abortion with surgical vacuum aspiration: Women's preferences and acceptability of treatment. British Medical Journal 1993 September 18;307(6906):714-7.

Creinin MD and Vittinghoff E. 1994. See n. 9.

Hausknecht 1995. See n. 9.

el-Refaey H and Templeton A. Induction of abortion in the second trimester by a combination of misoprostol and mifepristone: A randomized comparison between two misoprostol regimens. Human Reproduction 1995 February;10(2):475-8.

Wiebe ER. Comparing abortion induced with methotrexate and misoprostol to methotrexate alone. Contraception 1999 January;59(1):7-10.

_____. Oral methotrexate compared with injected methotrexate when used with misoprostol for abortion. American Journal of Obstetrics and Gynecology 1999 July;181(1):149-52.

11 Ferguson et al. 1993. See n. 10.

12 Henshaw 1994. See n. 10.

13  Guidozzi F, van der Griendt M, Israelstam D. Major complications associated with extra-amniotic prostaglandin F2 alpha termination of the mid-trimester pregnancy. South African Medical Journal 1992 August;82(2):102-4.

14  Grimes 1997. See n. 2, p. 795.

15  Wiebe ER. Abortion induced with methotrexate and misoprostol. Canadian Medical Association Journal 1996 January 15;154(2):165-70.

16  Belanger E, Melzack R, Lauzon P. Pain of the first trimester abortion: A study of psychosocial and medical predictors. Pain 1989 March;36(3):339-50.

17  Wiebe ER, Rawling M. Jannssen P. Comparison of 0.5% and 1.0% lidocaine for abortions. International Journal of Gynaecology and Obstetrics 1996 October;55(1):71-2.

18  Wiebe 1996. See n. 15.

19  Wiebe et al. 1996. See n. 17.

20  Creinin and Vittinghoff 1994. See n. 9, p. 1193.

21  Henshaw et al. 1994. See n. 10

22  Grimes 1997. See n. 2.

# Chapter 9

# Pain

Physical and psychological factors play a part in pain experienced by women during an abortion. Studies suggest that most women experience greater pain than predicted in pre-abortion counseling; however, pain is an underestimated and little-studied effect of the abortion procedure.

Exceptional levels of pain may indicate acute physical complications, though abortion practitioners who survey levels of pain may fail to note the possible connection to complications and, instead, assume that women who experience severe pain are psychologically unstable.

Depression after abortion appears to be strongly linked to the intensity of reported pain and reflects the frequent failure of abortion to relieve depression. There is no evidence, however, that a woman's risk of suffering pain is ever taken into consideration in pre-abortion counseling to recommend that she consider alternatives to abortion. Pain during abortion requires wider and more independent study.

# Pain

Little is known about the accuracy and extent of information given to abortion patients about the level of pain to expect. There are calls for further research into the experience of pain during abortion.[1] Consent forms give the impression that the sensation will resemble heavy menstrual cramps. But this is not what women report. Anecdotal evidence suggests that the pain levels during abortion can reach the severe range.

### McGill Pain Questionnaire

Pain can be viewed as one aspect of the body's physical reaction to injury or invasion, but it can also be viewed as a psychic response, that is, an expression of underlying psychological and emotional factors such as self-hate, isolation, ambivalence, depression, guilt, or fear. When dealing with the pain that accompanies abortion, these two responses often merge. Belanger and colleagues found that 97 per cent of the 109 women in a study at a Montreal abortion clinic experienced pain, and 61 per cent reported pain levels ranging from moderate to severe. The researchers used the McGill Pain Questionnaire, an instrument used in a variety of clinical settings, to measure pain. The total pain scores were then compared with pain scores for "other acute and chronic pain syndromes." It was found that the average abortion pain ranked higher than that experienced by people suffering from fractures, sprains, neuralgia, or arthritis, and was equal to that reported by amputees experiencing phantom limb pain and patients with cancer.[2]

Of particular interest are the demographic factors that separated those women who experienced severe pain from those who found the pain more tolerable. The factors isolated by these researchers were: age, education, pre- operative anxiety, depression, fear, ambivalence, low pain tolerance, and moral or social concerns. For example, with respect to the criterion of age, "...not all adolescents reported severe levels of pain, but they were nearly twice more likely than older patients to experience the more severe levels of pain recorded."[3]

The main finding of the study, however, was that pre-abortion depression emerged as the principal predictor of pain intensity. It is often suggested that pregnancy causes a woman to be depressed and because abortion removes this cause of depression she should feel relief. But Belanger and colleagues found that half the women who pre-abortion, had elevated depression scores on the Beck Depression Inventory "remained clinically depressed and anxious two weeks after the procedure."[4]

Of the 116 women invited to participate in the research, four refused and three others *"were too incapacitated to complete the assessments"* [emphasis added].[5] The article does not explain the incapacitation, but post-abortion medical complications could well have been the reason.

Belanger and colleagues concluded that women who meet the criteria of predisposing factors, particularly the ambivalent or depressed, may be most in need of counseling and "might benefit from having general anesthesia or additional narcotic analgesia."[6]

**Other Studies**
A Medline search for the topic of pain during or following abortion shows that since 1979, there have been only a few research initiatives designed to look specifically at the topic. One discursive chapter has appeared in a monograph prepared by a U.S. abortion clinic. Of the nine studies on pain, two besides Belanger and colleagues were from a single Canadian abortion practitioner (and an associate): Wiebe (1992) and Wiebe and Rawling (1995). These studies, together with those by Borgatta and Nickinovich, were undertaken by associates in abortion facilities or by employees of the Planned Parenthood Federation of America, all advocates of the easy availability of abortion.[7]

The researchers mentioned above have identified pain as a problem for their clients. Borgatta and Nickinovich report, *"We were surprised to note that the majority of women reported moderate or more discomfort during the procedure; we had not expected as many women to report severe pain"* [emphasis added].[8] Pre-abortion counseling falsely minimized the pain that their patients were about to experience. The pain of abortion was usually described to their patients in terms of "menstrual cramping that might be quite strong, lasting for five–ten minutes".[9] Would the patient understand this to mean a level of pain that was equivalent to a high score on the McGill Pain Questionnaire?

Wiebe and Rawling tested various analgesics during abortion and compared their efficacy in alleviating pain. In their study, they discuss the impact of these drugs both during the procedure and 30 minutes post-operatively. The main topic of their research, however, was the comparison of different drugs when applied to the pain experienced by abortion patients; their focus was not the measurement of the pain itself. When they tested waiting times on one group of clients, however, they found that "the lidocaine had stopped working because all of the women experienced moderate to severe pain". They concluded: *"Our patients are still experiencing a significant amount of pain so more research is needed in pain control in abortion"* [emphasis added].[10]

In 1996 Wiebe published a research paper on drug-induced abortion patients and found that these women report higher pain levels than women who undergo surgically-induced abortions. The Wiebe results corroborated those found in the research of the Swedish scientist Holmgren in 1992.[11] (For a fuller discussion of drug-induced or "medical" abortion see Chapter 8.)

Pain from surgical abortion can be caused by the procedure itself or by complications of the procedure such as infection, uterine damage, or cervical rupture. In retrospective *epidemiological* research, Holt, Daling and colleagues studied the effect of abortion history on future ectopic pregnancy rates. They found that women with a later ectopic pregnancy had experienced pain for one week more following a previous abortion (12.5 per cent), than women who did not have a future ectopic pregnancy.[12] This suggests that there may be a possible connection between pain after an induced abortion and future ectopic pregnancies. This finding should alert both women having an abortion – and their doctors – to possible future difficulties.

Unfortunately, there is little acknowledgement in the present literature that moderate to severe pain may be a symptom of a surgical complication. Rather, those women who require analgesics or have pain levels consistent with possible complications are said to be unable to tolerate pain as well as other women studied.[13]

It is an anomaly that in the study of pain, as in other areas of abortion research, the awareness that a woman may be predisposed to physical and psychological suffering never translates into a recommendation that she consider alternatives to abortion. This point will be discussed further in Chapter 11.

**Conclusion**

It is clear from the present research that women experience pain during and after abortion, especially those who report depression before the procedure. Contrary to what women are often told at abortion facilities – that they will experience pain similar to that of heavy menstrual cramping – pain is often reported that is as severe as that reported by cancer patients and the phantom pain experienced by amputees. Because pain after an abortion can be an indicator of an ectopic pregnancy and other negative sequelae, doctors need to be more attentive to post-abortion pain, and women need to be alerted to the fact that pain might indicate post-abortion complications. More independent research needs to be done in this area.

**Key Points Chapter 9**

- Pain during and after abortion has been inadequately studied.

- Women report pain levels that are usually much worse than suggested in pre-abortion counseling.

- Severe pain after abortion is strongly linked to depression before and after abortion.

- Pain can be a key indicator of serious medical complications, a fact not often told to women.

- Pain levels reported by women may be dismissed or minimized in surveys conducted by abortion practitioners.

- There need to be more independent studies on the connection of abortion to pain.

# Notes

1   Wiebe ER, Rawling M. Pain control in abortion. International Journal of Gynaecology and Obstetrics 1995 July;50(1).41-6.

Borgatta L, Nickinovich D. Pain during early abortion. Journal of Reproductive Medicine 1997 May;42(5):287-93.

2   Belanger E, Melzack R, Lauzon P. Pain of the first trimester abortion: a study of psychosocial and medical predictors. Pain 1989 March; 36(3):339-50.

3   Belanger 1989. See n. 2, p. 345.

4   Belanger 1989. See n. 2, p. 347.

5   Belanger 1989. See n. 2, p. 340.

6   Belanger 1989. See n. 2, p. 348.

7   Smith GM, Stubblefield PG, Chirchirillo L, McCarthy MJ. Pain of first-trimester abortion: its quantification and relations with other variables. American Journal of Obstetrics and Gynecology 1979 March;133(5):489-98.

Suprapto K, Reed S. Naproxen sodium for pain relief in first-trimester abortion. American Journal of Obstetrics and Gynecology 1984 December 15;150(8):1000-1.

Wells N. Pain and distress during abortion. Health Care of Women International July/Sept 1991;12(3):293-302.

Stubblefield PG. Control of pain for women undergoing abortion. Supplement, International Journal Gynecology and Obstetrics 1989;44(3)3:131-4.

Wiebe ER. Comparison of the efficacy of different local anesthetics and techniques of local anesthesia in therapeutic abortions. American Journal of Obstetrics and Gynecology 1992 July;167(1):131-4.

Wiebe and Rawling 1995. See n. 1.

Donati S, Medda E, Proietti S, Rizzo L, Spinelli A, Subrizi D, et al. Reducing pain of first trimester abortion under local anaesthesia. European Journal of Obstetrics and Gynecology and Reproductive Biology 1996 December 27;70(2):145-9.

Borgatta and Nickinovich 1997. See n. 1.

Baker A. Helping clients manage pain and fear of pain. In: *Abortion and Options Counseling: A Comprehensive Reference.* Granite City, Illinois: Hope Clinic For Women, 1995.

8   Borgatta and Nickinovich 1997. See n. 2, p. 292.

9   Borgatta and Nickinovich 1997. See n. 2, p. 288.

10   Wiebe and Rawling 1995. See n. 1, p. 43.

11   Wiebe ER. Abortion induced with methotrexate and misoprostol. Canadian Medical Association Journal 1996 January 15;154(2):165-70.

Holmgren K. Women's evaluation of three early abortion methods. Acta Obstetricia et Gynecologica Scandanavica 1992 December;71(8):616-23.

12   Holt VL, Daling JR, Voigt LF, McKnight B, Stergachis A, Chu J, et al. Induced abortion and the risk of subsequent ectopic pregnancy. American Journal of Public Health 1989 September;79(9):1234-8.

13   Creinin MD. Methotrexate and misoprostol for abortion at 57-63 days gestation. Contraception 1994 December;50(6):511-5.

# Chapter 10

# When Abortion Fails

Occasionally abortion fails, especially when it is drug induced. When this happens, either a second D&C or a more serious surgery may be attempted. The other alternative is a decision to continue the pregnancy and give birth to the baby. In the case of "selective reduction" where only some fetuses are aborted from a multiple pregnancy (usually the result of fertility treatments), the remaining fetuses can be endangered and the mother may be at risk of miscarrying. Deciding after a failed abortion whether to continue or to terminate the pregnancy often results in feelings of grief and guilt for which a woman may need counseling. In the past 45 years there have been only seven studies on failed abortion suggesting that there has probably been systemic underreporting of its effects on women and their children.

# When Abortion Fails

### Surgical Abortion

In the vast majority of cases of surgical abortion, a failed abortion – meaning that the fetus continues to survive or is not fully expelled – leads to a second surgery which itself raises the possibility of medical complications.

> "...patient [who] had a D & C abortion at ten weeks gestation later presented to ER [Emergency Room] with fever and bleeding; ultrasound indicated retained partial fetal parts."
>
> *Survey of Canadian Physicians on Women's Health after Induced Abortion*

Failed abortion is an extremely rare, but possible, result of induced surgical abortion. Nevertheless, in the United States alone, roughly 700 pregnancies a year continue following an initial abortion procedure, and that over the past 25 years about 17,500 women required either a second procedure, or a more serious surgery, or changed their mind and continued the pregnancy to term.[1]

A 1999 Canadian study by Hall reviewed the literature and found that when abortion fails and women choose not to undergo a second procedure, the children born may have "limb or digit abnormalities and congenital contractures." The review goes on to note, "However, it is likely there has been bias leading to the reporting of abnormal cases."[2] Given the fact that only seven studies in the past 45 years have addressed failed abortion, there may also be systemic underreporting as well.

Holt, Daling and colleagues noted that for 3.4 per cent of women in the study of ectopic pregnancy, the original abortion procedure did not succeed and a D&C was performed. In these cases the abortion failed because the clinic did not test for ectopic pregnancy[3] (see Chapter 4 on "ectopic pregnancy"). This failure to test for ectopic pregnancy can be life-threatening.

Infants are also known to survive late-term abortions.[4] This outcome is now a less frequent occurrence with the use of *KCL injections* (potassium chloride) in late-term abortion, to ensure that a viable fetus does in fact die. As Ferguson and colleagues state, "We use urea to be certain that we effect fetal death. It is unsettling to all personnel to deliver these fetuses when they are not stillborn".[5] In the Ferguson study, 34 per cent of the abortions were on fetuses over 22 weeks gestation. (Fetal viability in premature birth is currently 23-24 weeks, and rarely babies born at 21-22 weeks have been resuscitated.)

A recent Canadian court case has drawn attention to the plight of a child who suffered cerebral palsy as an abortion survivor. The child was born alive and left without oxygen or medical treatment for 40 minutes until a nurse took her to the neonatal intensive care unit. The hospital involved was found negligent and thus responsible for her disabilities, and was ordered to pay the plaintiff $8,700,000.[6] Holmes has also reported two known cases of infant malformation following prenatal exposure to cervical dilation and uterine curettage.[7]

Abortion can also fail in cases where multiple pregnancies are reduced to one or two desired fetuses. "Selective reduction" is now a common practice in large teaching hospitals. Hall has documented cases in Canada where the procedure killed the intended fetus but "puts the remaining fetus(es) at risk for vascular compromise" and elevates the risk of miscarriage (see also Chapter 13 on "Multifetal Pregnancy Reduction").

**Failed Drug-Induced or "Medical" Abortion**
Drug-induced or "medical" abortion has a higher failure rate than surgical abortion. When abortion is induced by the use of chemical *prostaglandins* or prostaglandin analogues, two possible scenarios may lead to failed abortion.

The first is the actual failure of the drugs to complete the abortion. Grimes reports the overall complete abortion rate from his *meta-analysis* of seven chemical (drug-induced) abortion studies from 1991 to 1994 as 93.9 per cent.

He goes on to say, "Failed abortion is an infrequent but important complication of medical abortion. These women should undergo suction curettage as soon as the diagnosis is made".[8] Similarly, Collins and Mahoney noted that "...prostaglandins and their analogues must be given in doses yielding unacceptably high levels of side effects... [With a] lower dose...some failures will occur and these women will then need abortion by other methods".[9] Women may even be unaware that the abortion is incomplete and may only later seek medical help when infection develops.

The second scenario is the woman's own decision-making process: Drug-induced abortion requires at least two infusions of drugs at two separate office visits and may require up to two weeks to complete. During this time a woman may change her mind and decide to continue with the pregnancy. Holmes and Fonseca and colleagues have found that "Exposure during pregnancy to the synthetic prostaglandin misoprostol has also been associated with the occurrence of terminal transverse limb defects and scalp defects."[10] Likewise, Gonzalez identified Brazilian children suffering from limb deficiencies as a result of exposure to misoprostol in early pregnancy.[11]

However, Grimes records that "... some women with a failed abortion choose to continue the pregnancy and a small number of normal infants have been born after exposure to mifepristone in early pregnancy."[12] (For a fuller discussion of drug-induced or "medical" abortion, see Chapter 8.)

**Psychological Issues**
The woman who seeks abortion is often promised a relatively painless and simple procedure to eliminate a pregnancy that she does not wish to carry to term. Failed abortion may involve her in a number of unanticipated outcomes. If she changes her mind about "medical" abortion and a child is born with anomalies, maternal grief and guilt may be anticipated and counseling may be necessary. If a second abortion procedure is successful at a late stage of fetal development, where the woman knows that procedures are chosen to ensure that an anticipated live birth cannot occur, grief and guilt may likewise ensue. (See Chapters 11 and 12 for more information.)

## Conclusion

Though rare, there are some instances when both surgical and drug-induced abortions do fail, putting a woman's health at risk (and, need we add, her child's as well?) When this happens, there are decisions to be made about what alternative to pursue: continue the pregnancy or have a second attempted abortion? There are both psychological and ethical questions involved, in addition to purely medical and scientific ones. More study needs to be done in this area with its many medical and psychological implications for both mother and child(ren).

## Key Points Chapter 10

- Failure of abortion, though infrequent, is a complication of the procedure.

- The woman can decide to attempt another abortion or to continue her pregnancy.

- Children born after a failed abortion may have limb or digit abnormalities and other congenital problems, though a number of infants with no defects are born.

- Drug-induced abortions are more likely to fail than surgical abortions partly because drug dosages which would ensure that the fetus is stillborn would yield in the mother "unacceptably high levels of side effects" (see note 9).

- Maternal grief and guilt are concerns after a failed abortion.

- More research is needed in this area.

## Notes

1 Fielding WL, Lee SY, Friedman EA. Continued pregnancy after failed first-trimester abortion. Obstetrics & Gynecology 1978 July;52(2):56-8.

Steier A, Bergsjo P. [Failed induced abortion. Pregnancy continuing after induced abortion]. Tidsskr Nor Laegeforen. 1992 August 20;112(19):2538-40.

Hall JG. Arthrogryposis associated with unsuccessful attempts at termination of pregnancy. American Journal of Medical Genetics 1996 May 3;63(1):293-300.

2 Hall 1996. See n. 1, p. 293.

3 Holt VL, Daling JR, Voigt LF, McKnight B, Stergachis A, Chu J, et al. Induced abortion and the risk of subsequent ectopic pregnancy. American Journal of Public Health 1989 September;79(9):1234-8.

4 Shaver J. Gianna: *Aborted...and Lived to Tell About It.* Colorado Springs, CO: Focus on the Family Publishing, 1995.

5 Ferguson JE 2d, Burkett BJ, Pinkerton JV, Thiagarajah S, Flather MM, Martel MM, et al. Intraamniotic 15(s)-15-methyl prostaglandin F2 alpha and termination of middle and late second-trimester pregnancy for genetic indications: A contemporary approach. American Journal of Obstetrics and Gynecology 1993 August;169((2 Pt 1)):332-9;discussion 339-40, p. 340.

6 Hospital pays $8.7M settlement: Premature baby was abandoned with dead foetuses. The National Post 1999 July 31;Sect. A:1.

7 Holmes LB. Possible fetal effects of cervical dilation and uterine curettage during the first trimester of pregnancy. Journal of Pediatrics 1995 January;126(1):131-4.

8 Grimes D. Medical abortion in early pregnancy: A review of the Evidence [Review]. Obstetrics & Gynecology 1997 May;89(5 Pt 1): 790-6, p. 793.

9 Collins FS, Mahoney MJ. Hydrocephalus and abnormal digits after failed first-trimester prostaglandin abortion attempt. Journal of Pediatrics 1983 April;102(4):620-1, p. 621.

10 Holmes 1995. See n. 7, p. 132.

Fonseca W, Alencar AJ Pereira RM, Misago C. Congenital malformation of the scalp and cranium after failed first trimester abortion attempt with misoprostol. Clinical Dysmorphology 1993 January;2(1)76-80.

11   Gonzalez CH, Vargas FR, Perez AB, Kim CA, Brunoni D, Marques-Dias MJ, et al. Limb deficiency with or without Mobius sequence in seven Brazilian children associated with misoprostol use in the first trimester of pregnancy, American Journal of Medical Genetics 1993 August 1;47(1):59-64.

12   Grimes 1997. See n. 8.

Chapter 11

# Psychological Risk Factors

Although more research on the psychological effects of abortion on women needs to be done, it is clear that women experience varying degrees of emotional distress. Both internal and external risk factors come into play, and women particularly at risk of future psychological problems include those who had psychiatric or psychological problems before the abortion, those who are in dysfunctional or abusive relationships (either present or past), those who hold religious or philosophical values in conflict with the procedure, those who are not sure how they feel about their pregnancy and lack support systems, and those who are in adolescence at the time of an abortion and lack the ability fully to understand future implications.

When women at any age are pressured by those around them to have an abortion they are likely to experience more distress around the decision, as well as guilt, anxiety and depression. In countries where counseling and psychological and practical help are offered to pregnant women, they are less likely to make the decision to abort. Unfortunately, most abortion facilities in North America offer no such counseling opportunities, nor do they make women aware of the possible negative psychological impact the procedure could have on them. It is not clear how likely women will be able to give informed consent under these circumstances.

# Psychological Risk Factors

### Shortcomings in the Psychological Outcome Literature

North-American researchers and practitioners of abortion tend not to identify psychological problems for women after abortion because they do not expect them. Rather, they assume that women, anxious about an unwanted pregnancy, will be relieved after the procedure. As a consequence, they minimize any damage abortion does to women's psychological health, and attribute negative psychological effects either to women's immaturity or to their pre-existing psychological problems.[1]

As in many other areas of abortion research, conclusive findings are difficult to arrive at owing to short-term follow up, subjective measurements, lack of volunteers for research studies (because many women do not want to recall their abortion(s)), researchers' politically motivated agendas, and stereotypes about the kind of women who exhibit negative psychological traits. As deVeber and colleagues observe:

> In the search for evidence of deep-seated, long-term adverse reactions to the abortion experience, the small-scale studies provide what the large projects lack: they examine reactions over years and probe for reactions in a variety of behavioural and symptom areas. Studying 50 postabortive women in psychotherapy, Kent and colleagues found that, although none had entered therapy because of adverse emotional reactions to abortion, they expressed deep feelings of pain and bereavement about the procedure as treatment continued. Typically the bereavement response emerged during the period when the patient was recovering from the presenting problem.[2]

Until information that is now only available in anecdotal women's stories can be subjected to critical analysis, it will be difficult to assess the risks abortion poses to women's psychological health.

**Risk Factors: Introduction**

There is a general consensus that women who exhibit certain pre-existing characteristics are at greater risk for post-abortion problems.[3]

In 1977, Belsey established the following high-risk criteria for British women undergoing induced abortion.[4] Women who exhibited any, some, or all of these factors would experience negative emotional reactions following abortion:

- Poor or unstable relationships
- Socially isolated (few friends)
- History of unemployment
- Psychosocial instability
- Contraceptive failure

While these factors have been generally accepted in the literature, over time other factors have been added. Dunlop added the following factors:[5]

- Pressure or coercion in decision-making
- Previous psychiatric condition
- Medical reasons for the abortion, such as genetic abnormalities

Shusterman isolated additional factors:[6]

- Anger at pregnancy
- Low intimacy with partner
- Dissatisfaction with abortion decision

More recent studies have included factors such as religiosity, feelings of loss immediately after abortion, and age.[7]

The risk factors that are reported depend in large measure on the focus of the research studies. Research that is directed toward psychological factors will isolate the pre-existing psychological and psychiatric issues that affect post-abortion adjustment, while studies that focus on interpersonal relationships will determine the relationship factors that affect women after abortion. Since no one study can address all social and psychological factors, the list of factors included as pre-existing risks may be expected to grow and change over time and across disciplines.

**Internal or Personal Risk Factors**
Internal factors are the pre-existing risk conditions that have a significant impact on post-abortion well-being. McAll and Wilson speak to this in their discussion of negative emotional reactions following abortion "...it seems probable that because of their internal origin they may persist as repressed conflicts that can surface later in life if the person is stressed by later events."[8]

Internal or personal factors are part of a woman's personality development, and may contain components of genetics, past experience, and personal value systems. But they are still an integral part of the individual; they cannot be considered external even if they originated outside of the person and have been accommodated into the personality.

Included in this group are: Psychiatric or psychological history; history of abusive and/or dysfunctional relationships; religious values; ambivalence about the abortion decision; and age.

**1. Psychiatric or Psychological History**
Women who suffer from diagnosed psychological or psychiatric disorders or conditions before abortion will have emotional difficulties following abortion, as a sampling of the literature shows:

> ...among women who had a termination, the rate of psychiatric illness in those with a previous history of psychosis was higher than the rate in those with no history of psychiatric illness....[9]

> ...women who...have pre-existing psychiatric problems...are more likely to have emotional difficulty.[10]

Pre-existing psychiatric conditions, including depression, have been found to be associated with post-abortion problems: "...pre-abortion depression had both direct and indirect...effects on adjustment"[11] Severe grief reactions in women who aborted because of fetal abnormality were found to be linked to previous mental health treatment.[12]

David reported that an examination of admission rates to psychiatric hospitals showed 50 per cent significantly higher rates for women following abortion than for women who delivered.[13] The psychiatric admission rates for separated, divorced, and widowed women were nearly four times greater among those who aborted than among those who delivered. Most recently, a very large-scale study in California, using record linkage, found that over a four-year period women who aborted had a 72 per cent higher rate of psychiatric admission than women who delivered their babies.[14]

The Planned Parenthood Federation of America reports that ten per cent of women who abort will experience lingering depression. They go on to note that pre-existing psychiatric disturbances correlate with these negative emotional reactions.[15]

The prevailing interpretation of this finding is that the problems that these women experience is the result of their pathology and not the abortion itself. The "emotional harm some women experience post-abortion is not attributable to the abortion, but to their pre-abortion psychological fragility".[16] Abortion is seen as one of many stressful life events that will trigger their instability.

Zolese and Blacker analyzed follow-up studies of psycho-logical sequelae and interpreted Greer as follows: "Two-thirds of those undergoing psychiatric treatment following abortion had in fact had psychiatric treatment before, so the cumulative incidence of new cases in the two-year period was only 6.5 per cent."[17]

But one limitation of this kind of research is the problem of long-term follow up. To measure psychiatric disorder as a complication of abortion requires identifying those women who have been retained in a follow-up sample who have used specific psychiatric services either as outpatients or inpatients. It is, therefore, only in jurisdictions where there is continuity of service that such information is available. In the United States and increasingly in Canada, where the majority of abortions occur in freestanding clinics, there is little continuity. Only those individuals who are especially willing to participate in research can even be traced.

It must also be remembered that pre-existing risk factors are not mutually exclusive; several characteristics may apply to the same woman. For example, women with psychiatric histories may experience unstable relationships, live more chaotic lives, and be exposed to other factors which may exacerbate post-abortion reactions. Such a loading of factors has not been fully analyzed to determine their interactive effects. It may be premature to conclude that the identified psychiatric problem is the only relevant factor, or even the main one, in a particular case.

In the newly-emerging literature on post-abortion healing, therapists have isolated other factors in women's histories that may predispose them to post-abortion guilt and depression. Of particular note are early relationship disorders such as parental abandonment or unresolved conflicts in the family of origin.

**2. Abusive and/or Dysfunctional Relationships**
A 1998 research paper by Glander and colleagues looked at the relationship between domestic violence and abortion. Their focus was comparative, to determine the level of abuse reported by women who had recently undergone an outpatient abortion. The results of the self-administered questionnaire indicated that 39.5 per cent of participants (the total participation rate was 81 per cent) identified themselves as having a history of abuse. Abused women were less likely to inform their partners or involve the fathers in the abortion decision. "Relationship issues were significantly more likely to be stated as the primary reason for abortion by women with a history of abuse than nonabused women."[18]

The presence of relationship dysfunction has been identified by researchers as a strong indicator of pre-abortion depression. These researchers also call for family assessment for any woman reporting abortion-related depression since "the association between depressive symptoms and denial might reflect a lack of perceived social support, engendered by unsatisfactory family relationships."[19]

Researchers have found this issue to be particularly significant in the relationships of adolescents who abort.[20] Barnet and Freudenberg considered the relationship outcomes for unmarried but co-habiting women who aborted and found that prior to abortion their relationships were characterized by "significantly more conflict and were less harmonious than in the control group." Following abortion, when separations occurred, more of the women who had aborted initiated the breakup than did the women in the control group and the majority of these women reported that the abortion was implicated in the decision.[21]

Women who have a history of abusive relationships are likely to experience what some researchers have called "poor obstetrical history." The researchers include in this category a previous premature or low birthweight child and two or more abortions. They found that abused women were less likely to have a recorded birth as an outcome of pregnancy (i.e., they were more likely to have either a miscarriage or abortion), and that abuse was a significant predictor of poor obstetric history. They conclude, "women with a history of abuse are more likely to tolerate abuse in future relationships."[22]

Physical or sexual abuse causes a severe rupture in a woman's perception of her own self-worth. Mannion and colleagues found that when abortion is sought as part of a pattern of accepting abusive relationships, it may cause women to internalize abusive or profoundly dysfunctional relationships from the past or present, and may make it more difficult to break the cycle. For example, "Mary" and "Liane" tell their stories of abuse as children:[23]

*Mary*: I was quite sexually permissive, believing very wrongly that my worth to men lay in pleasing them physically. I was taught [through the abuse] that if I could make them happy sexually, they would stay forever.

*Liane*: I had been sexually abused for two years by a family friend when I was nine and ten years old, lost my virginity by rape in high school and had an overall poor self-image. This feeling did not start with the abortion. It started with the abuse at age nine...The abortion merely intensified this feeling.

Torre-Bueno focuses on the nature of what she calls shame following abortion. She distinguishes between guilt and shame by saying that shame is internal and reflects the collapse of self-esteem, leading to feelings of worthlessness and stupidity. She describes a patient she calls Michelle who had been molested by her cousin and by a school teacher and had never felt strong enough to follow through with prosecuting them. "These events left her feeling flawed and pathetic and the abortion confirmed for her that she was a powerless, shameful person." Torre-Bueno records that her therapy was unsuccessful because the patient was unable to confront the role that shame played in her life.[24]

Rue notes that "Abuse in relationships complicates both the abortion decision and its aftermath...[the aborting woman] may feel there is simply no other 'choice' or even feel coerced, as many women feel today in abusive relation-ships... 'Learned helplessness' is a fundamental aspect of a battered woman's functioning that is repetitively reinforced in an abusive relationship. Consequently, without a thorough exploration of her relationship in pre-abortion counseling, this woman's abortion decision-making is likely to be passive, highly conflicted and burdened by feelings of hopelessness."[25]

Women who have histories of abuse may present two pre-existing high risk characteristics: possible coercion or ambivalence about the abortion and reinforced feelings of shame or powerlessness. These characteristics can result in post-abortion psychosocial and social difficulties, not the least of which is the continuation of the cycle of abuse.

### 3. Religious Values

Although the literature on the psychological outcome of abortion does not deal much with the issue of abortion among women with strong traditional religious convictions, it appears that for them, abortion can lead to both psychological and spiritual damage.

Research on adolescent abortion patients has suggested that religious affiliation and church attendance did not stop young women from choosing abortion.[26] A Canadian study on unplanned motherhood found that:

> ...few mothers regard religion as a factor influencing a woman's decision in a crisis pregnancy...Nor do agencies regard religion as a factor of importance in any of the three dimensions in question: the likelihood of pregnancy, the abortion and the parenting decision.

In this study, only one out of five social service agencies reported that clergy played any determining role in women's decisions about their pregnancies.[27]

While the religious background of young women may not alter the original decision to abort, it is an important precursor of post-abortion distress. Dirks concluded that women from religious denominations which strongly opposed abortion were more likely to experience depression following abortion.[28]

Tamburrino and colleagues, noting that "Research has not adequately addressed how women cope with religious conflict after abortion, or whether religion is experienced as another stress factor or as a support system," studied religion as a psychosocial variable in women who describe themselves as *dysphoric* (depressed, lacking a sense of well-being) one to fifteen years following an induced abortion. The women in this sample experienced regret, guilt, and sadness, and 46 per cent "have changed their religion to Evangelical or Fundamentalist Protestant denominations...to help themselves cope with their post-abortion feelings."[29]

One difficulty with research in this area is that a distinction is not always made between religion as an extrinsic factor (the woman feels that she has violated the beliefs of others to whom she may be attached) and religion as an intrinsic factor (the woman feels that she has violated her own beliefs). Some researchers and therapists report that a woman from a religious background may suffer intense guilt over abortion if it is incompatible with her intrinsic value system. The guilt is a personal response to the violation of a value that she herself has believed and accepted but has not been able to act upon.[30]

This dissonance between the choice for abortion and accepted beliefs – for example, beliefs about the sanctity of human life – may lead to the onset of later disorders. These difficulties often arise as women mature and are able to evaluate their earlier actions in light of a more adult understanding of their faith. Women may seek resolution in one of several possible ways:

**a. Denial and Repression**
These tools are often used to accommodate psychologically incompatible ideas. Denial can become pathological when women use drugs, alcohol, or sexual promiscuity as a way to avoid confronting an underlying problem. When repression is used to suppress unpleasant thoughts and feelings about a previous abortion, they remain unresolved and can lead to future psychological problems.

**b. Isolation**
When post-abortal women feel unaccepted, unworthy, or hypocritical in continuing the affiliation with their denomination or faith community, feelings of isolation develop. The director of a counseling program that assists women with spiritual healing puts it this way:

The abortion is for many an experience of the first serious perceived sin. She believes that she has committed the unforgivable sin, leaving her isolated from God...She realizes that she has victimized an innocent being and she must take responsibility for the choice and the outcome...This spiritual woundedness crosses denominational lines.[31]

These women may still attend services and appear to be part of the community, but they often carry the burden of guilt and grief, viewing their sin as unforgivable, which places them emotionally outside that community.

**c. Rejection of the Previously Accepted Value System**
Delegitimizing of the previously accepted morality is a third way of coping with psychic distress. This last response is suggested by some therapists as an appropriate way of coping. Authors such as Torre-Bueno view the post-abortion distress of religious women as a problem with the faith or denomination rather than as a factor internal to the women themselves. It is their contention that because these churches or religious systems are philosophically opposed to abortion they are burdening women with "religious guilt".[32] To avoid such "religious guilt," they suggest that women re-evaluate their commitment to that denomination and develop their own personal spirituality that accepts their choice. This prescription amounts to changing their religious affiliation, which the women did in Tamburrino's sample above, but the difference is that in this case the change will probably be to an affiliation that accepts abortion rather than one that repudiates it.

It is worth noting that women who express philosophical, though not necessarily religious, opposition to abortion are also at risk for developing post-abortion symptoms. Franz and colleagues observed, "For women who view abortion as morally wrong prior to the procedure, undergoing an abortion may initiate a life-time of suffering. This may be particularly true for younger women."[33]

## 4. Ambivalence

Ambivalence exists when a woman is unsure if the abortion decision is the correct one. Ambivalence is an important factor in the decision-making process because the majority of crisis pregnancy decisions are marked by ambivalence. A 1994 study of unmarried single parents in Canada found that "...in a crisis pregnancy women do change their mind about the direction they will take."[34] When this ambivalence was measured by Decision Shift, there was a "...significant shift toward investment in the life of the child," and toward the parenting option. Social service agencies dealing with single mothers reported that 51 per cent of those women who were ambivalent were likely to move from abortion to parenting, while another 40 per cent occasionally made that shift. On the other hand, only seven per cent of those who originally considered parenting were likely to move toward abortion and ten per cent would occasionally make such a move. Few women make the choice to abort or to parent without experiencing some degree of uncertainty. If this uncertainty is not resolved before the abortion, it will often surface later as regret and guilt. In the Canadian research, for those who opted to parent, there appeared to be a qualitative difference in how that choice was perceived. The social workers dealing with women experiencing crisis pregnancies interpreted the decision to abort in the face of ambivalence as a result of negative influences, and one agency response stressed that women who are abandoned or are dominated, most often choose abortion even though they might want to carry to term. Osler and colleagues and Husfeldt and colleagues found that "ambivalent women run a greater risk of suffering negative emotional sequelae such as depression and guilt."[35] In short, women who are feeling ambivalent about their pregnancy are much less likely to resort to abortion if they receive positive encouragement and support, particularly from their male partners.

Ambivalence in making the decision to abort has also been isolated in the published works of Trost, Holmgren, Lemkau, and Bracken.[36] At the time of the decision, at least 25 per cent of all women and perhaps as high as 55 per cent are uncertain that abortion is the right choice. These ambivalent women are seen by Husfeldt as a separate cohort from those for whom the decision seems straightforward and unambiguous.[37] The researchers established that ambivalence could be affected by external socio-economic factors. Ambiguous women report significantly more often they would have continued their pregnancy "...if the partner had wanted the baby or if personal finances had been better." Following abortion, as women consider the possibility of acting without the support of their partner or as their financial circumstances improve, the past abortion decision may come to be viewed as a negative event.

It would appear that the socio-economic and interpersonal circumstances of ambivalent women are the main forces impelling them toward abortion. Hamark and colleagues found that, while only eight per cent of women were ambivalent when they arrived at the abortion clinic, 43.1 per cent reported initial positive or mixed feelings about the pregnancy.[38] This finding is consistent with the results of the Holmgren research which established that 42 per cent of women giving birth also had negative or mixed feelings about their pregnancy.[39] Indeed, ambivalence can occur in pregnancies that are defined as wanted and planned, and Tornbom notes that the initial unwanted or unplanned nature of pregnancies does not exclude welcome or acceptance at the time of birth, just as planning does not exclude ambivalence.[40]

When women are ambivalent, they are likely to be influenced by the views of others or by social attitudes generally. Pressures to abort for relational, financial, or social reasons may make the decision subtly coerced. The combination of ambivalence and coercion can lead to dissatisfaction and, ultimately, to psychological distress. The survey by Husfeldt and colleagues reported that 30 per cent of the women who aborted felt doubtful about the decision up to the time of the abortion. "Ambivalent women more often felt exposed to social pressure and some felt that the abortion was not their own choice...The ambivalent women more often stated that it was their partner who decided on abortion...Only a minority initially wanted abortion when the pregnancy was established...."[41] Hamark and colleagues also found "unstable relationships to be an important motive for abortion".[42] Counseling often helps in such situations.

In North America, where such counseling is not mandated or available as part of the medical system, attempts to resist the external pressure may not lead to a re-evaluation of the decision but may lead to a delay in making it. Such delays make the abortion procedure more difficult and the post-abortion distress more apparent. As Peppers found, "...where external control is strong the decision may be laden with ambivalence, anxiety, and concern for subsequent consequences. Indeed these external factors appear to be the most frequently mentioned reasons for delaying the abortion beyond the first trimester of pregnancy...The longer the pregnancy continues the greater the grief response."[43] It is at the point when ambivalent women are exposed to external pressure that they perceive a lack of control. In the research of Franco and colleagues, women who experienced negative emotional reactions on or about the date that the aborted child would have been born – known as Anniversary Reactions – often reported ambivalence about the decision to abort.[44]

This expression of ambivalence was also detected in the work of Allan and Astbury. They established that: "Too ready acceptance of women's endorsement of knowing the procedure is safe and simple may obscure important areas of ambivalence...all but one woman endorsed that she knew that a 'termination is a very safe and simple procedure.' Despite this, half the sample endorsed being really scared and 40 per cent agreed they were scared that a termination might damage them emotionally or physically."[45]

Based on the information gathered by researchers, the clinical experience of therapists, and the information from women themselves, it is clear that the presence of ambivalence at the time of an abortion is a risk factor for significant post-abortion dysfunction. What remains to be determined are the exact internal psychological processes that produce ambivalence. Tornbom has determined that ambivalence can occur in pregnancies that do not end in abortion and that wanted or planned pregnancies are not the same as welcome pregnancies.[46] Similarly, unwanted or unplanned pregnancies may well elicit feelings of ambivalence, but women who choose not to abort often describe the resulting birth as welcome.

## 5. Age

Abortion during the formative adolescent years carries with it problems that are significantly different from those experienced by mature adults. American figures show that one in three abortions are performed on teenagers, while recent British research establishes that abortion occurs in "69 per cent of conceptions to under sixteens...[and] 37 per cent of conceptions in those aged sixteen to nineteen."

The literature suggests that this group of aborters are at greater risk for subsequent physical, as well as psychological, problems. Age is the one predisposing factor that affects both medical outcome and emotional adjustment.

Coleman and colleagues studied the cognitive and developmental difference between adolescent females and their adult counterparts.[47] As well as exhibiting less intellectual, moral, and emotional maturity, adolescents are more likely to have unrealistic views of the future. Even if goals are articulated, the adolescent may be too immature to undertake the long-term planning required to reach them. Adolescents live in the present. Their decisions are egocentric; while their network of friends and peers may be wide, it is usually composed of other equally immature persons. Such relationships lack the depth required to provide appropriate support for young women experiencing crisis pregnancies.

Adolescents often view themselves as affected by events but not in control of them. Things like pregnancy are seen as having "happened to" them rather than as the outcome of choices. When cognitive immaturity is coupled with limited ability to plan ahead, a teenager is predisposed to have an abortion. The adolescent is not able to conceptualize the long-range implications of the abortion decision nor to take responsibility for them; thus, abortion seems to be an easy solution and thoughts of negative after-effects are not as frequent as in adults making the decision.[48]

While young women may lack a conscious understanding of the long-term outcomes of the abortion decision, the impact of that decision is real nonetheless. It can profoundly affect their cognitive development. Deutsch found lower levels of self-esteem in adolescents who aborted, while a Canadian study of women, post-abortion, found that "absence of affect [expression of emotion] ...especially of teenagers, was so marked as to be judged an adverse reaction in itself."[49] Kent and Linares compared adolescents who aborted a second pregnancy with two matched cohorts – teenagers who were pregnant for a second time but went on to give birth, and teenagers with no repeat pregnancy. They found that depressive symptoms among those who had abortions were nearly twice as frequent as among those who give birth, and nearly 60 per cent higher than among those who were not pregnant.[50]

Research makes it clear that important life-decisions, such as having an abortion, taken at a young age, can affect basic personality development. This becomes apparent from comparative data between adolescent and adult aborters. An American retrospective study conducted in 1988 determined that there were "significant personality trait differences between those who abort in adolescence and those who abort as adults."[51] Clinical scores indicated pathology in many of the adolescent samples. Dysfunctional levels were observed for antisocial traits, paranoia, drug abuse, and psychotic delusions. As well, the adolescent group also reported more suicide attempts.

A 1985 American study of high school students in a midwestern state found six to tenfold increases in suicide attempts when the adolescent had had an abortion.[52] The main factors underlying teen suicide attempts are anger, anxiety, and impulsiveness. The precipitating events are often relationship breakup, family disorder, and poor decisions in academic, social, or moral areas. In the year following an abortion, 90 per cent of adolescent relationships end, and if the decision to abort is taken to maintain a relationship, the ensuing split will often elicit emotions of anger, hurt, or abandonment.

Within the adolescent group are young women who experience external pressure to abort from peers, family, boy-friends, medical professionals, or counselors If young women experience such pressure, their abortion choice may be characterized by lack of informed consent and a perceived lack of control.

Even if adolescents are given full and accurate information, their immature cognitive processes may impede their understanding. Discussion of possible long-term consequences requires the ability to plan ahead, not a skill many adolescents possess. It also requires that information regarding medical and psychological sequelae be understood.

A Canadian study of Sexual Abuse Prevention Programs found that young people may verbally register information, but that being aware of facts does not necessarily lead to anticipated behavior changes.[53] Similar studies of adolescent smoking behavior and contraceptive usage confirm that, for immature persons, behavior change is less likely to follow from the acquisition of factual information.

**Conclusion**

Women who have a psychiatric history, live in abusive relationships, believe abortion is morally wrong, are ambivalent, or are adolescents are more likely to have serious problems coping with abortion. But for reasons that are not altogether clear, the presence of such a history is seldom considered by abortion clinic personnel or abortion researchers to be a reason to recommend against abortion.

Some clinicians may argue that the social impact of giving birth is worse for women than having an abortion. But that proposition is not based on documented findings. In any event, it is doubtful that information from abortion research about negative psychological sequelae is routinely shared with women who are having an abortion. This raises the issue of informed consent. By withholding information, is the clinician acting in the patient's best interest or in the perceived interests of society? It is also worth noting that all five of the higher risk categories noted above have to do with situations in which considerable pressure may be exerted on the woman to undertake a course of action she does not believe to be in her best interests. This factor of coercion may account for many women coping poorly after an abortion.

**Key Points Chapter 11**

• Women who have abortions are at risk of emotional difficulties after the procedure, especially those with pre-existing factors such as relationship problems, ambivalence about their abortion, adolescence, previous psychiatric or emotional problems, pressure by others into making a decision to abort, or religious or philosophical values that are at odds with aborting a pregnancy.

• The prevailing interpretation of post-abortion grief, depression, guilt, anger, and anxiety in abortion clinics and research studies in North America is that they are due, not to the procedure, but to a woman's pre-existing disposition to psychological problems.

• Where support through counseling is offered (for example, in Sweden) to pregnant women who are not sure if they should or can carry their pregnancy to term, they are more likely not to abort.

• Given the evidence that women in certain risk groups are more emotionally vulnerable after an abortion, should abortion clinics and medical facilities consider recommending against abortion in their cases? This question has becomes crucial given recent findings that women who abort are much likelier to commit suicide.

• Informed consent for the psychological well-being of women, post-abortion, is an issue which health care professionals should address.

## Notes

1  deVeber LL, Ajzenstat J, Chisholm D. Postabortion grief: psychological sequelae of medical abortion. Humane Medicine 1991 August;7(3):203-9.

2  deVeber 1991. See n. 1, pp. 204-205.

Kent I, Greenwood RC, Loeken J, Nicholls, W. Emotional sequelae of elective abortion. BC Medical Journal 1978 April;20(4):118-19.

3  deVeber 1991. See n. 1, p 206.

4  Belsey EM, Greer HS, Lal S, Lewis SC, Beard RW. Predictive factors in emotional response to abortion: King's termination study--IV. Social Science and Medicine 1977 January;11(2):71-82.

5  Dunlop JL. Counselling of patients requesting an abortion. Practitioner 1978 June;220:847-52.

6  Shusterman LR. Predicting the psychological consequences of abortion. Social  Science and Medicine 1979 November;13A(6):683-9.

7  Tamburrino MB, Franco KN, Campbell NB, Pentz JE, Evans CL, Jurs SG. Postabortion dysphoria and religion. Southern Medical Journal 1990 July;83(7):736-8.

Congleton GK, Calhoun LG. Post-abortion perceptions: a comparison of self-identified distressed and nondistressed populations. International Journal of Social Psychiatry 1993 Winter;39(4):255- 65 Winter 1993;39(4):255-65.

Turell Susan C, Armsworth Mary W, Gaa John P. Emotional response to abortion: A critical review of the literature. Women & Therapy 1990;9(4):49-68.

Franz W, Reardon D. Differential impact of abortion on adolescents and adults. Adolescence Spring 1992;27(105):161-72.

8  McAll K, Wilson WP. Ritual mourning for unresolved grief after abortion. Southern Medical Journal 1987 July;80(7):817-21, p. 817.

9  Gilchrist AC, Hannaford PC, Frank P, Kay CR. Termination of pregnancy and psychiatric morbidity. British Journal of Psychiatry 1995 August;167(2):243-8, p. 244.

10  Rosenfeld JA. Emotional responses to therapeutic abortion. American Family Physician 1992 January;45(1):137-40, p. 137.

11  Cozzarelli C. Personality and self-efficacy as predictors of coping with abortion. Journal of Personality and Social Psychology 1993 December;65(6).1224-36, p. 1224.

12  Hunfeld JAM, Wladimiroff JW, Passchier J. Pregnancy termination, perceived control, and perinatal grief. Psychological Reports. 1994 Feb;74(1):217-218.

13  David HP. Post-abortion and post-partum psychiatric hospitalization. Ciba Foundation Symposium 1985;115·150-64,

14  Cougle, JR, Reardon, DC, Rue VM,  Shuping MW, Coleman PK, Ney PG. Psychiatric admissions following abortion and childbirth: A record-based study of low-income women. Archives of Women's Mental Health 2001;3(4)Supp.2:47.

15  The Emotional Effects of Induced Abortion. Fact Sheet. New York: Planned Parenthood Federation of America, May 2000.

16  Rue V. *Postabortion Trauma*. Lewisville, Texas: Life Dynamics, 1994; p. 7.

17  Zolese G, Blacker CV. The psychological complications of therapeutic abortion. British Journal of Psychiatry 1992 June;(160):742-9; p. 745.

Greer HS, Lal S, Lewis SC, Belsey EM, Beard RW. Psychosocial consequences of therapeutic abortion King's termination study III. British Journal of Psychiatry 1976 January;128:74-9.

18  Glander SS, Moore ML, Michielutte R, Parsons LH. The prevalence of domestic violence among women seeking abortion. Obstetrics & Gynecology 1998 June;91(6):1002-6; p. 1004.

19  Bluestein D, Rutledge CM. Family relationships and depressive symptoms preceding induced abortion. Family Practice Research Journal 1993 June;13(2):149-56; p153.

Ney PG, Fung T, Wickett AR, Beaman-Dodd C. The effects of pregnancy loss on women's health. Social Science and Medicine 1994 May;38(9): 1193-200.

20  Rosenfeld 1992. See n. 10.

Major B, Cozzarelli C, Sciacchitano AM, Cooper ML, Testa M, Mueller PM. Perceived social support, self-efficacy, and adjustment to abortion. Journal of Personality and Social Psychology 1990 September;59(3):452-63.

21 Barnett W, Freudenberg N, Wille R. Partnership after induced abortion: a prospective controlled study. Archives of Sexual Behavior 1992 October;21(5):443-55; p.443.

22 Curry MA, Perrin N, Wall E. Effects of abuse on maternal complications and birth weight in adult and adolescent women. Obstetrics & Gynecology 1998 October;92(4 Pt 1):530-4; p. 553.

Parker B, McFarlane J, Soeken K. Abuse during pregnancy: effects on maternal complications and birth weight in adult and teenage women. Obstetrics & Gynecology 1994 September;84(3):323-8.

23 Mannion M. Abortion and healing: A pastoral church responds in word and sacrament. In: Mannion M, editor. *Post-Abortion Aftermath: A Comprehensive Consideration: Writings Generated by Various Experts at a 'Post-Abortion Summit Conference'* Kansas City: Sheed and Ward, 1994: 106-18.

24 Torre-Bueno A. *Peace After Abortion*. San Diego, California: Pimpernel Press, 1997.

25 Rue 1994. See n. 16, p.63.

26 Silber T. Abortion in adolescence: the ethical dimension. Adolescence 1980 Summer;15(58):461-74.

Ortiz CG, Vazquez Nuttall E. Adolescent pregnancy: effects of family support, education, and religion on the decision to carry or terminate among Puerto Rican teenagers. Adolescence 1987 Winter; 22(88):897-917.

27 Bierling G, Cassidy E, Carter E. Agency and maternal perceptions of the decision to parent. Joseph Koterski SJ, ed. *Life and Learning IV*. Fourth University Faculty for Life Conference; Fordham University. Washington, D.C.: University Faculty for Life; 1995; p. 297.

28 Dirks MJ. Psychological Outcomes of Abortion: An Exploration of Knowledge, Conflict, and Expectancies [Doctoral Dissertation]: University of Cincinnati, 1979.

29 Tamburrino et al. 1990. See n. 7, pp. 736-7.

30 Thorn V. Project Rachel: Faith in action, A ministry of compassion and caring. In: Mannion M, editor. *Post-Abortion Aftermath*. Kansas City, MO: Sheed and Ward, 1994: 144-63.

31 Thorn 1994. See n. 30, p. 153.

32  De Puy C, Dovitch D. *The Healing Choice: Your Guide to Emotional Recovery After an Abortion*: Fireside, 1997; p. 142.

33  Coleman PK, Franz W, Reardon D. The Salience of Pressure to Obtain an Abortion as a Predictor of Post-Abortion Adjustment in Adolescents and Adult Women [Unpublished Manuscript].1998; p. 16.

34  Ajzenstat J, Cassidy E, Carter E, Bierling G. *Going It Alone: Unplanned Single Motherhood in Canada*. Toronto: The de Veber Institute, 1994.

35  Osler M, Morgall JM, Jensen B, Osler M. Repeat abortion in Denmark. Danish Medical Bulletin 1992 February;39(1):89-91.
*

Husfeldt C, Hansen SK, Lyngberg A, Noddebo M, Petersson B. Ambivalence among women applying for abortion. Acta Obstetricia et Gynecologica Scandanavica 1995 November;74(10):813-7; p. 813.

36  Trost J. Abortions in relation to age, coital frequency, and fecundity. Archives of Sexual Behavior 1986 December;15(6):505-9.

Holmgren K, Uddenberg N. Ambivalence during early pregnancy among expectant mothers. Gynecologic and Obstetric Investigation 1993;36(1): 15-20.

Lemkau, JP. Post-Abortion Adjustment of Health Care Professionals in Training. American Journal of Orthopsychiatry. 1991 January;61(1):92-102.

Bracken, MB, Klerman, LV, Bracken, M. Coping with Pregnancy Resolution among Never-Married Women. American Journal of Orthopsychiatry. April 1978 April;48(2):320-334.

37  Husfeldt 1995. See n. 35, p. 815.

38  Hamark B, Uddenberg N, Forssman L. The influence of social class on parity and psychological reactions in women coming for induced abortion. Acta Obstetricia et Gynecologica Scandanavica 1995 April;74(4):302-6.

39  Holmgren K, Uddenberg N. Ambivalence during early pregnancy among expectant mothers. Gynecologic and Obstetric Investigation 1993;36(1):15-20.

40  Tornbom M, Ingelhammar E, Lilja H, Svanberg B, Moller A. Decision-making about unwanted pregnancy. Acta Obstetricia et Gynecologica Scandanavica 1999 August;78(7):636-41.

41  Husfeldt 1995. See n. 35, p. 816.

42  Hamark 1995. See n. 38, p. 305.

43  Peppers LG. Grief and elective abortion: Breaking the emotional bond? Omega-Journal of Death and Dying 1987-1988;18(1):1-12.; p. 9.

44  Franco KN, Tamburrino MB, Campbell NB, Pentz JE, Jurs SG. Psychological profile of dysphoric women postabortion. Journal of the American Medical Women's Association 1989 July-August;44(4):113-5.

45  Allanson S, Astbury J. The abortion decision: reasons and ambivalence. Journal of Psychosomatic Obstetrics and Gynecology 1995 September;16(3):123-36; p. 130.

46  Tornbom 1999. See n. 40.

47  Coleman et al. 1998. See n. 33.

48  Franz W. Post-abortion trauma and the adolescent. In: Mannion M, editor. *Post-Abortion Aftermath*. Kansas City: Sheed and Ward, 1994: 119-30.

49  Deutsch MB. Personality Factors, Self Concept, and Family Variables Related to First Time and Repeat Abortion-Seeking Behavior in Adolescent Women [Doctoral Dissertation].: The American University, 1982.

Kent et al. 1978. See n. 2, p.118.

50  Kent et al. 1978. See n. 2.

Linares LO, Leadbeater BJ, Jaffe L, Kato PM, Diaz A. Predictors of repeat pregnancy outcome among black and Puerto Rican adolescent mothers. Journal of Developmental and Behavioral Pediatrics 1992 April;13(2):89-94.

51  Campbell, NB, Franco K, Jurs S. Abortion in Adolescence. Asolescence 1998 winter; 23(92):813-823;p.821.

52  Garfinkel, B, Hoberman HM, Parsons JH, Walker, J. Stress, Depression and Suicide: A Study of Adolescents in Minnesota. Responding to High Risk Youth, Minnesota Extension Service, University of Minnesota (1986). 43-55.

53  Gentles I, Cassidy E. Evaluating the Evaluators: Child Sexual Abuse Prevention-Do We Know It Works? in Christopher R. Bagley and Ray J. Thomlison, eds., *Child Sexual Abuse: Critical Perspectives on Prevention, Intervention, and Treatment*. Toronto: Wall and Emerson, 1991. 27-40

Chapter 12

# Abortion after Prenatal Testing *

In advanced industrial countries prenatal testing in order to detect fetal abnormalities has become routine. The amount of genetic information that has become available through such testing has expanded enormously within the past few years. There are a number of ways of carrying out these tests, yet for each of them there is a danger of inaccurate results, and for some of them there is the additional hazard of injury to the fetus. Pregnant women and their partners are often unprepared for the news that they are carrying a "defective" fetus. An abortion agreed to in haste and under coercive pressure, can have devastating consequences, not only for the parents, but for other children. Is enough being done to inform women about the implications of prenatal testing, and to provide them with alternative choices to abortion when tests prove positive?

* We are indebted to Dr Bridget Campion for her invaluable help in preparing this chapter.

# Abortion after Prenatal Testing

Selective or genetic abortions are undertaken not because the pregnancy itself is unwanted but because some fetal attribute discovered through prenatal diagnosis has made the particular fetus unwanted. According to one study, "as many as four out of every 1000 recognized pregnancies are terminated in the second trimester for fetal abnormality"[1] as discovered during prenatal diagnostic testing.

Prenatal diagnosis is increasingly seen as a routine part of prenatal care, although it seems rarely to be linked explicitly to abortion, at least in the minds of pregnant women and their partners. Yet an abortion following the detection of a fetal anomaly can be devastating for all concerned. Additionally, even the diagnostic tests carry risks to fetal well-being quite apart from abortion.

### Testing for Fetal Abnormality

Over the past two decades, little emphasis has been placed on the psychological outcome for women who abort a child owing to genetic disorders following prenatal diagnosis. But one significant change in the past decade has been the growing amount of available genetic information about individual fetuses. This information increases the likelihood that a woman will opt for abortion, perhaps at a late stage in her pregnancy.

Since the early 1980s, *amniocentesis* has been used to diagnose chromosomal anomalies such as Down Syndrome or Tay-Sach's disease after the sixteenth week of pregnancy. The introduction of ultrasonography has also allowed physicians to identify the presence of neural tube defects (spina bifida).

In the mid 1990s, the application of the technique of *chorionic villi sampling* has led to further advances in early detection.

Through prenatal diagnosis it is now possible to detect medical conditions such as cystic fibrosis and late or adult-onset diseases such as Huntington's Chorea or multiple sclerosis. Further, it is now possible to test for what is known as "genetic susceptibility" or predisposition for conditions such as breast cancer or Alzheimer's disease.

## Methods of Prenatal Diagnosis

There are four types of prenatal diagnosis commonly offered to women.

**1. Ultrasonography ("ultrasound"):**
Through the use of sound waves, ultrasound provides a visual picture of the developing fetus. It is a test used to detect anomalies that are physically distinctive – defects of limbs and internal defects of the abdomen, chest, and heart. Neural tube defects, such as anencephaly, can also be diagnosed quite reliably by the fourteenth to sixteenth week of pregnancy. Ultrasound may also be used to confirm the presence of more that one fetus in the womb or measure the progress of fetal growth.

**2. Maternal Serum Alpha Fetoprotein Screening (MSAFP):**
Raised alpha fetoprotein levels in the pregnant woman's blood may mean that the fetus has a neural tube defect. The test is usually done in the fifteenth to seventeenth week of gestation with results available up to two weeks later. Because MSAFP has a high ratio of false-positives,[2] the test is usually followed by an ultrasound or amniocentesis to confirm the presence of an anomaly in the fetus.

**3. Amniocentesis**
Amniocentesis normally involves inserting a needle into the uterus through the abdomen and withdrawing fluid. This may be a therapeutic intervention, as when a pregnant woman suffers from polyhydramnios – that is, an excess of amniotic fluid. For diagnostic purposes, however, amniotic fluid is withdrawn in order to test for the presence of chromosomal abnormalities or neural tube defects in the fetus. Amniocentesis is usually performed at sixteen to

20 weeks' gestation, with the results being available three to four weeks later. The risk of miscarriage with amniocentesis, while small (one per cent), is nevertheless real.[3] As well, there is the possibility that the fetus may be hit by the needle.

**4. Chorionic Villi Sampling (CVS):**
In this relatively new procedure, the villi are used to provide chromosomal information about the fetus. The test can be done in the first trimester, with the results available within one or two days. However, because placental rather than fetal material is used, CVS is not as accurate as amniocentesis. Because it is performed so early, it cannot be used to detect anomalies that develop later in the pregnancy (e.g. neural tube defects). CVS carries with it a 3.2 per cent risk of miscarriage[4] and the danger of "limb reduction" in the fetus. In one study of 394 fetuses, four genetically "normal" babies nevertheless had damage to their limbs; in another study of 289 pregnancies, five fetuses were similarly affected. These deformities were attributed to CVS.[5] However, proponents of CVS believe that its advantage lies in the early detection of fetal anomalies which allows for the early termination of those pregnancies.

**Parents Unprepared for Diagnosis**
There appears to be dissonance between the practitioner's understanding of the purpose of prenatal diagnosis and the pregnant woman's perception of the procedure. While the practitioner may offer or even insist on the diagnostic tests as a way of preventing the birth of a "defective" child, pregnant women seek them out for reassurance that their babies are well and healthy.[6] For many expectant couples, the link between testing and abortion, at least initially, does not exist.[7] This may be in part because genetic counselors do not make this link explicit to their clients. In her study of the effects of prenatal diagnosis on the dynamics of pregnancy, Barbara Katz Rothman found that, while genetic counselors might presume that selective abortion would follow the detection of an anomaly, rarely did they offer any information about actual abortion procedures. Indeed, some did not even include a discussion of abortion in the first counseling

158

session.[8] Even when birth defects and abortions are explicitly discussed, couples seem to "deny this possibility, and when faced with the reality, react as though they were hearing for the first time that birth defects can occur."[9] The pregnant woman and her partner simply do not link this outcome to prenatal diagnosis.

**Quick Decision**

Despite the shock and grief they may experience upon hearing the news of a fetal anomaly, the pregnant woman and her partner are usually urged to make the decision to terminate quickly.[10] Behind this urgency is the physician's desire to avoid complications of "late" terminations of pregnancy. Because of the delays involved in amniocentesis, abortions may occur in the second and even third trimesters of pregnancy. In health care settings, the issue of such late abortions has raised ethical and legal questions.[11] In one early study, most of the terminations occurred within 72 hours of the woman receiving the news of the abnormality.[12] This hardly allows enough time for the couple to become informed about parenting children born with that anomaly and thus consider carrying through with the pregnancy.

**Methods of Termination**

The method of termination chosen will depend on the stage of pregnancy. CVS, with its results available in the first trimester, may be followed by dilation and curettage, the type of abortion normally done at an early stage of pregnancy.[13] Later terminations following amniocentesis may be carried out by dilation and evacuation or by the instillation of urea or saline into the uterus, to kill the fetus and initiate labor.[14] While D&E may be relatively fast and physically painless for the pregnant woman, the destruction of the fetus makes post-mortem examination almost impossible. Similarly, instillation procedures that kill the fetus make fetal tissue unsuitable for later examination.[15] This type of abortion may take up to 40 hours.[16] More commonly, women undergoing late termination of pregnancy have labor induced through the use of prostaglandins.[17] It is a procedure that has the advantage of delivering the fetus intact, therefore making the baby suitable for post-mortem examination.

Unless urea is injected into the womb prior to delivery, the procedure carries the possibility of delivering the baby alive, normally not a desired outcome.[18] The labor itself can be lengthy and intense[19] but because of a desire not to interfere with the labour, analgesics are usually not administered.[20] According to one study, "virtually all of the women experienced the termination procedure as one where they felt sick, painful, or frightened."[21]

**Sequelae of Genetic Termination of Pregnancy**
While couples may not be completely aware of the physical aspects of genetic abortions, they usually know even less about the accompanying and subsequent psychological and emotional distress of the procedure.[22] In interviews conducted by White-Van Mourik and colleagues and by Zeanah and colleagues *all of the study subjects* found the pregnancy termination to be a traumatic experience.[23] Rayburn and Laferla support the finding, observing that, "Terminating a pregnancy because of a major fetal malformation is often a shattering experience, and time for adjustment may be prolonged."[24] This is true for both "early" as well and "late" genetic abortions.[25] Indeed, there may be instances in which an early abortion may present more difficulties than a later abortion. One study subject reported this to be so because "there was no fetus to see and hold" after an early termination.[26] Boss speculates that "it is possible that the 'privacy' of first trimester prenatal diagnosis and selective [genetic] abortion may actually increase the unresolved 'disenfranchised' grief since so few people know about the person's loss."[27]

Researchers offer various explanations for this phenomenon. In almost all cases, pregnancies terminated for genetic anomalies were pregnancies in which maternal attachment had begun,[28] even as women may have hoped to avoid such attachment.[29] Many of the women choosing or urged to undergo prenatal diagnosis were older and, as some authors speculate, the pregnancy may have been seen to be one of a declining number of opportunities to have a child.[30] As well, unlike a miscarriage, a genetic termination occurs because the woman chooses or consents to it. According to Kolker and Burke, "genetic abortions are especially poignant because the parents take an active part in the baby's death."[31] Blumberg and colleagues speculate that "Perhaps the role of decision making and the responsibility associated with selective abortion explains [sic] the more serious depression following [the abortion]."[32] Whatever the reason, as Boss observes, "Prospective parents are rarely prepared...for the extent of the psychological trauma experienced after a selective [genetic] abortion."[33] According to Brown, after having a genetic abortion, "It took several weeks to recover physically; emotional scars are raw two years later."[34]

**Grief, Guilt, Depression**
The extent and intensity of grief can be a surprise to many couples.[35] Iles and Gath found that nearly one half of the women in their study had symptoms of grief six months after the abortion and almost one third continued to grieve thirteen months after the termination.[36] Seller and colleagues discovered that "the loss of a fetus can cause intense grief reactions, often commensurate with those experienced over the loss of a spouse, parent, or a child."[37] Zeanah and colleagues found that neither the method of termination nor the type of anomaly seems to have affected the intensity of grief, and Kolker and Burke found that women grieved abortions following both CVS and amniocentesis.[38] White-Van Mourik and colleagues observed that, with abortions following ultrasound and maternal serum alpha fetoprotein testing, there was "more confusion, numbness and subsequently more prolonged grief reactions...." They suggest that, with these "relatively non-invasive procedures...less thought is usually given by the women to preparation for an abnormal finding."[39]

Following genetic termination of pregnancy, women endure the normal but difficult symptoms of grief, such as psychosomatic disturbances, guilt and anger, as well as the symptoms characteristic of an abruptly ended pregnancy in which the fetus dies – distress upon seeing pregnant women or newborn babies, continuing to feel pregnant, and experiencing more pronounced stress around the due date and anniversaries.[40] Recovery can take a very long time[41] and, because of the nature of genetic abortions, the grief may be accompanied or complicated by other factors.

Guilt and shame are often experienced after a genetic abortion. In one study, this was the case for one-third of subjects.[42] In another, researchers found that, more than a year after the abortion, 31 per cent of the women who had terminated their pregnancies for fetal indications continued to feel guilt and anger.[43]

Following a genetic abortion, the guilt and shame may be two-pronged. On the one hand there is a sense of failure elicited by the fact of the fetal anomaly. Parents may feel that they are to blame for their child's imperfection.[44] Sixty-one per cent of woman and thirty-two percent of men felt this way in one study.[45] In another study, 43 per cent of the women suffered from this sense of guilt.[46]

On the other hand, there is the guilt generated by having made the decision to terminate the pregnancy.[47] In one study, "forty per cent of the women and nine per cent of the men" felt this way.[48] One researcher found that many women are reluctant to admit that they have had a genetic abortion and will tell relatives and friends that they had suffered a miscarriage instead.[49]

A very common form of psychological disturbance following a genetic abortion is depression.[50] Taking into account some study subjects' strong denial of feelings, Blumberg and colleagues speculate that "the actual incidence of depression following selective abortion may be as high as 92 per cent among women and as high as 82 per cent among the men studied."[51] In another study, researchers found that, six months after the abortion, almost half of the study subjects suffered from depression and anxiety and that ten of 48 women were receiving psychiatric treatment.[52] The researchers concluded that it was not the case that women were simply relieved not to be giving birth to or raising a child with an anomaly.[53] According to Donnai and colleagues, "women undergoing termination of a planned or wanted pregnancy after prenatal diagnosis constitute a high risk group, vulnerable to depression and social disruption."[54]

**Grief, Whether Pregnancy Had Been Planned or Unplanned**

The assumption of many researchers is that genetic abortions are the terminations of planned or "wanted" pregnancies.[55] In this respect, researchers contend that genetic abortions differ from elective terminations of pregnancy.[56] Further, the assumption of many researchers is that the grief and depression that often follow genetic abortions occur precisely because the pregnancy was planned and "wanted".[57] In many cases, maternal attachment may even have begun.[58] Thus researchers have compared genetic abortions to miscarriages and stillbirths insofar as they evoke grief and depression arising from the loss of an anticipated and hoped-for baby.[59]

The sequelae following genetic terminations of pregnancy may not be so easily explained, however. Research indicates, first, that not every pregnancy terminated because of fetal indications is a "wanted" or planned pregnancy. In the study by Iles and Gath, 23 per cent of pregnancies aborted for genetic reasons were unplanned as were 27 per cent of the pregnancies in the White-Van Mourik study. As well, two per cent of women remained "ambiguous" about their pregnancies in the latter study.[60]

Second, and more importantly, research indicates that grief and depression are not confined to the termination of planned and "wanted" pregnancies.[61] The "ambiguous" subjects of the White-Van Mourik study "felt very guilty about the intervention two years after the event."[62] Reardon's study shows a clear link between depression and the abortion of "unintended" pregnancies.[63] Similarly, work by Brown links grieving and elective abortions, not normally considered to be terminations of "wanted" pregnancies.[64]

While grief and depression often follow genetic terminations of pregnancy, it is a mistake to attribute this reaction solely and simply to the "wantedness" of the pregnancy.

**Living Children**

The decision to abort for genetic reasons can have a negative impact on living children. Although it is not often considered a factor in the initial decision-making process, the abortion of a sibling can have emotional consequences for children in a family. Children are affected by the anxiety of parents over the abortion and react to the absence of the baby (whose presence they will have been aware of from the third or fourth month of pregnancy).

Furlong and Black studied the impact of genetic abortion on families and found that even very young children react to their parents' distress and may have difficulty understanding and coping with the outcome. They show that young children are unable to deal with the complexity of the decision.[65] In the presence of prenatal life, young children do not separate the concept of "fetus" from the concept of "baby". The conceptual difference between the two is a medical and social construct of adults and is not easily understood by children whose approach to the world is concrete.

The couples who participated in the Furlong and Black research adopted one of three approaches in explaining the abortion to their children. The first was a partial explanation that avoided discussing the role of their own choice. The children who received such an explanation expressed sadness, disappointment, and guilt and one child wrote an essay on the event as the worst thing that had ever happened to him. Parents of very young children chose to give no explanation and yet observed behavioral changes such as motor regression in their children. Those parents who chose the third option – to give a complete explanation – did not find that it solved the problem. Rather, they reported marked and disturbing reactions. Garton reports that "Abortion can produce a deep, subtle (and often permanent) fracture of the trusting relationship that once existed between a child and parent."[66] Looking at this problem from a psychodynamic perspective, Ney and Peeters have identified a number of *"post-abortion survivor syndromes"*. They conclude that: "There are terrible conflicts that arise from these situations, and these have an impact on the individual and society."[67]

**Public Opinion versus Medical Opinion**
At present, in the general population, there appears to be a gap between acceptance of testing for disorders and acceptance of abortion of the affected fetus. When a similar group of Canadian adolescents was presented with already com-

pleted prenatal test results, the researchers Curtis and Standing found that "females are consistently more opposed to abortion than are males and both sexes show a considerable opposition to abortion in absolute terms". But Drake, Reid and Marteau note that "Health professionals hold more positive attitudes towards termination of pregnancy for a fetal abnormality than do lay groups."[69] Under the present circumstances, this could lead to "stimulating a demand for services" rather than responding to a perceived need.

Prenatal diagnosis, already accepted as part of obstetrical care, is expanding to include many conditions, disorders, and personality traits. With these new opportunities for aborting affected pregnancies come issues about informed consent and possible social coercion to abort.

As noted, health professionals are more in favor of abortion for genetic reasons than the general public. If women choose to abort as a result of medical pressure then the decision will be conflicted and a violation of their personal autonomy. Indeed, Feitshans raises issues of autonomy and informed consent and also asks: "Does genetic testing of a foetus empower women or pose an unanticipated threat to autonomy? To address these issues there is a need to articulate a feminist perspective on genetic testing and possibly to legislate protection for women's rights during prenatal care."[70] Furthermore there is a negative presumption in the medical milieu regarding children with these conditions. There is an imbalance of information, with little provided that is favorable to children with special needs.

**Informed Consent**

Generally speaking, practitioners must have the patient's consent before undertaking any treatment. To make an informed choice, the patient must have the pertinent information, including the benefits and risks of the treatment, explained in a way that can be understood by her; she must be deemed competent to make this particular decision; and the choice must be voluntary. Given current practices, there is some question as to whether the criteria for informed choice are met when women choose genetic abortions.

**a) Information:**

As Kolker and Burke note, "To make a truly informed decision, clients need to be aware not only of the risk of miscarriage entailed in the two procedures [CVS and amniocentesis]
but also of the consequences of the abortion experience. Yet
counselors rarely discuss this prior to the test and the diagnosis."[71] While genetic counselors may simply assume that
clients come to the initial sessions with ready knowledge,
Kolker and Burke point out that ignorance may in fact
underlie clients' tendency to ask few questions about genetic
terminations of pregnancy. Because clients do not make a
ready link between prenatal diagnosis and abortion, because
they have little or no knowledge of the procedures or of the
aftermath, they do not know what they should be asking.
This ignorance is an obstacle to informed choice.[72] As Brown
points out, learning that there is a fetal anomaly is not the
only information that is needed. "We had only one isolated
piece of information, not a whole crystal ball. How were we
to know what would be best?"[73] Additionally, there appears
to be little or no positive information given about the choice
of parenting a child with a given condition.

**b) Competence:**

A further obstacle to informed choice is the state in which
parents find themselves upon learning of the fetal anomaly.
Most are in shock initially and, as Brown writes, "a person
reeling from shock, numbed by a sudden catastrophe,
cannot think."[74] Nevertheless, patients are urged to make
the decision quickly, often before they have completely
recovered from the shock. In a study undertaken by White-
Van Mourik, 21 per cent of the study participants agreed to
an abortion even as they had uncertainty about the decision
because they were experiencing numbness and shock. In
their cases, "the decision was made about an event which
felt unreal."[75]

**c) Voluntariness:**

Genetic abortions involve two separate but related choices:
prenatal testing and abortion. A study presented at the
American Society of Human Genetics in 1997 found that *36
per cent of obstetricians did not mention to their patients that*

166

*prenatal testing is voluntary.* The National Institutes for Health (NIH) note: "Care should be taken to ensure that the decision to have testing is completely voluntary "[76]

Despite current emphasis on the principle of respect for patient autonomy and the practice of informed consent, studies suggest that, for many women, there was not always a sense of having had a choice in the matter. Jones and colleagues found that, for 93 per cent of the women studied, the genetic termination of pregnancy was something that simply had to be done.[77] The pressure to abort can be subtle. Even as genetic counselors consciously attempt to be non-directive in their sessions, many nevertheless believe in the efficacy of genetic terminations of pregnancy.[78] More overtly, some physicians will insist that their patients agree not to continue the pregnancy in which a fetal defect has been found before undertaking the amniocentesis.[79] Coercion is not only an obstacle to informed choice but is a contributing factor in post-abortion distress. (See also Chapters 11 and 15.)

**Conclusion**
Prenatal testing is expanding rapidly, as ever more genetic markers are discovered and women are urged to undergo these tests. It seems that there can be enormous pressures applied to mothers to go through with terminations if an anomaly is found.[80] Couples are not prepared for the depression and guilt that frequently ensue. Nor are they usually informed about the help that is available for raising children with special needs. For an informed choice to be truly available pregnant women and their partners need to be told about the possible impact of abortion on them and their other children, and they also need to have information about the care of children with special needs.

**Key Points Chapter 12**

•   Prenatal diagnosis is increasingly seen as a routine part of prenatal care, yet in the minds of pregnant women and their partners it is rarely linked explicitly to abortion.

•   The growing amount of available genetic information about individual fetuses over the past decade has increased the likelihood that a woman will opt for abortion, perhaps at a late stage in her pregnancy.

•   When testing reveals a fetal anomaly the pregnant woman and her partner are usually urged to make the decision to terminate quickly.

•   Terminating a pregnancy because of a major fetal malformation is often a shattering experience for women. The grief, guilt, and depression experienced after a genetic abortion can come as a complete surprise to many couples.

•   These negative experiences occur whether the pregnancy has been planned or unplanned.

•   The decision to abort for genetic reasons can also have a negative impact on living children.

•   Positive information needs to be given about the choice of parenting a child with special needs resulting from physical or mental handicaps.

## Notes

1  Elder SH, Laurence KM. The impact of supportive intervention after second trimester termination of pregnancy for fetal abnormality. Prenatal Diagnosis 1991;11:47-54, p. 47.

2  Rayburn WF, Barr M Jr. The malformed fetus: Diagnosis and pregnancy management. Obstetrics and Gynecology Annual 1985;14:112-126, p. 116.

3  Boss JA. First trimester prenatal diagnosis: Earlier is not necessarily better. Journal of Medical Ethics 1994;20.146-151, p. 146.

4  Boss 1994. See n. 3, p. 146.

5  Boss 1994. See n. 3, p. 147.

6  Green JM. Obstetricians' views on prenatal diagnosis and termination of pregnancy: 1980 compared with 1993. British Journal of Obstetrics and Gynaecology 1995 March;102(3):228-232, p. 231.

Mander R. Loss and Bereavement in Childbearing. Oxford: Blackwell Scientific Publications, 1994, p. 44.

7  Mander 1994. See n. 6, pp. 44-45.

8  Rothman Barbara Katz. *The Tentative Pregnancy: How Amniocentesis Changes the Experience of Motherhood.* Revised. New York: W.W. Norton and Company, 1993, pp. 36-47.

Kolker A, Burke BM. Grieving the wanted child: Ramifications of abortion after prenatal diagnosis of abnormality. Health Care for Women International 1993 November-December;14(6):513-26, p. 515.

9  Jones OW, Penn NE, Shuchter S, Stafford CA, Richards T, Kernahan C, Gutierrez J, Cherkin P. Parental response to mid-trimester therapeutic abortion following amniocentesis. Prenatal Diagnosis 1984;4:249-256, p. 250.

10  Rayburn WF, Laferla JJ. Mid-gestational abortion for medical or genetic indications. Clinics in Obstetrics and Gynaecology 1986;13:71-82, p. 72.

Rothman 1994. See n. 8, pp. 192-3.

Blumberg BD, Golbus MS, Hanson KH. The psychological sequelae of abortion performed for a genetic indication. American Journal of Obstetrics and Gynecology 1975;122:799-808, p. 806.

11  Green 1995. See n. 6, p. 232

Hunfeld JAM, Wladimiroff JW, Passchier J, Venema-Van Uden MU, Frets, PG, Verhage F. Emotional reactions in women in late pregnancy (24 weeks or longer) following the ultrasound diagnosis of a severe or lethal fetal malformation. Prenatal Diagnosis 1993;13:603-612, p. 603.

12  Donnai P, Charles N, Harris R. Attitudes of patients after "genetic" termination of pregnancy. British Medical Journal 1981;282:621-622, p. 622.

13  Rayburn and Laferla 1986. See n. 10, p. 71.
Kolker and Burke 1993. See n. 8, p. 515.

14  Rayburn and Laferla 1986. See n. 10, p. 73.
Rothman 1993. See n. 8, p. 195.

15  Rayburn and Laferla 1986. See n. 10, p. 78.

16  Lorenzen J, Holzgreve W. Helping parents to grieve after second trimester termination of pregnancy for fetopathic reasons. Fetal Diagnosis and Therapy 1995 May-June;10(3):147-56, p. 149.

17  Rayburn and Laferla 1986. See n. 10, p. 81.
Rayburn and Barr 1985. See n. 2, p. 119.
Rothman 1993. See n. 8, p. 195.

18  Rayburn and Barr 1985. See n. 2, p. 119.

19  Jones et al. 1984. See n. 9, p. 253.
Rothman 1993. See n. 8, pp. 194-200.
Kolker and Burke 1993. See n. 8, pp. 516-7.

20  Kolker and Burke 1993. See n. 8, pp. 516-7.

21  Jones et al. 1984. See n. 9, p. 253.

22  Boss 1994. See n. 3, p. 147.
Kolker and Burke 1993. See n. 8, p. 516.

23  White-Van Mourik MCA, Connor JM, Ferguson-Smith MA. The psychological sequelae of a second trimester termination of pregnancy for fetal abnormality over a two year period. Birth Defects: Original Articles Series 1992;28:61-74, p. 71.

Zeanah CH., Dailey JV, Rosenblatt MJ, Saller, DN Jr. Do women grieve after terminating pregnancies because of fetal abnormalities? A controlled investigation. Obstetrics & Gynecology 1993;82:270-275, p. 275.

24 Rayburn and Laferla 1986. See n. 10, p.80.
Blumberg et. al. 1975. See descriptions, n. 10, pp. 803-805.

25 Kolker and Burke 1993. See n. 9, p. 519, p. 520, p. 524.
Rothman 1993. See n. 8, p. 261.

Black RB. A 1 and 6 month follow-up of prenatal diagnosis patients who lost pregnancies. Prenatal Diagnosis 1989;9:795-804, p. 801.

26 Seller M, Barnes C, Ross S, Barby T, Cowmeadow P. Grief and mid-trimester fetal loss. Prenatal Diagnosis 1993;13:341-348, p. 344.

27 Boss 1994. See n. 3, p. 147.

28 Lorenzen and Holzgreve 1995. See n. 16, p. 154.
Kolker and Burke 1993. See n. 8, p. 519.
Seller et al. 1993. See n. 26, p. 347.

29 Lorenzen and Holzgreve 1995. See n. 16, p. 154.

30 Kolker and Burke 1993. See n. 8, p. 524.

Iles S, Gath D. Psychiatric outcome of termination of pregnancy for foetal abnormality. Psychological Medicine 1993 May;232:407-13, p. 407.

31 Kolker and Burke 1993. See n. 8, p. 524.

32 Blumberg et al. 1975. See n. 10, p. 805.

33 Boss 1994. See n. 3, p. 147.

34 "Brown, Judy." (pseudonym) The choice. Journal of the American Medical Association 1989;262:2735.

35 Kolker and Burke 1993. See n. 8, p. 522.

36 Iles and Gath 1993. See n. 30, p. 411.

37 Seller et al. 1993. See n. 26, p. 346.
Mander 1994. See n. 6, p. 47.

38 Zeanah 1993. See n. 23, pp. 273-4;
Kolker and Burke 1993. See 8, p. 523.

39 White-Van Mourik 1992. See n. 23, p. 72.

40 Iles and Gath 1993. See n. 30, see Table 3, p. 410.
Seller et al. 1993. See n. 26, p. 343.

41  Kolker and Burke 1993. See n. 8, p. 522.
White-Van Mourik 1992. See n. 23, p. 72.

42  Jones et al. 1984. See n. 9, p. 254.

43  Iles and Gath 1993. See n. 30, p. 411.

44  Blumberg et al. 1975. See n. 10, p. 806.
Kolker and Burke 1993. See n. 8, p. 520.

45  White-Van Mourik 1992. See n. 23, pp. 69-70.

46  Jones et al. 1984. See n. 9, p. 254.

47  Mander 1994. See n. 6, p. 46.
Seller et al. 1993. See n. 26, p. 343.

48  White-Van Mourik 1992. See n. 23, p. 70.

49  Seller et al. 1993. See n. 26, p. 343.

50  Donnai et al. 1981. See n. 12, p. 622.
Blumberg et al. 1975. See n. 10, p. 805.

51  Blumberg et al. 1975. See n. 10, p. 805.

52  Lloyd J, Laurence KM. Sequelae and support after termination of
pregnancy for fetal malformation. British Medical Journal 1985;290:907-909,
p. 908.

53  Iles and Gath 1993. See n. 30, p. 412.
Mander 1994. See n. 6, p. 44.

54  Donnai et al.1981. See n. 12, p. 622.

55  Elder and Laurence 1991. See n. 1, p. 47.
White-Van Mourik 1992. See n. 23, p. 69.
Donnai et al. 1981. See n. 12, p. 622.

56  Rayburn and Laferla 1986. See n. 10, p. 72.
Kolker and Burke 1993. See n. 8, p. 524.

57  Rayburn and Laferla 1986. See n. 10, p. 72.
Blumberg 1975. See n. 10, p. 805.
Kolker and Burke 1993. See n. 8, p. 520.

58  Lorenzen and Holzgreve 1995. See n. 16, p. 154.
Kolker and Burke 1993. See n. 8, p. 519.
Seller et al. 1993. See n. 26, p. 347.

59  Zeanah 1993. See n. 23, p. 274.
Kolker and Burke 1993. See n. 8, p. 524.
Iles and Gath 1993. See n. 30, p. 412.

60  Iles and Gath 1993. See n. 30, p. 409.
White-Van Mourik 1992. See n. 23, p. 63.

61  Neugebauer R, Kline J, Shrout P, et al. Major depressive disorder in the 6 months after miscarriage. Journal of the American Medical Association 1997 February; 277(5):383-8, p. 387.

62  White-Van Mourik 1992. See n. 23, p. 63.

63  Reardon DC, Cougle JR. Depression and unintended pregnancy in the National Longitudinal Survey of Youth: a cohort study. British Medical Journal 2002 January 19; 324:151-152.

64  Brown D, Elkins TE, Larson DB. Prolonged grieving after abortion: A descriptive study. The Journal of Clinical Ethics 1993 (4):118-123.

65  Furlong RM, Black RB. Pregnancy termination for genetic indications: the impact on families. Social Work in Health Care 1984, Fall;10(1):17-34.

66  Garton J. The cultural impact of abortion and its implications for a future society. In: Mannion M, editor. Post-Abortion Aftermath. Kansas City: Sheed and Ward, 1994: 88-99; p. 91.

67  Ney P, Peeters A. Hope Alive: Post Abortion and Abuse Treatment. A Training Manual for Therapists. Victoria, B.C.: Pioneer Publishing, 1993; pp. 29-33.

68  Curtis M, Standing L. The decision to abort: No sex-role bias, and little enthusiasm. Social Behavior & Personality. 1992;20(4):237-242, p. 239.

69  Drake H, Reid M, Marteau T. Attitudes towards termination for fetal abnormality: comparisons in three European countries. Clinical Genetics 1996 March;49(3):134-40, p. 139.

70  Feitshans IL. Legislating to preserve women's autonomy during pregnancy. Medical Law (South Africa) 1995;14(5-6):397-412, p. 397.

71  Kolker and Burke 1993. See n. 8, p. 515.

72  Kolker and Burke 1993. See n. 8, p. 516.
Blumberg et al.1975. See n.10, p. 808.

73  "Brown" 1989. See n. 24, p. 2735.

74 "Brown" 1989. See n. 24, p. 2735.

75 White-Van Mourik, 1992. See n. 23, p 64.

76 Genetic testing for cystic fibrosis. National Institutes of Health Consensus Development Conference Statement on Genetic Testing for Cystic Fibrosis. Archives of Internal Medicine 1999 July 26;159(14):1529-39, p. 1534.

77 Jones et al. 1984. See n. 9, p. 253.

78 Rothman 1994. See n. 8, pp. 46-7.

79 Green 1995. See n. 6, p. 228.
Mander 1994. See n. 6, p. 44.

80 Mander 1994. See n. 6, p. 45.

Chapter 13

# Multifetal Pregnancy Reduction

Reproductive technologies, specifically *in vitro fertilization* (*IVF*), have made it possible for infertile couples to have children; ironically, IVF often brings these couples face to face with abortion: Assisted reproduction often results in the implantation of multiple embryos, and the subsequent expectation by medical staff that the number of fetuses will be reduced in a process known as multifetal pregnancy reduction (MFPR), by which selected fetuses are terminated by means of heart puncture.

The justification for aborting fetuses in these cases is that it will increase the chances of carrying at least one embryo to term, but the research on which this is based is usually carried out by the practitioners and advocates of the procedure. Furthermore, analysis of the results has not shown MFPR to actually improve the chances for a healthy birth. Many critics call for a curb to limit the number of embryos fertilized and implanted.

There is also the question of whether MFPR involves "informed consent" on the part of the parents because the medical profession has tended to assume that parents would not want several babies and doctors may not present parents with a choice about how many babies they can keep. The aftermath of MFPR for some parents, now becoming apparent as they seek therapy, is feelings of pain, frustration, sadness, and guilt and a sense that they have been coerced by the medical staff into aborting some of their babies. Up to this point, there are few studies looking into the impact of multifetal abortions on family life with the surviving babies. It is clear that further research needs to be done on the wider impact of MFPR.

## Multifetal Pregnancy Reduction

Just as reproductive technologies have changed obstetrical practice, so too have they led to a type of abortion which affects a different population of pregnant women from those who do not want to be pregnant. These women want very much to have a child, and it is ironic that they and their partners who are suffering the problems of infertility must often come face-to-face with abortion.

There is a large literature detailing the psychological distress experienced by couples who wish to have children but who cannot conceive naturally. The following quotation captures the feeling poignantly:

> You can't have a baby – a numbness beyond despera-
> tion. Baby lust – do you know how it feels to want a
> baby so much that every other activity in life, everything
> you've worked for and planned for – jobs, friends, fami-
> ly, marriage, seem hollow as a tin can? To be in emo-
> tional pain so extreme that when you see a pregnant
> woman's stomach or a newborn baby the pain becomes
> physical?[1]

Laffont and Edelmann concluded that long-term infertility that is treated by *in vitro fertilization (IVF)* superimposes cycles of hope and disappointment on the already depressed and vulnerable psyche of couples who are having difficulty conceiving.[2] The process can take up to nine cycles of treatment because few couples conceive on the first attempt. Indeed, the overall success rate of IVF is a matter of continuing controversy. Oddens and colleagues found that for women involved in this treatment psychological well-being may deteriorate after unsuccessful treatment cycles.[3] Both partners experience psychological swings during treatment, and Boivin and colleagues observed that "Spouses appeared equally...to respond...with ambivalent feelings involving emotional distress and positive feelings of hope and intimacy."[4] But the literature suggests that women report greater negative reactions to IVF failures than men. The

176

coping mechanisms utilized by some women to face the cycles of failure, identified by Lukse and Vacc,[5] are the same denial and desensitization often seen in post-abortion psychopathology.

Following this cyclical emotional roller coaster, the fortunate couple may find themselves pregnant. In increasing numbers, however, these pregnancies are "higher order" with three or more implanted fetuses. "The international rates of triplet or higher order pregnancies after assisted reproduction are 7.3 per cent at conception."[6] In order to deal with such pregnancies, women must put themselves in the care of high-risk obstetrical experts who know the latest research on the new technologies used in the management of multiple pregnancies.

One of these new and highly recommended approaches is known as *Multifetal Pregnancy Reduction (MFPR)* – a form of abortion in which the most accessible fetuses are terminated by a needle stab through the heart and the overall pregnancy number is reduced to twins or a singleton. The dead fetuses remain in utero until the delivery of the living ones. This approach was developed by genetic researchers, some of whom are active participants in the prenatal diagnostics aspects of the *Human Genome Project*.

While many researchers end their studies with a call for curbs on the number of embryos that are implanted (which would reduce the likelihood of higher order multiple births to near-natural levels),[7] many other continuing studies are committed to the improvement of the techniques for MFPR. What is interesting about the studies in this area is the high degree of overlap between researchers. The twelve most prolific writers in this field all cite each other and often collaborate on research.[8] This self-referral or "incestuous citation"[9] is similar to that found in the general abortion literature. As in the other abortion areas the majority of these researchers are themselves practitioners of the MFPR procedure and some have the distinction of being not only practitioners but also advocates for and cited as experts on the probity of the procedure.

The procedure for aborting some of the fetuses in multiple pregnancies has been improved and expanded to the point that all major teaching hospitals in North America and Western Europe now routinely offer couples MFPR as an option for management of multiple pregnancies. One problem, however, is that the couple who never imagined themselves actually having a single child, and who have succeeded thanks to advanced IVF techniques, may feel themselves to be faced with what auto dealers call a "mandatory option" in dealing with their unexpected bounty. For many couples their new situation is very uncomfortable, not least because the gestational age at which these abortions are occurring has steadily increased to the point where Evans and colleagues are supporting the use of the technique into the third trimester (or after 26 weeks of pregnancy).[10]

The use of this technique is often a logical outcome of the psychology of desperation of infertile couples, and itself produces a logic described by Berkowitz and colleagues:

> The medical justification for performing multifetal pregnancy reduction is philosophically similar to the "lifeboat analogy"...it is justifiable to sacrifice some "innocent" fetal lives to increase the chances of survival or decrease the risk of serious morbidity in the survivors of the procedure.[11]

**Compared to Genetic Abortions**

In an attempt to make the use of MFPR a more readily-accepted part of obstetrical practice, the literature links the procedure to the already well-tolerated practice of abortion for genetic or fetal abnormality. The proponents of this technique believe the linkage addresses two important concerns: First, they conclude that patients will not tolerate multiple births, so the use of MFPR will avoid the "trauma"[12] of the abortion of a wanted pregnancy on the grounds that if reduction is not offered, the patient will choose to abort all the embryos. Second, MFPR will lead to the ultimate goal of having their own child. This principle of Ethical Justification has also been articulated by Chevernak and colleagues who express it in terms of three goals:

1.  achieving a pregnancy that results in a live birth of one or more infants with minimal neonatal morbidity and mortality;

2.  achieving a pregnancy that results in the birth of one or more infants without antenatally detected anomalies;

3.  achieving a pregnancy that results in a singleton live birth.[13]

The research literature assumes that parents faced with the potential birth of three to seven children at once are "free" to choose to abort most of them to achieve a family size of their choice. Individuals acting out of desperation, however, are not "free", and without freedom there is no true choice. The psychological impact of coercive choice is well documented in the decision-making literature. Miller delineated several models that apply to the decision to abort[14] and Cassidy expanded upon these in relation to decision-making in abortions for fetal abnormality.[15] The consensus among psychologists is that major life decisions based on perceived or overt coercion result in significant psychological distress.

In North America, the prevailing model for making medical decisions is based on the concept of "personal autonomy" and informed consent which have become cornerstones for the ethical acceptability for all medical procedures.[16] Often however, the decisions taken by couples to reduce the number of fetuses can be seen as lacking true personal autonomy because of parental desperation, medical coercion, and a lack of informed consent.

**Lack of Informed Consent**
A couple's capacity to give full assent is badly compromised due to the pre-existing psychological trauma brought on by long-term infertility and the IVF process itself. As the number of these multifetal abortions grows, the families involved are now coming forward to discuss pursuant issues which are only just beginning to be dealt with in the clinical therapy

and post-abortion healing literature. Kluger-Bell describes a family of triplets whose IVF resulted in a quad pregnancy. As her client notes "...I really didn't feel like I had a whole lot of choice about reducing it. And I was pretty much told by the doctors, 'Oh, well, you're not going to *carry* that many babies.' And most likely it would have to be reduced to two. And not knowing anything about it, we thought that was just the way it was." It was only when this family firmly expressed their desire to have all four babies that the doctors agreed to leave three. The MFPR was successful, "but emotionally there's still an ache that will probably always be there. We had been trying for so many years to create life, it was very contradictory and painful...no one ever said we could *consider* keeping all four...why wasn't that an option?"[17]

Ninety-nine per cent of the women who go through fetal reduction had achieved pregnancy through infertility treatment. Therefore, they represent a group which Tabsh describes as "...highly motivated to have a successful pregnancy outcome. They tend to be compliant with the medical plan for their care..."[18] and will therefore, as Macones and Wapner imply, assent to whatever approach will most likely assure them of a healthy child. In general, women seeking such an outcome will do anything the medical experts deem necessary.[19]

Ironically, until 1995, the attitude of infertility patients towards multiple births had never been investigated. Gleicher and colleagues found that the medical profession's implementation of MFPR was made without input from patient populations:

> It can therefore be no surprise that the survey reported here about patient attitudes is in strong conflict with the rather universally accepted practice patterns of minimizing multiple pregnancy rates...[infertile patients] express a considerable desire for multiple births...The medical profession so far has assumed that the decision to minimize multiple births...was reflective of patient desires. This study suggests otherwise.[20]

The ethical justification for MFPR is the desperate desire of parents to have a healthy baby. But what is the psychological price?

To desperate people, the avenue that promises the greatest hope may appear to be the morally best option, especially if pregnancy reduction is presented as the medically appropriate decision – the decision that will guarantee them one live baby. To refuse such an option requires freedom from coercion and access to other management approaches that provide alternatives. It is clear that these couples do not meet the criterion for free choice and, indeed, the actual level of coercion in this procedure is striking in the recent literature on surrogacy.

**Medical Outcomes of Multifetal Pregnancy Reduction**
The main rationale for MFPR is clearly the birth of at least one healthy child. Does MFPR guarantee this? This seems to be a matter of debate. Groutz and colleagues found that "Contrary to previous studies we found a higher incidence of pregnancy complications after MFPR compared with spontaneous twins...."[21] Souter and Goodwin did a *meta-analysis* of all 83 of the articles published on the procedure since 1989 and found that "there is a general consensus that reducing triplets to twins results in significant secondary benefits: lower cost and fewer days in hospital and a decrease in a variety of moderate morbidities associated with prolonged hospitalizations and preterm delivery for mother and baby. However, it is not clear that couples are more likely to take home a healthy baby, if they undergo multifetal pregnancy reduction."[22]

A recent Swedish study also identified the presence of post-procedure full miscarriage in 21 per cent of the cases undertaken in that country, a further eighteen per cent died in the womb or shortly after birth, or were born with defects.[23] Likewise, Elliott has suggested that studies of properly managed triplet pregnancies "show an equal or better outcome with nonreduced triplets compared with selective reduction."[24]

181

**Psychological Outcomes of MFPR**

Given the difficulties inherent in the MFPR procedure, it is not surprising that even following the achievement of the goal of parenting a child, couples who have participated in MFPR decisions experience the grief and emotional distress concomitant with the loss of a child. Follow-up studies of these families point to the fact that the parents do not experience significant psychiatric disturbance, and that "the birth of healthy children helps reduce the traumatic impact of fetal reduction".[25] What is not stressed in the literature, however, are the following observations:

1.  There is significant attrition and refusal rates in study samples.
2.  Couples who miscarried the whole pregnancy following the procedure are unwilling to participate in follow up.
3.  There is no study of the full psychological impact on the children who are described by practitioners as "the surviving fetuses."

Given these limitations, the studies that do address the psychological outcomes find that a significant proportion of their sample experience psychological distress following the procedure. The affective reactions are immediate, and intense grief reactions are characterized by repetitive and intrusive thoughts and images of the terminated fetus(es).

Schreiner-Engel and colleagues report that twenty per cent of those willing to participate in follow up experienced long-term *dysphoria*. "Their continued feelings of guilt appeared due to a wishful belief that some better solution should have been found." The characteristics of the most disturbed group were those who were young, religious, came from larger families, wanted more than two children, and viewed the ultrasound of the pregnancy more frequently. The authors conclude that "seeing multiple viable fetuses on repetitive sonograms may interfere with the ability of women to maintain an intellectualized or emotionally detached stance toward the multifetal pregnancy."[26]

Interestingly, the researchers assume that women who have undergone the stress and emotional impact of infertility and subsequent treatment can – and somehow should be able to – be detached from the one thing that has been a driving force in their lives, pregnancy. This expectation goes against all that is known about maternal-infant attachment and psychosocial understanding of the nature of pregnancy.[27]

Garel and colleagues had a 44 per cent interview refusal rate among reduction patients. Of those who agreed to be seen at one and two years post-procedure, one-third reported "persistent depressive symptoms related to the reduction, mainly sadness and guilt. The others made medical and rational comments expressing no emotion."[28]

In these reactions, the link becomes apparent between the lack of affect as an outcome of elective abortion and a similar lack of emotion among women who undergo abortion in the form of MFPR. Another issue of concern is the psychological impact this will have on parenting interactions with surviving children. About such parents, McKinney and colleagues noted: "Conscious and unconscious responses to the procedure included ambivalence, guilt, and a sense of narcissistic injury, increasing the complexity of their attachment to the remaining babies."[29] No research has been done on the long-term implications of parental distress on the psychological development of these children nor have any studies addressed the dynamics of *Post-Abortion Survivor Syndrome.*

**Conclusion**
There is still a great deal of research to be done in the area of the effects of multifetal pregnancy reduction on parents and on the surviving children of the pregnancy. What research has been done suggests similar reactions to induced abortion; namely, feelings of grief and loss, minimized somewhat by the carrying to term of at least some of the fetuses. Certainly, to enable parents to make decisions about such births, more research needs to be undertaken in this area, and subsequent findings need to be shared with them in order for their consent to be truly informed in compliance with current criteria for medical procedures.

**Key Points Chapter 13**

• For couples who cannot conceive a child, there is a very strong motivation to do whatever is medically recommended in order to have a child, whether using in vitro fertilization (IVF) or multifetal pregnancy reduction (MFPR). With either method there is the possibility of coercion by medical personnel.

• IVF is often used in cases of long-term infertility, and sometimes as many as nine cycles of treatment are needed for conception to take place, often resulting in three or more implanted fetuses.

• An approach doctors currently recommend to ensure a living birth in multifetal pregnancies is MFPR, a form of abortion (a needle stab to the heart) to reduce the number of fetuses. This procedure does not guarantee that the remaining fetuses will remain healthy, but it usually results in at least one live birth.

• Parents' reactions to the loss of some of the fetuses conceived are similar to those experienced after abortion for genetic reasons: sadness, guilt, and depression.

• Too often MFPR is assumed by the medical and research community to be what the parents want without obtaining true informed consent or giving them a choice about the number of fetuses to be kept alive.

• More research needs to be done into the effects of MFPR on couples and on their future family life with the surviving babies. This research should be carried out by investigators not already involved in performing and advocating this procedure.

## Notes

1 Blomain K. Customer Review of *An Empty Lap: One Couple's Journey to Parenthood*, by Jill Smolowe. [http://www.amazon.com/exec/obidos/tg/stores/detail/-/books/0671004379/customer- reviews/107-9690183-1333303], 1997 October 31.

2 Laffont I, Edelmann RJ. Psychological aspects of in vitro fertilization: A gender comparison. Journal of Psychosomatic Obstetrics & Gynecology 1994 June;15(2):85-92.

3 Oddens BJ, den Tonkelaar I, Nieuwenhuyse H. Psychosocial experiences in women facing fertility problems--a comparative survey. Human Reproduction 1999 January;14(1):255-61.

4 Boivin J, Andersson L, Skoog-Svanberg A, Hjelmstedt A, Collins A, Bergh T. Psychological reactions during in-vitro fertilization: Similar response pattern in husbands and wives. Human Reproduction 1998 November;13(11):3262-7, p. 3262.

5 Lukse MP, Vacc NA. Grief, depression, and coping in women undergoing infertility treatment. Obstetrics & Gynecology 1999 February;93(2):245-51.

6 Cohen J. How to avoid multiple pregnancies in assisted reproduction. Human Reproduction 1998 June; 13(Supplement 3):197-214; discussion 215-8; p. 197.

7 Cohen 1998. See n. 6.

8 Cassidy, Elizabeth. Multifetal Pregnancy Reduction (MFPR): The psychology of desperation and the ethics of justification. In *Life and Learning IX: Proceedings of Ninth Annual Meeting, University Faculty for Life in Trinity International University 1999*, ed. Koterski, J.W. 331-46. Washington, D.C.: University Faculty for Life, 2000.

9 Crutcher M. *Lime 5: Exploited by Choice*. Denton, Texas: Life Dynamics, 1996.

10 Evans MI, Goldberg JD, Horenstein J, Wapner RJ, Ayoub MA, Stone J, and colleagues Selective termination for structural, chromosomal, and Mendelian anomalies: international experience. American Journal of Obstetrics and Gynecology 1999 October;181(4):893-7.

11 Berkowitz RL, Lynch L, Stone J, Alvarez M. The current status of multifetal pregnancy reduction. American Journal of Obstetrics and Gynecology 1996 April;174(4):1265-72; p. 1270.

12  Evans MI JM, Quintero RA, Fletcher JC. Ethical issues surrounding multifetal pregnancy reduction and selective termination. Clinical Perinatology 1996 September;23(3):437-51.

13  Chervenak FA, McCullough LB, Wapner R. Three ethically justified indications for selective termination in multifetal pregnancy: A practical and comprehensive management strategy. Journal of Assisted Reproduction and Genetics 1995 September;12(8):531-6; p. 531.

14  Miller WB. An empirical study of the psychological antecedents and consequences of induced abortion. Journal of Social Issues 1992 Fall;48(3) pp. 67-93.

15  Cassidy E. Psychological Decision-Making Models: An Extension of Miller's Abortion Decision Models to Miscarriage and Genetic Abortion in Light of the Human Genome Project [Unpublished Conference Paper]. University Faculty for Life, 1997 June.

16  Beckwith FJ. Absolute autonomy and physician-assisted suicide: Putting a bad idea out of its misery. Joseph Koterski SJ, ed. Life and Learning VII. Seventh University Faculty for Life Conference; 1997; Loyola College, Baltimore. Washington, D.C.: University Faculty for Life; 1998.

17  Kluger-Bell K. *Unspeakable Losses: Understanding the Experience of Pregnancy Loss, Miscarriage, and Abortion.* New York: W.W. Norton, 1998.

18  Tabsh KM. A report of 131 cases of multifetal pregnancy reduction. Obstetrics & Gynecology 1993 July;82(1): 57-60.

19  Macones GA, Schemmer G, Pritts E, Weinblatt V, Wapner RJ. Multifetal reduction of triplets to twins improves perinatal outcome. American Journal of Obstetrics and Gynecology 1993 October; 169(4):982-6.

20  Gleicher N, Campbell DP, Chan CL, Karande V, Rao R, Balin M, et al. The desire for multiple births in couples with infertility problems contradicts present practice patterns. Human Reproduction 1995 May;10(5):1079-84.

21  Groutz A, Yovel I, Amit A, Yaron Y, Azem F, Lessing JB. Pregnancy outcome after multifetal pregnancy reduction to twins compared with spontaneously conceived twins. Human Reproduction 1996 June;11(6):1334-6; p. 1334.

22  Souter I, Goodwin TM. Decision making in multifetal pregnancy reduction for triplets. American Journal of Perinatology 1998 January;15(1):63-71; p. 63.

23  Radestad A, Bui TH, Nygren KG, Koskimies A, Petersen K. The utilization rate and pregnancy outcome of multifetal pregnancy reduction in the Nordic countries. Acta Obstetricia et Gynecologica Scandanavica 1996 August;75(7):651-3.

24  Elliott JP. Multifetal reduction of triplets to twins improves perinatal outcome. American Journal of Obstetrics and Gynecology 1994 July;171(1):278.

25  McKinney M, Downey J, Timor-Tritsch I. The psychological effects of multifetal pregnancy reduction. Fertility and Sterility 1995 July;64(1):51-61, p. 59.

26  Schreiner-Engel P, Walther VN, Mindes J, Lynch L, Berkowitz RL. First-trimester multifetal pregnancy reduction: acute and persistent psychologic reactions. American  Journal of Obstetrics and Gynecology 1995 February;172(2 Pt 1):541-7; pp. 545, 546.

27  Campion B. An argument for continuing a pregnancy where the fetus is discovered to be anencephalic. In *Life and Learning IX: Proceedings of Ninth Annual Meeting, University Faculty for Life in Trinity International University 1999,* ed. Koterski, JW. Washington, D.C.: University Faculty for Life, 2000.

28  Garel M, Stark C, Blondel B, Lefebvre G, Vauthier-Brouzes D, Zorn JR. Psychological reactions after multifetal pregnancy reduction: A 2-year follow-up study. Human Reproduction 1997 March; 12(3):617-22; p. 617.

29  McKinney MK, Tuber SB, Downey JI. Multifetal pregnancy reduction: psychodynamic implications. Psychiatry Winter 1996;59(4):393-407; p. 393.

Chapter 14

# Behavioral Outcomes, Suicide, Healing

14

After an abortion, a number of behavioral and social outcomes which threaten women's health, their relationships,
and their ability to cope have been observed. Teenage girls
and women who have already experienced abuse or psychological problems are especially vulnerable. Post-abortion
behaviors tend to be self-destructive and include suicide,
both actual and attempted; deliberate self-harm such as
mutilation and other punishments; unconscious self-harm in
the form of substance abuse, smoking, and various eating
disorders; and unstable, often abusive and battering, relationships.

Recent research reveals that the suicide rate following
abortion is six times greater than that following childbirth,
and three times the general suicide rate – sobering figures
which should be of great concern to advocates of women's
health and well-being. Self-destructive behaviors are ways
in which women often deny or minimize the emptiness and
pain they are experiencing. Abortion supporters tend to
downplay these outcomes. There is a recognized pattern of
abuse-abortion-abuse (including repeat abortions), which
needs more study if women are to be helped from continuing the cycle of self-abuse and abuse of their children.

Frequently, women seek support to recover from post-abortion distress years after their abortion. Project Rachel, The
Healing Choice, and The National Office for Reconciliation
and Healing are among the many therapeutic options that
have evolved in the wake of widely-practiced abortion.

# Behavioral Outcomes, Suicide, Healing

It is commonly thought that most women emerge psychologically unscathed from the abortion experience and that rather than regretting their decision, they would make the same decision again; any distress they do experience is thought to be minor and short-lived. Thus, Brenda Major and colleagues found that only 1.4 per cent of the 442 women they studied for two years following abortion reported post-traumatic stress disorder.[1]

On the other hand, the British authors of a major review article concluded that "marked, severe or persistent" psychological or psychiatric disturbances occur in approximately ten per cent of women.[2]

Many studies are hampered by inadequate sample size, unsatisfactory study design, the reluctance of many women to be interviewed about their abortions, and political bias (See Chapter 17). As we shall see below, one objective and revealing approach to finding out the real consequences of abortion may lie in large-scale record linkage studies extending over periods of many years. Nevertheless, even if the true incidence of severe psychological distress is no greater than one to ten per cent, it means that many hundreds of thousands or millions of women have been affected over the past 30 years in North America alone.

Bearing in mind the reported magnitude of the problem, it is noteworthy that researchers have recently established that a high proportion of women conceal or deny that they have had abortions. Concealment is particularly common among non-white and unmarried women. The U.S. National Longitudinal Survey of Youth, begun in 1979, found that women who aborted had significantly higher depression scores ten years after their abortion than those who bore their children. After controlling for a wide range of variables, Cougle and colleagues ascertained that post-abortive women were 41 per cent more likely than non-aborting women to score in the "high-risk" range for clinical depression. In response to a self-assessment question, aborting women

190

were 73 per cent more likely to complain of "depression, excessive worry, or nervous trouble of any kind" an average of seventeen years later.[3] In a Canadian study of 50 postabortive women in psychotherapy, Kent and colleagues found that, "although none had entered therapy because of adverse emotional reactions to abortion, they expressed deep feelings of pain and bereavement about the procedure as treatment continued. Typically the bereavement response emerged during the period when the patient was recovering from the presenting problem."[4]

Several behavioral and social outcomes from abortion have been identified that should be of concern to physicians or counselors. They include self-destructive behaviors such as suicide (actual and attempted); deliberate self-harm (mutilation, punishment); and unconscious self-harm, including substance abuse, increased smoking, and eating disorders.

There is also considerable evidence that childhood abuse may be a predisposing factor in abortion. Although this outcome may at first glance seem surprising, it is less so when the practitioner considers that the young woman with a history of sexual abuse may not connect sex acts with pregnancy, at least not in the same way that a woman might who has not experienced sex until she is physically mature. Sexual dysfunction or psychological numbing can follow abortion. In some cases, women may have repeat abortions hoping to quell the anxiety associated with previous ones, a phenomenon that will be explained later in this chapter.

**Self-Destructive Behaviors**
In the sociological literature, women who engage in activities which are unhealthy or which undermine their well-being are considered to be engaging, either consciously or unconsciously, in self-destructive behaviors. When their behaviors threaten their health, their ability to cope, or their relationships, they may come into contact with the healthcare system or seek out therapists or counselors. Under care, previous abortions may be identified as contributing to their problem in one of two ways: First, the women may readily admit to having had an abortion or, second, because of the comfort level and feeling of safety

in the ongoing therapeutic relationship with a counselor, they may find that they can discuss the sensitive topic of a previous abortion. However, the information that has been gathered about this is anecdotal.

A quantitative way of studying a connection between destructive lifestyle issues and abortion is through the analysis of studies that do not address reproductive issues as such but, as part of the overall study or survey questionnaire, ask background questions on fertility. The presence of abortion in a woman's history may not be seen as central to the original research, but the analysis of the abortion component of the data may provide insights into long-term relationships between abortion and lifestyle choices. This mathematical or statistical construct lacks the individual woman's perspective or story, but it does provide clinicians with information on the possible connection of present symptoms to past abortion experiences.

Self-destructive behaviors associated with abortion are symptoms of what Brende describes as "self-fragmentation" and part of a "traumatic matrix". This fragmentation may also predispose a person to "unstable and destructive (sadistic, masochistic, abusive and battering) relationships".[5]

A teenager engaged in these behaviors is more vulnerable and at the same time is likely to show insufficient self-awareness to recognize or admit the root cause of her difficulty. The egocentrism of youth, often identified in developmental literature, allows adolescents to take risks without awareness of consequences and also allows them to project onto others blame for any self-destructive behavior. Franz explains the adolescent response in the following way:

> The girl who has had an abortion may find it very difficult to admit to having any psychological problems. She will be inclined to blame others for her unhappiness, because she couldn't possibly be a victim of such problems. She will deny that she has a problem or that she could develop one. If she is engaging in self-destructive behavior, she will deny that the root cause may be her abortion experience.[6]

**1. Suicide: Actual or Attempted**
In 1995, Gilchrist studied psychiatric morbidity following abortion and found that Deliberate Self-Harm (DSH) was a statistically significant 70 per cent more prevalent among "women with no previous psychiatric history who had an abortion...." In the definition of Deliberate Self-Harm used by these authors, the women's actions can be categorized as suicide attempts. Eighty-nine per cent were drug overdoses, and it is difficult to determine whether they were accidental (unconscious) or deliberate attempts to end their lives. Following a trend that is quite common in post-abortion literature, the researchers attempted to debunk their own results by stating that "The findings on DSH are probably explicable by confounding variables." They also noted that the rate of DSH for women who abort dropped after the first year following abortion. A finding that they did not stress was that there was an opposite trend for adolescents, namely women who aborted under the age of nineteen.[7]

Using death records from hospitals and government death certificates Gissler and colleagues established that the suicide rate following childbirth and the suicide rate in the year following an abortion were dramatically different:

**Table 14-1**
**Suicide rate per 100,000 women in Finland, 1987-1997**[8]

| | |
|---|---|
| Associated with childbirth | 5.9 |
| Associated with miscarriage | 18.1 |
| Associated with abortion | 34.9 |
| Mean annual rate for all women | 11.3 |

This prestigious study, based on the records of almost 600,000 women, discovered *a suicide rate among women who aborted nearly six times greater than among women who delivered their babies.*

Gissler and her colleagues also reviewed the hospital records to establish the reasons given for abortion by women who later committed suicide. They found that the reasons "did not differ from those for all abortions; over 80 per cent were performed because of social reasons."[9] The researchers established that the suicide rate following abortion is six times greater than that for women following childbirth and three times the general suicide rate. They concluded both that "childbearing prevents suicide", and that the increased risk for suicide after abortion may indicate "the harmful effects of abortion on mental health"[10] "Rather than being a relief, an abortion for them may be additional proof of their worthlessness and might contribute to suicidality and to the decision to commit suicide."[11] The researchers also noted that only eleven per cent of the suicides following pregnancy had this connection reported in the death certificate. They conclude that there is a massive underreporting of suicide as an outcome of pregnancy, particularly following abortion.

An interesting feature of this Finnish study is the connection of abortion/suicide and social class. They note that, along with the negative effect of abortion on emotional well-being, there are also higher post-abortion suicide rates for women in the lower social classes. In Scandinavia in 1995, a study of abortion by Hamark and colleagues reported that the repeat abortion rate was highest for women in the poorest socio-economic group. They concluded that with unrestricted elective abortion, it was poorer women who had multiple abortions. This was the case before abortion on demand and continues to be so: "The class distribution was consistently uneven, with the majority within the indigent group." Disadvantaged women are overrepresented in both the abortion and suicide statistics.[12]

**Suicide and Pregnancy, Childbirth, Stillbirth and Abortion**
Conversely, an Irish study found that the psychological effects of being refused an abortion did not put women at risk of suicide: "the risk of suicide is low in pregnancy and suicide is a rare outcome of refused abortion".[13]

In the United States, suicide is the third leading cause of death among fifteen- to 24- year-olds. This age group also has the fastest growing suicide rate in the country. How many of the women in this group have committed suicide following abortion? No one knows for sure. Appleby does not address abortion as a variable but found that among women who gave birth, the standardized mortality ratio was one-sixth of that projected by the researcher. "The low ratio was less pronounced, but still present, in teenage mothers and in unmarried mothers." These are the groups of women for whom pregnancies are often unplanned and whose children are considered unwanted by society, but of whom Appleby observed, "Motherhood seems to protect against suicide." At the same time, "The low ratio was not found after stillbirth, which was associated with a rate six times that in all women after childbirth."[14] Both stillbirth and abortion involve the death of a child. Both can have devastating effects on the woman. Clearly, more research is needed to specify the relationship between female suicide, stillbirth, and abortion.

In Chapters 11 and 12, it was noted that women with any history of psychiatric or psychological problems are at greater risk for negative reactions following abortion. It was also reported that adolescents have different developmental and cognitive issues which predispose them to post-abortion distress. When these two factors are combined, the outcome can be, as noted by Tishler, that young women with any history of psychiatric difficulties are vulnerable to "emotional stress and potential suicide...Should the patient's perceived death of the fetus during abortion be punished by suicide?"[15] Campbell, Franco and Jurs suggest that adolescents do think their act is punishable by suicide. They report that teenagers are significantly less likely to attempt suicide before an abortion than adult women, but more than twice as likely as adult woment to attempt it after abortion (29 per cent compared to thirteen per cent).[16] Adolescents may, however, be less likely to recognize abortion as a factor. Franz notes that until  adolescents develop more mature reasoning patterns they may continue to deny the effect of abortion on their lives.[17]

Reardon studied a self-selected sample of women who had elective abortions and who later experienced negative psychological *sequelae*. Among these women, "60 per cent had experienced suicidal ideation, 28 per cent had attempted suicide and eighteen per cent had attempted suicide more than once, often several years after the event." He concludes that "actual data suggests that abortion is far more likely than pregnancy and childbirth to drive an unstable woman to suicide." Reporting statistics from a chapter of Suiciders Anonymous, he goes on to say that 1400 of 1800 post-abortion women who sought help from the support group were between the ages of fifteen and 24.[18]

Suicide attempts often follow years of denial, repression, and depression. "Perhaps one reason for the strong abortion/suicide link exists in the fact that in many ways abortion is like suicide. Just as a suicidal person is crying out for help when she tells others she wishes she were dead, so a woman who is distressed over a pregnancy is crying out for help when she tells others she is considering abortion".[19]

A recent study addressing suicide and abortion was conducted in Wales among a population of 408,000 between 1991 and 1995. Morgan and colleagues studied hospital admissions for attempted suicide among women, post-abortion, post-miscarriage, and postnatal. They concluded that in women who abort, "attempted suicide may be a consequence of the pregnancy rather than some underlying mental illness." For women who miscarried or delivered, risk of suicide dropped after the event, while for women who aborted the risk increased from insignificant prior to the abortion to significant after the procedure: "Our data suggest that a deterioration in mental health may be a consequential side effect of induced abortion." They found that the relative risk of suicide after induced abortion was 3.25; in other words, *women who had induced abortions were 225 per cent more likely to commit suicide than women admitted for normal delivery.*[20]

Similarly, Michels reports on women who mutilate themselves and later recognize the connection between such behavior and earlier induced abortion.[21]

A recent American record-linkage study came up with results similar to those uncovered by Morgan and colleagues in Britain. Medical records were linked to death certificates for 173,279 low-income women who underwent a state-funded delivery or induced abortion in 1989. Four years later the annual suicide rate was found to be *160 per cent higher (7.8 compared to 3.0) among the aborting women than among the delivering women.*

**Table 14-2**
**U.S. annual suicide rate per 100,000 women**
**aged 15 - 44**[22]

| | |
|---|---|
| All women | 5.2 |
| Women who aborted | 7.8 |
| Women who delivered their baby | 3.0 |

In all three countries, the U.S., Britain and Finland, abortion sharply increases the likelihood of suicide. Conversely, carrying a baby to term sharply reduces the risk of suicide.

**2. Deliberate Self-Harm**
The cycle of self-loathing and self-punishment, although not thoroughly explored in the post-abortion research literature, is often painfully expressed in the personal stories of women who are attempting to recover and to find healing after an abortion.

Michels integrated the stories of women seeking post-abortion support into a psychological context and analyzed the emotional structures women developed to try to cope following their abortions. She points out that the mechanisms of coping were often methods of sublimating grief which were in themselves self-destructive. In the case of Jane, who was able to articulate her fear in terms of her possible self-harm, "I was very fearful of myself and didn't trust myself. I thought I might even kill myself."[23]

Even Sue Nathanson, self-described supporter of "abortion rights," says (after her own abortion) that "The inner torment is so unbearable that the only peaceful state I can imagine is death." She does not act on this feeling but attempts to use exercise as a way of both avoidance and self-abuse: "...Perhaps I can die if I keep going in this heat...I cannot drive my physical body to death. I am a Frankenstein who has transformed myself into a monster that will not die."[24]

### 3. Unconscious Self-Harm
To cope with the dissonance and pain following abortion, women may also engage in activities that are intrinsically unsafe. The mechanisms involved are extremely complex and can reflect the disorder of a chaotic, abusive, or neglected background. They can also reflect psychological coping strategies that allow the individual to remain functional by forgetting or ignoring the abortion experience. The following factors are known ways of externalizing internal conflicts and disorders:

### a. Substance Abuse
Reardon and Ney note that "Women who aborted a first pregnancy were five times more likely to report substance abuse than women who carried to term".[25] For the woman who wishes to ignore, forget, or minimize unresolved psychic issues resulting from an elective abortion, the use of drugs and alcohol can provide a ready vehicle for avoidance. Brende sees substance abuse as part of the constellation of self-destructive behaviors that are part of the woman's attempt to cope with her decision to abort, and describes this coping strategy as follows: "...victims develop repetitive

symptoms with splitting and dissociation as mental defenses; often using alcohol, tranquilizers or other substances".[26]

Raphael observed that self-destructive behaviors have their origins in guilt surrounding the loss of the baby.[27] Speckhard, in a Ph.D. thesis, undertook in-depth interviews with 30 women post-abortion and found that 61 per cent reported increased alcohol consumption while 58 per cent reported increased drug use. Speckhard attributed this increase to the stress from the abortion. Only ten per cent reported any substance use/abuse before their abortion. The conclusions from this research are based on the assumption that substance abuse is a reactive response to distress, lack of personal control, or a lack of positive self-esteem.[28]

Drower and Nash found that eleven per cent of the women in their abortion sample reported increased alcohol and tobacco use while sixteen per cent had increased their use of tranquilizers.[29] Frank and colleagues found that cocaine users differed significantly from non-users on a number of obstetrical risk factors. Twenty-eight per cent of cocaine users had undergone two or more abortions compared to twelve per cent of non-users.[30]

While Frank and colleagues do not discuss the causative factors (for example, do more cocaine users abort or do women who have abortions turn to cocaine use to help them cope psychologically?), Mensch and Kandel found a correlation between illegal drug use, pregnancy, and a *five-fold* positive relationship between teenage users and abortion: "...illicit drug use increases the likelihood of an abortion by a factor of 5."[31]

In a population-based study, Klassen and Wilsnack found that among 917 women in the U.S. Midwest, 26 per cent of those who described themselves as moderate to heavy drinkers had previously undergone an induced abortion.[32]

What seems to occur in the cycle of abortion and substance abuse is a cross-over between cause and effect. For some women, the problems that lead to substance abuse also lead to abortion while, for others, substance abuse becomes a way of coping with the emotional consequences of an abortion. Most studies do not attempt to establish cause-and-effect relationships in such circumstances, but Reardon and Ney did find that those women who had reported repeat abortions had higher rates of substance abuse than those who had had only one abortion.[33]

### b. Smoking

Lydon and colleagues report that Canadian women who reported being committed to their pregnancy displayed their commitment through a reduction of the use of cigarettes. Those who decided to continue their pregnancy smoked fewer cigarettes a month after a positive pregnancy test.[34] Obel established that a prior induced abortion is a risk factor for increased cigarette use in subsequent pregnancies,[35] and a study by Thomas and Tori found that women who aborted or relinquished children were more likely to have a history of substance abuse.[36]

### c. Eating Disorders

The use of food as a tool for *sublimation* or repression/denial is well known in the literature on anorexia and bulimia. The connection between abortion and such eating disorders has not been adequately explored. Psychiatric case profiles have linked the cycle of multiple pregnancies and abortions to eating disorders such as bingeing and purging. Personal accounts of post-abortion behavior strongly support the clinical research on unconscious self-harm. Women often report the use of substances as a means of dealing with pathological grief – that is, grief that cannot be integrated into normal life. As is common in the study of post-abortion problems, the stories have often surfaced in healing programs or support groups, such as Project Rachel and The Healing Choice. These groups are discussed at the end of this chapter (see "Healing"). The impact of these stories is gripping:

*"Wendy"*: I developed anorexia shortly after my abortion, but I never connected the two. I disowned my body. I became an eighty pound skeleton A totally non-sexual, non-woman.[37]

*"Jane"*: I was becoming anorexic and didn't care about my appearance or health.[38]

**Childhood Abuse and The Abortion Cycle**
Sometimes, a history of induced abortions can be related to childhood abuse. Wyatt and colleagues studied revictimization of women who were sexually abused as children and found that "women who were sexually abused in childhood and revictimized in adulthood... as well as those with more than one incident in both childhood and adulthood were most likely to report high rates of unintended and aborted pregnancies...." The sex act itself is often perceived in isolation from the consequences...."Just as they may perceive sex and its consequences as separate issues, survivors of sexual abuse may not consider that one of the risks of engaging in sex is becoming a parent and may choose, instead, to terminate unintended pregnancies...."[39]

In the epidemiological literature and clinical case histories the abuse/abortion/personality disorder correlations are so strong that psychiatrist Ney developed a therapeutic treatment program which addresses these issues. Called Hope Alive: Post Abortion and Abuse Treatment, this inpatient program is based on the conclusion that "people who have had an abortion are more likely to abuse their children and people who have been abused are more likely to have an abortion...Abortion results in more post-partum depression and therefore less bonding, less touching and less breast feeding...It should be noted that one of the earliest arguments was that aborting unwanted children would diminish the incidence of child abuse. Statistics show precisely the opposite; that is, with more frequent abortions, all kinds of child abuse have increased." Ney and Peeters add that "Child mistreatment and abortion are both cause and effect, one of the other. Abortion also runs in families, with mothers and grandmothers for three to four generations having had abortions often for the same reasons."[40]

Ava Torre-Bueno, a clinical social worker and Planned Parenthood volunteer, describes the effect of physical abuse on the guilt women feel following abortion. Women who have suffered abuse internalize responsibility for the feelings of others, usually due to their perception that their actions are the cause of other people's problems. The guilt of these women becomes pathological and encompasses those around them: "Sarah felt guilty about everything...Her guilt wasn't only about harming herself by having her abortion it was just how she felt about everything."[41]

What Torre-Bueno does not explore with this client is the underlying motivation for the abortion. She gives the usual reasons that young adults provide for their abortion – too young, not financially self-sufficient – but does not delve into the role the damage from abuse played in her decision. Torre-Bueno may be committed to the assumption that post-abortion guilt is rooted in systemic clinical pathology, not in the abortion itself, but why was the young woman's motivation to abort not explored? In ignoring this question, a pre-abortion counseling process might miss the presence of abuse or a chaotic personality, which if recognized would obligate the therapist to consider the possible outcome of pathological guilt and to question the choice to abort.

In particular, anecdotal counseling stories from this literature lack discussion of the recognition of *borderline personality disorder*, a condition characterized by impulsive and self-destructive behaviors of the kind potentially magnified by abortion.

Therapists such as Torre-Bueno help post-abortion women deal with the consequences of their choice, but will not suggest that the choice itself might have been inappropriate. The most they can say is that the resulting feelings are part of an underlying problem, usually related to the family of origin. In this model, abortion is only a trigger or stress. However, while abortion may not be the main causative factor in post-abuse effects, it is certainly an avoidable one.

If the literature on abortion and abuse is accurate, of the 1,300,000 women in the U.S. who abort yearly, 25 per cent have a background of abuse. Indeed, if the proportion of abuse victims in the aborting population is higher than non-victims then this number could be significantly larger. Thus, 325,000 North American women may be experiencing the psychological impact of abuse and abortion. Without appropriate therapy, the abuse cycle can continue into further generations, assuming that the women have live births at some point. These women, in turn, may be physically abusive with their children and/or not act to protect their female children from sexual abuse.

Crawford and Mannion put it this way: "Several studies now show that many aborted women were victims of sexual abuse as children. They who were the victims of violence, now become perpetrators. How? Why? Does not this knowledge of the women's history or similar insights demand even greater compassion and commitment to help heal?"[42]

The mechanisms at work in this transmission of self-destructive behaviors from one generation to the next seem to be mediated in part by the parent-child attachment.[43] Cole and Woolger found that this was particularly true of the child-rearing practices of women who had been victims of incest as compared to women whose abuser was extra-familial.[44]

What is applicable about this research is the emphasis on the parent-child bond which is, by definition, severed in the abortion decision. As Benedict, White and Cornely put it, "it is apparent that reproductive history and the circumstances surrounding past pregnancies may provide important clues in eliciting more precisely what family dynamics may be related to subsequent maltreatment." Their study also found that women who are abusive have more stillbirths and abortions.[45]

**Sexual Dysfunction**
Following abortion, women may suffer from sexual dysfunction. For some women, the abortion experience leads to a fear for the possibility (or the impossibility) of future

pregnancy. As Torre-Bueno puts it, they "become convinced that they will never be able to get pregnant, or they may fear another pregnancy so much that they become afraid of having sex. This fear may look more like a sudden or slow loss of interest in sex."[46]

In addressing psycho-spiritual healing following abortion, Crawford and Mannion found that in structured clinical interviews, both verbal and written, a patient whose profile included sexual dysfunction also included chaotic relationships.[47]

## Psychic Numbing: The Absence of Affect
In a Greek study Naziri and Tzavaras found that women experienced a feeling of guilt following abortion and that this is an "unavoidable consequence of the violation of some prohibitions concerning particularly female sexual fulfillment and/or the possibility of pregnancy without becoming a mother...To whom and to what is this feeling [of guilt] directed?...the answer to this question led us to distinguish two tendencies among the women interviewed: Either they felt guilty toward their family or immediate environment or they felt guilty toward themselves."[48]

This study also found that guilt was linked to aggressiveness and to anxieties about bodily integrity. "Before the operation women often felt 'a big anxiety' and immediately after the operation 'an emptiness', 'a cold feeling'". These same feelings are also found among women following *multifetal pregnancy reduction (MFPR)* (see Chapter 13) and are identified by Kent as a clinically pathological outcome.[49] Many women who tell their own abortion stories use the terms "numb" and "disconnected" both of which describe an acute phase of post-abortion psychological dysfunction.

A recent Canadian study also found that guilt (ambivalence about the decision), as well as thoughts of suicide, helped to explain why "being involved in a first-trimester abortion can be highly distressing" for women.[50]

**Repeat Abortion**

Although repeat abortion is sometimes considered to be caused by an inability to find a comfortable contraceptive routine, it can, in fact, have deeper psychological motives. Some research suggests that it is an attempt to find an abortion situation that relieves anxiety. As reported by Naziri and Tzavaras, "Repetition of the act (even on an impressive number of occasions) does not alleviate the pain and the anxiety brought on by the experience; repeated abortion leads neither to adjustment nor to a solution to the anxiety."[51]

Regarded from a clinical and psychoanalytical viewpoint, these researchers consider repeat abortion as related to unresolved Oedipal conflicts of the faltering image of the father figure because of absence or indifference. "Unwanted pregnancies then unveil the steady unconscious incestuous desire and at the same time the attempt to fill the narcissistic rift which the absent or indifferent father had caused."[52]

From the nonanalytic approach to psychology, repeat abortion can be seen as the outcome of a woman's grief surrounding the original abortion. If a woman has buried or repressed feelings of grief after multiple abortions, Rue noted that, "...reenactment of the first abortion trauma can become an organizing feature." For some, grief can lead to attempts to replace the aborted child with a baby, and for others, "...the resurfacing of the trauma in a subsequent pregnancy is too threatening and compels another abortion. When multiple abortions occur, the traumatizations and resulting psychological impairment can be overwhelming."[53]

Congleton and Calhoun discovered that the mechanisms that cause or trigger distress following a first abortion may be part of the pattern of behavior that results in repeat abortion.

Within the group of all women who abort, those who have repeat abortions have higher scores on measures of disturbance such as paranoid thoughts, phobic anxiety, and problems with sleep. Other correlations with repeat abortion rates appear to be: unstable relationships marked by lack of a partner or satisfaction with partner, a lack of perceived control in their lives, and less reported religious affiliation and social connectedness.[55]

Here are the conclusions of four separate studies on repeat abortions:

    i   When asked about psychological problems and contacts with the social welfare service, women having another abortion differ significantly from women having a first abortion. [They] also evaluate their relationship with their partner more negatively.[56]

    ii   Most women having repeat abortions seem to have a psychological vulnerability and demonstrate current and previous problems. Poor self-esteem and lack of assertiveness seem predominant, especially in relationships with men.[57]

    iii   Patients having a repeat abortion are more often dissatisfied with themselves, more often perceive themselves as victims of bad luck, and more often express negative feelings toward the current abortion than women who are obtaining abortions for the first time.[58]

    iv   On the other hand two studies, one from Montréal and the other from Copenhagen, reported no major differences between women having their first abortion, and those having repeat abortions.[59]

During the 1990s, one half of the abortions in the United States and approximately 40 per cent in Canada were repeat abortions. In studies of social and personal factors pre-diposing women to repeat the abortion experience, researchers have found that in any given group of abortion seekers, the numbers of women who report at least one previous abortion ranges as high as 60 per cent in older women. Soderberg and colleagues found that in women 24 or younger "...a history of previous abortion was the factor most strongly correlated with the decision to undergo abortion." American research suggests that 50 per cent of women currently obtaining an abortion have already undergone the procedure at least once.

**Abortion and Poverty**
In Sweden where socioeconomic data are collected on abortion patients, Hamark found that women from "indigent areas" were younger, more likely to have had previous abortions, and least likely to respond positively immediately following the abortion. What is startling about the Swedish experience is that abortion has the greatest negative impact on the poor. "So far, we have demonstrated that socioeconomic conditions have an impact on abortion prevalence, thereby confirming the persistence of the situation when abortion laws were restrictive." Swedish women most likely to suffer the medical sequelae and psychological problems following repeat abortion are poor. The extent to which repeat abortion is part of the cycle of poverty needs to be more fully explored.

**Abortion and Crime**
Much attention has been given to the claim by Donohue and Levitt that "legalized abortion has contributed significantly to recent crime reduction."[62] This claim has been vigorously contested by a number of social scientists. David Murray, the director of the Statistical Assessment Service, a non-partisan think-tank in Washington, stated that "the study poses an intriguing argument, but does not stand up to scrutiny." He went on to observe that "using the authors' hypothesis, crime rates in other countries with abortion access should have seen a similar dip in crime. But in Great Britain, which liberalized abortion in 1968, violent crime has risen dramatically in the past decade."[63] In a recent major paper Lott and Whitley severely criticize Donohue and Levitt's methodology and assumptions, concluding that "There are many factors that reduce murder rates, but the legalization of abortion is not one of them". They add, "We find evidence that legalizing abortion increased murder rates by around 0.5 to seven per cent."[64]

**Healing**
One sociological development that has followed in the wake of widely available abortion is a plethora of therapeutic groups for women seeking post-abortion support. Although support groups are particularly common in the United States

they appear to exist across cultures and religious denominations. "In Japan since the 1950s special mourning rooms
have been established in temples for those who are seeking
to grieve and atone for...abortions. The same is true in
Taiwan where 'baby spirit' programs have been established
in temples to help parents...There are support groups for
aborted women in Ireland, England, Switzerland, South
Africa, Australia, New Zealand, Uruguay and Hong Kong to
name only some."[65]

In North America as well, many organizations have established self-help groups run for and by women struggling
after an abortion. "Crisis pregnancy counselling agencies
and family service organizations provide post-abortion
counselling, often by women who have had abortions."[66]
Some groups are faith-based as part of a community out-
reach service. Still others are psycho-therapeutic, offering to
help women integrate their abortion experience into their
lives. Project Rachel, founded in 1984 by the Roman Catholic
Archdiocese of Milwaukee, is probably one of the largest of
them. Its London, Ontario chapter describes Project Rachel
as a "post-abortion program offered by certified counsellors
and trained clergy representing a variety of Christian
denominations."[67]

A woman who seeks out Project Rachel goes through a
process which involves telling her story and grieving her
loss. Forgiveness is at the heart of this therapy: forgiveness
of everyone involved in her abortion, forgiveness of herself,
and finally, discernment of how to move on and make a
positive impact on her world.

The National Office of Post-Abortion Reconciliation and
Healing, Inc. is a group dealing with post-abortion issues
and their impact on women. It networks with researchers
and professional counselors, provides training and operates
an "800" referral line. It also sponsors an annual conference
on abortion's aftermath and its resolution called "The
Healing Vision".[68]

Among abortion advocates there now exist some emotional recovery programs such as "The Healing Choice". In the introduction to their book of the name title, Candace De Puy and Dana Dovitch explain the rationale for this program:

> Psychological studies show that only 10 per cent of the 1.4 million American women who undergo abortions every year experience emotional trauma following the procedure and these women were most often psychologically unstable prior to their pregnany. Unfortunately, most studies dismiss the other 90 per cent of women as if they had no reaction whatsoever. Because the majority of women move forward with their lives, any normal grief, confusion or ambivalence they might feel is dismissed.
>
> In reality, women who find themselves confronted with the decision to abort do not always walk away from the experience unscathed, even though they move forward with their lives. As psychotherapists, we see such women in our practices every day.[69]

All of these and other therapeutic programs try to address the significant distress experienced by some women after an abortion. Insofar as post-abortion distress represents an unexpected outcome of pregnancy termination, the fact that some women do undergo psychological anguish after an abortion suggests that women should be informed about its possibility beforehand. After the fact, it is also important that these therapeutic options be made more public and available. "Indeed, what we are dealing with is the need we have to make sense of our parenting history, that is, to acknowledge, take ownership for, and grieve the loss of each pregnancy experience, whether it ends in abortion, miscarriage or stillbirth. This is a human need."[70]

**Conclusion**

A number of self-destructive behaviors are identified after a woman has had an induced abortion, but for reasons that are seldom apparent, these are not usually regarded as a reason to avoid the procedure. Given the seriousness of post-abortion behavioral dysfunction among some women, which includes suicide, mutilation, substance abuse, and abusive behavior in family and partner relationships, it would make sense for the medical and helping professions to take a greater interest in finding ways to help women avoid these harmful tendencies. Repeat abortion as a means of relieving anxiety about a previous abortion is also a problem but, again, there is little knowledge as yet on how to prevent this outcome. Various therapeutic options for unresolved bereavement have evolved. Their purpose is to facilitate a means of healing for those women who continue to be affected emotionally after an abortion.

**Key Points Chapter 14**

• It is becoming clear, as women who have had abortions present themselves for therapy, that previous abuse sometimes leads to the decision to abort.

• After an abortion, women are more likely to display self-destructive behaviors including suicide and attempts at suicide; mutilation and various forms of punishment (including repeat abortions and sterilization); drug, alcohol and tobacco abuse; and eating disorders as a way of denying or minimizing the guilt, pain and numbness they feel.

• Women who abort often have trouble bonding with the children of future pregnancies and have a higher chance of eventually abusing them, which leads to a cyclical pattern of abuse-abortion-abuse.

• It seems clear, given the frequency of negative behavioral outcomes for women after abortion, that more thought needs to be given to appropriate therapy for women (and their children) who are at risk.

• Many women seek support in recovering from post-abortion distress, often years after the abortion. Project Rachel, The Healing Choice, and The National Office for Reconciliation and Healing are among the many therapeutic options that have evolved in the wake of widely-practised abortion.

## Notes

1  Major B, Cozzarelli C, Cooper ML, Zubek J, Richards C, Wilhite M, Gramzow RH. Psychological responses of women after first-trimester abortion. Archives of General Psychiatry 2000 Aug;57:777-786.

2  Zolese G, Blucker CVR. The psychological complications of therapeutic abortion. British Journal of Psychiatry 1992;160:742-749, p. 742.

3  Cougle JR, Reardon DC, Coleman PK. Depression associated with abortion and childbirth: A long-term analysis of the NLSY cohort. Archives of Women's Mental Health 2001;3(4)Supp.2:105.

4  deVeber LL, Ajzenstat J, Chisholm D. Postabortion Grief: Psychological sequelae of medical abortion. Human Medicine 1991;7(3):203-209; p. 205.

5  Brende JO. Fragmentation of the personality associated with post-abortion trauma. Newsletter of the Association for Interdisciplinary Research in Values and Social Change July/August 1995; 8(3):1-8; p. 6.

6  Franz W. Post abortion trauma and the adolescent. In *Post-Abortion Aftermath,* ed. Mannion M, Kansas City: Sheed and Ward, 1994: 119-30, p. 126.

7  Gilchrist AC, Hannaford P, Frank P, Kay CR. Termination of pregnancy and psychiatric morbidity. British Journal of Psychiatry 1995 August;167(2):243-8; p. 243.

8  (a) Gissler M, Hemminki E, Lonnqvist J. Suicides after pregnancy in Finland, 1987-94: register linkage study. British Medical Journal 1996 December 7;313(7070):1431-4.
   (b) Gissler M, Hemminki E, Lonnqvist J. Letters: Suicides after Pregnancy - Authors' Reply. British Medical Journal 1997 March 22;314(7084):902-3

9  Gissler 1996. See n. 8(a), p. 1432.

10  Gissler 1996. See n. 8(a), p. 1433.

11  Gissler 1997. See n. 8(b), p. 903.

12  Hamark B, Uddenberg N, Forssman L. The influence of social class on parity and psychological reactions in women coming for induced abortion. Acta Obstetricia et Gynecologica Scandanavica 1995 April;74(4):302-6; p. 305.

13  Clare AW, Tyrrell J. Psychiatric aspects of abortion. Irish Journal of Psychological Medicine 1994 June;11(2): 92-8, p.92.

14  Appleby L. Suicide during pregnancy and in the first postnatal year. British Medical Journal 1991 January 19; 302(6769):137-40; p. 137.

15  Tishler CL. Adolescent suicide attempts following elective abortion: a special case of anniversary reaction. Pediatrics 1981 November;68(5):670-1; p. 671.

16  Campbell N, Franco K, Jurs S. Abortion in adolescence. Adolescence Winter 1988;23(92):813-23.

17  Franz W. See n. 6.

18  Reardon D. *Aborted Women, Silent No More.* Chicago: Loyola University Press, 1987; p. 129.

19  Reardon D. The abortion/suicide connection. Springfield IL. The Post-Abortion Review Summer 1993;1(2); p. 1

20  Morgan CL, Evans M, Peters JR. Suicides after pregnancy. Mental health may deteriorate as a direct effect of induced abortion. British Medical Journal 1997 March 22;314(7084):902; discussion 902-3.

21  Michels N. *Helping Women Recover From Abortion.* Minneapolis, MN: Bethany House, 1988.

22  Reardon DC, Ney PG, Scheurer FJ, Congle JR, Coleman PK. Suicide deaths associated with pregnancy outcome: A record linkage study of 172,279 low income American women. Archives of Women's Mental Health 2001;3(4)Suppl.2:104

23  Michels 1988. See n. 21, p. 104.

24  Nathanson S. *Soul Crisis: One Woman's Journey Through Abortion to Renewal.* New York: New American Library, 1989, pp. 148, 150.

25  (a) Reardon D. Substance Abuse Subsequent to Abortion. Presented to the Society of Catholic Social Scientists, Second Annual Conference, 1994 November 4.
    (b) Reardon DC, Ney PG. Abortion and subsequent substance abuse. American Journal of Drug and Alcohol Abuse 2000 February;26(1):61-75; p. 61.

26  Brende. See n. 5, p. 5.

27  Raphael B. *The Anatomy of Bereavement.* New York: Basic Books, 1983.

28  Speckhard A. *The Psycho-Social Aspects of Stress Following Abortion.* Kansas City, MO: Sheed & Ward, 1987; p. 51.

29  Drower SJ, Nash ES. Therapeutic abortion on psychiatric grounds. Part I. A local study. South African Medical Journal 1978 October;54(15):604-8.

30  Frank DA, Zuckerman BS, Amaro H, Aboagye K, Bauchner H, Cabral H, et al. Cocaine use during pregnancy: prevalence and correlates. Pediatrics 1988 December;82(6):888-95.

31  Mensch B, Kandel DB. Drug use as a risk factor for premarital teen pregnancy and abortion in a national sample of young white women. Demography 1992 August;29(3):409-29; p. 409.

32  Klassen AD, Wilsnack SC. Sexual experience and drinking among women in a U.S. national survey. Archives of Sexual Behavior 1986 October;15(5):363-92.

33  Reardon and Ney 2000. See n. 25(b).

34  Lydon J, Dunkel-Schetter C, Cohan CL, Pierce T. Pregnancy decision making as a significant life event: a commitment approach. Journal of Personality and Social Psychology 1996 July;71(1):141-51.

35  Obel EB. Pregnancy complications following legally induced abortion. Acta Obstetricia et Gynecologica Scandanavica 1979;58(5):485-90.

36  Thomas T, Tori CD. Sequelae of abortion and relinquishment of child custody among women with major psychiatric disorders. Psychological Reports 1999 June;84(3 Pt 1):773-90.

37  De Puy, C and D Dovitch. *The Healing Choice: Your Guide to Emotional Recovery After an Abortion.* N.Y.: Fireside, 1997; p. 58.

38  Michels 1988. See n. 21, p. 47.

39  Wyatt GE, Guthrie D, Notgrass CM. Differential effects of women's child sexual abuse and subsequent sexual revictimization. Journal of Consulting and Clinical Psychology 1992 April;60(2):167-73; p. 171.

40  Ney P, Peeters A. *Hope Alive: Post Abortion and Abuse Treatment. A Training Manual for Therapists.* Victoria, B.C.: Pioneer Publishing, 1993; p. 28.

41  Torre-Bueno A. *Peace After Abortion.* San Diego, California: Pimpernel Press, 1997; p. 43.

42  Crawford D, Mannion M. *Psycho-Spiritual Healing After Abortion.* Kansas City: Sheed and Ward, 1989; p. 66.

43  Alexander PC. Application of attachment theory to the study of sexual abuse. Journal of Consulting and Clinical Psychology 1992 April;60(2): 185-95.

Egeland B, Jacobvitz D, Sroufe LA. Breaking the cycle of abuse. Child Development 1988;59:1080-8.

Main M, Goldwyn R. Predicting rejection of her infant from mother's representation of her own experience: Implications for the abused-abusing intergenerational cycle. Child Abuse and Neglect 1984;8(2):203-17.

44 Cole PM, Woolger C. Incest survivors: The relation of their perceptions of their parents and their own parenting attitudes. Child Abuse and Neglect 1989;13(3):409-16.

45 Benedict MI, White RB, Cornely DA. Maternal perinatal risk factors and child abuse. Child Abuse and Neglect 1985;9(2):217-24; p. 223.

46 Torre-Bueno. See n. 41, p. 27.

47 Crawford and Mannion. See n. 42.

48 Naziri D, Tzavaras A. Mourning and guilt among Greek women having repeated abortions. Omega: Journal of Death & Dying 1992-1993;26(2):137-44; p. 139.

49 Kent I, Greenwood RC, Loeken J, Nicholls W. Emotional sequelae of elective abortion. BC Medical Journal 1978 April;20(4):118-9.

50 Lauzon P et al. Emotional distress in couples involved in first-trimester induced abortions. Canadian Family Physician 2000 October;46:2033-2040.

51 Naziri and Tzavaras. See n. 48 p. 142.

52 Naziri and Tzavaras. See n. 48, p. 143.

53 Rue V. *Postabortion Trauma*. Lewisville, Texas: Life Dynamics, 1994; pp. 67-8.

54 Congleton GK, Calhoun LG. Post-abortion perceptions: a comparison of self-identified distressed and nondistressed populations. International Journal of Social Psychiatry 1993 Winter;39(4):255- 65 Winter 1993;39(4):255-65.

55 Freeman EW, Rickels K, Huggins GR, Garcia CR, Polin J. Emotional distress patterns among women having first or repeat abortions. Obstetrics & Gynecology 1980 May;55(5):630-6.

Tornbom M, Ingelhammar E, Lilja H, Moller A, Svanberg B. Repeat abortion: a comparative study. Journal of Psychosomatic Obstetrics and Gynecology 1996 Dec;17(4):208-14.

Osler M, Morgall JM, Jensen B, Osler M. Repeat abortion in Denmark. Danish Medical Bulletin 1992 February;39(1):89-91.

Leach J. The repeat abortion patient. Family Planning Perspectives 1977 January-February;9(1):37-9

56  Tornbom 1996. See n. 55, p. 213.

57  Tornbom M, Moller A. Repeat abortion: a qualitative study. Journal of Psychosomatic Obstetrics and Gynecology 1999 Mar;20(1):21-30; p. 28.

58  Leach, See n. 55, p. 37.

59  Berger C, Gold D, Andres D, Gillett P, Kinch R. Repeat abortion: is it a problem? Family Planning Perspectives 1984 March-April;16(2):70-5.

Osler et al. See n. 55.

60  Soderberg H, Andersson C, Janzon L, Sjoberg NO. Continued pregnancy among abortion applications. A study of women having a change of mind. Acta Obstetricia et Gynecologica Scandanavica 1997 November;76(10):942-7; p. 946.

61  Koonin LM, Strauss LT, Chrisman CE, Parker WY. Abortion surveillance--United States, 1997. Morbidity and Mortality Weekly Report, Centers for Disease Control, Surveillance Summaries 2000 Dec 8;49(11):1-43.

62  Donohue JJ, Levitt S. The impact of legalized abortion on crime. Quarterly Journal of Economics 2001 May; 116(2):379-420.

63  Chipman J. Study claims abortion cuts crime. The National Post 2001 May 17;Sect. A:1.

64  Lott JR, Whitley J. Abortion and Crime: Unwanted Children and Out-of-Wedlock Births [Working Paper #254]. Yale Law School, Program for Studies in Law, Economics, and Public Policy; 2001 May 15.

65  Thorn V. Project Rachel: Faith in action, a ministry of compassion and caring. In Post-Abortion Aftermath, ed. Mannion M, Kansas City, MO: Sheed and Ward, 1994: 144-63; pp. 159-60.

66  deVeber 1991. See n. 4, p. 207.

67  Project Rachel, Box 2400, London, Ontario Canada N6A 4G3.

68  National Office of Reconciliation and Healing, PO Box 074777, Milwaukee, Wis. 53207-0477; 1-800-5WE-CARE.

69  De Puy and Dovitch 1997. See n. 37, pp. 13-14.

70  Thorn 1994. See n. 65, p. 160.

Chapter 15

# Abortion and Interpersonal Relationships

Abortion can have a significant impact on every relationship a woman has; not only is her relationship with her partner affected, so are her relationships with the other members of her family and her other children.

After an abortion, the rate of marital breakups and relationship dissolution is anywhere from 40 to 75 per cent, often related to the breakdown of intimacy and trust. In addition, many women experience depression, guilt, and anger related to feelings of having been let down by their partner which, in turn, lead to communication problems and, frequently, sexual dysfunction. If their partners have manipulated or coerced them into having an abortion, women tend to feel angry and betrayed, and men, typically, feel a loss of control and pride especially if they were not consulted.

When a young girl is coerced into having an abortion by her parents, there is often a breakdown in the parent-child relationship; coping mechanisms include denial and avoidance with the end result often being an inability on the young woman's part to enter into maturity and act as an independent adult. Or, if a girl has an abortion without her parents' knowledge, she ends up in a cycle of lies and cover-ups which emotionally strain all her relationships.

Suppression of mourning which occurs in many of these situations often has marked negative effects on relationships with future children, some women reporting emotional numbing and inability to bond maternally. Living children in a family where there is an abortion are also negatively affected, frequently exhibiting fear, anxiety, and sadness at the loss of their sibling.

**Note:**
It is beyond the scope of our book to deal with the massive question of sex-selection abortion, which has resulted in a deficit of at least 100 million women in the world, according to one widely-accepted estimate.[1]

---

# Abortion and Interpersonal Relationships

Abortion never occurs within a relationship vacuum. Whether the abortion is shared or not, many significant others can be impacted.[2]

There is a general tendency to assume that the only interpersonal relations that are compromised by an abortion are those of the woman and her partner. Although these are the most obvious in the aftermath of abortion, other relationships can be severely strained as well. The most dramatic of these are relationships within the family in general: parent-child relations and sibling interactions.

### Marital Breakup and Relationship Dissolution
Between 40 and 50 per cent of couples break up following abortion. This can be attributed to several factors. Some arise from the experience of abortion in the lives of women, while others arise from the actions and reactions of the male partners. All can lead to a breakdown of intimacy and relationship failure.

Sherman found that 48 per cent of his sample reported that their relationship with their partner had been significantly altered by the abortion.[3] For younger women, the failure of the relationship after the abortion is often forced by parents who may also have been the prime movers in the abortion itself. They act to protect their daughter or themselves and judge that forcing an end to their daughter's relationship is the way to achieve this goal. But these actions may produce not only broken partnerships but damaged parent/child relations as well.

**Women's Reactions**

In 1992, Barnett and colleagues studied women from stable partnerships who had abortions and later reported being separated. In 80 per cent of the separated group, the breakup was initiated by the female partner, and 60 per cent reported an indirect connection between the abortion and the subsequent separation. None of these couples were married at the time of the abortion nor did any marry each other subsequent to the event. Relationships were reported to be initially worse, with more conflict and less mutual trust.[4]

When post-abortal women initiate separation, there are several possible mechanisms at work. The most simplistic and least psychologically likely is the popular assumption that the relationship was just temporary anyway and that the abortion was a life event that triggered the end of an already doomed partnership. Sometimes this may be the case, but usually more deep-seated factors seem to be at play. The abortion is indeed a trigger but not just a psychically simple, uncomplicated event.

Teichman found that there was a significant link between depression in post-abortion women and their relationship with their partners. Although this is not an unusual finding, what is startling is the way in which the two factors affected each other. Teichman established that the quality of the couple's relationship affected the level of depression experienced by the woman. The support of a stable relationship helped in coping with abortion. Unmarried women reported significantly higher levels of anxiety and depression. Unbalanced relationships, that were either too enmeshed or too disengaged, had the effect of elevating depression. However, the conclusion that emotional distress and discomfort are reduced after the abortion is devastatingly undermined by the fact that only 22 per cent of the women invited to participate in the study agree to do so.[5] One can only speculate about the emotional state of the 78 per cent who refused to talk about their abortions.

## Psychological Damage and Guilt

A woman experiencing emotional distress in the form of guilt feelings may attempt to lay the blame for the abortion on her boyfriend or husband. She may feel that the man did not provide sufficient support for her to continue the pregnancy. He may have kept silent, thinking he had no right to comment, whereas she wanted him to accept the responsibility of fatherhood and protect and cherish her and their child. Following the abortion, she may be unable to remain in a relationship in which she perceives the man has abandoned her. As Torre-Bueno puts it, "If your partner was supportive of your decision to have an abortion, and then is surprised to find himself feeling angry, depressed or grief-stricken, you might feel guilty. You also might find yourself feeling angry, betrayed and confused."..."You may be feeling guilty about hurting your husband or boyfriend because you did talk to him about the pregnancy and he wanted to keep the baby."[6]

Women experiencing post-abortion depression were studied by Firestein and colleagues. They determined that the most prolonged symptoms occurred in relationships where "pregnancy by the fiancé before marriage with subsequent abortion [was followed] by marriage."[7] The dissonance caused by the rejection of the first child of this now legitimately constituted family unit can lead to profound depression. Without proper therapeutic intervention, it can also lead to marriage dissolution.

The guilt a woman is feeling may impact on her ability to relate to the object of her blame – her partner. This can lead to a complete breakdown of communication and intimacy.

### Sexual Relations

Women who feel shame or anger may have problems with sexuality following abortion. Twenty per cent of Barnett's sample reported a reduction in libido two to three months after the abortion. Reisser explains the collapse of intimacy in the following way: "One of the most important factors in the breakup of a committed relationship following abortion is the disillusionment experienced by the woman...Women still respond powerfully to men who wholly love them and who are entirely committed to the family. When a partner fails in these tasks, a woman often feels deserted, and eventually disengages emotionally."[8] The feelings of abandonment lead to emotional disengagement which in turn manifests itself as female sexual dysfunction.

**Anger at Male Coercion**

A woman may feel betrayed at having been coerced by her partner to abort against her better judgment. In this case, she feels that she has compromised her own feelings and has been manipulated by a man who is supposed to be her "lover". The damage done to her self-perception may be immense and life in such a relationship may be emotionally untenable.

Shostak quotes a male Planned Parenthood counselor: "The men who seek abortion counseling are usually motivated by one of the following reasons: a need for information or education; a need for venting feelings; or a need to attempt to persuade their partner to have an abortion."[9] If, as we have seen (in Chapter 11), 23 per cent of women having an abortion in North America are pressured into it by their partners, this amounts to about 300,000 (out of 1.3 million) per year in the U.S., and 27,000 (out of 120,000) in Canada.

That these estimates may be too low is suggested by two articles. The first found that half the twelve men interviewed admitted that they had applied or would apply pressure on their partners to have an abortion.[10] The second noted that among women who had psychological difficulties after their abortion, more than one-third felt they had been coerced into their decision.[11] Well over half of the abortions had first been suggested by boyfriends or spouses. Afterwards many expressed vivid anger towards boyfriends, parents, and physicians who they felt had coerced them.

Morabito refers to the concept "seduction into abortion" which she views as a type of manipulation of the relationship and the woman, where deception, sometimes unwitting, is at play on the part of her partner/husband/boyfriend.

As one of the partners of a post-abortion woman put it, "Maybe I sort of knew that my support was what she needed to make the decision not to have a child."[12]

Because such manipulation shows a detachment from the needs and feelings of women, mature adult relationships may be impossible to sustain after an abortion. Mature relationships are based on honesty and mutual concern. Male coercion to abort is a form of manipulation whose purpose is to avoid responsibility and commitment. Under the guise of choice, men can walk away from fatherhood and commitment. Abortion highlights the breakdown between sex and commitment, and coercion to abort is an expression of this breakdown.

**Male-Initiated Breakups**
Because little academic research has been done to study the effects of abortion on men, the accounts of their reactions come from stories and clinical interviews. As a result, there is little statistical information on the effect of abortion on relationship dissolution and very seldom from a man's perspective.

In one study, unmarried male inmates, whose girlfriends aborted, overwhelmingly chose to end the relationship. They identified the abortion as the main cause of the breakup and suggested that they were the ones who initiated it.

Shostak identified a constellation of factors underlying male-initiated relationship breakdown: guilt and remorse along with post-abortion sexuality and contraception: "I found it [the abortion] affected my feelings for her more than I could control" was a common reaction.[13] For men who had been involved in relationships that were originally committed ones, the renewal of sexual intimacy is a way to reaffirm love. But, as previously noted, many women have sexual difficulties after abortion. "If his masculinity has been threatened during the decision-making process, resuming the sexual relationship assures him that all is well. But the resistance with which his sexual overtures will usually be met can instead provoke feelings of further emasculation and failure."[14]

At a more profound psychodynamic level is the nature of fatherhood lost. As Strahan puts it, "Abortion thwarts the most basic of paternal impulses – a man's instinct to protect his children." He goes on to note that in interviews, post-abortal men report that abortion and the fathering of children are issues of control and pride. In such cases, Strahan states that "the abortion violates the very essence of masculinity." Within the context of ethnic diversity, there are racial differences in male reactions, as stated in Chapter 16. Some males, he points out, consider that an abortion is a loss of a "sense of heritage and the importance of perpetuating" themselves. In some cases, the man identifies with the child who no longer exists and this form of identification can shatter the couple identification and precipitate a collapse in the relationship.[15] Inability to communicate these feelings of loss and self-identification means, as Reisser notes, that "the partner who is expressing grief and anger now unconsciously begins to self-protect from further pain, and the trusting vulnerability required for intimate interpersonal relationships is withheld."[16] It is therefore not surprising that Franco and colleagues found that only seven of the 66 single women in their study later married the father.[17]

**Parents and Abortion**
A frequent image in both clinical and popular literature is that of a young pregnant teenager being taken to an abortion clinic by her concerned but controlling parents. The focus of concern in research studies is usually the young woman and her reactions to the abortion situation. Seldom do researchers consider the impact that such a choice has on the fabric of family life. As Rue explains, "When an abortion decision is neither voluntary nor informed and when pre-abortion counseling does not address these issues as well as the relational context of the pregnancy, emotional traumatization is inevitable."[18] A subject from Ervin's study speaks:

> *Rachel*: "... my mom said if I was going to have the baby I couldn't stay at the house and see my brothers and sisters...his mom came to the house and tried to talk them [my parents] out of the abortion, but they wouldn't listen to her...my mother kept telling me I had cost them $800."[19]

Where there is ambivalence and coercion surrounding an abortion, a breakdown in the parent-child bond is inevitable. Young women feel they must repress and deny any negative effects because they need to preserve the belief that their family did what was best for them. When it is over, the abortion is often not mentioned again; it is as if it had never happened. Ultimately, this strategy is cognitively incompatible with healthy relationships. The parents sought the abortion because of the conviction that this was the right decision for their daughter and yet, by never mentioning it, by never discussing it, they give their daughter the clear signal that it was wrong.

From a developmental perspective, this type of situation can be very destructive to adolescent females. They are being told that they are not mature enough to make their own decisions. They are told that parents know best and therefore any feelings of regret or guilt must be repressed. Such messages reinforce the adolescent's perception of herself as not responsible for her actions, thereby allowing her to project blame onto her parents and away from herself. In the end, this impedes her ability to mature and act as an independent adult. As "Trudy" puts it:

> She [my mother] told me, "Trudy, I've made an appointment for you at the doctor's office, and he's going to take care of your problem"...I didn't go to work the next day. I lost my mind...I did blame myself a little bit. I blame my mom...we never talked about the abortion.[20]

Crawford and Mannion see the breakdown in relationships following abortion as a symptom of a psychological numbing and avoidance response in which the woman, unconsciously, attempts to disassociate from the events and people surrounding the abortion. "The parent...who thought to be helpful by helping to pay for the abortion or even by going with the woman to the abortion clinic might later be very confused and perplexed when the woman rejects her: 'I stood by her during the abortion. Why is she rejecting me?' The woman herself may look on the experience with great disappointment and anger [thinking], 'Why didn't they speak up and have the courage to tell me I was going to kill my baby?'"[21]

## Lack of Parental Support

What about the parents for whom abortion is morally unacceptable and who are unable to provide support for their daughter during the abortion? Their failure to stand by and accept a decision to abort has been seen by some commentators as a cause of post-abortion distress. The position of such parents may contribute to post-abortion distress, but so also may the choice to abort have an overall, but little studied, effect on the family.

Lack of support can occur before the adolescent becomes pregnant. Because teenagers operate at a concrete and ego-centric level of cognitive development, they tend to see the world only in terms of themselves. Franz describes such a teenager: "She sees everything in terms of her own agency and causation." If parents are not clear about their beliefs and values, and do not teach their children that their love will not be withdrawn if the children become pregnant, then situations arise in which the adolescents make decisions to abort based on their egocentric view of parent-child love. Fear that their behavior will cause their parents great distress may be based on inadvertent or inappropriate comments by the parents. In a 1985 study by Ervin, one teenager said, "Mom also threw in how she would have a nervous break-down if I ever became pregnant and Dad would have a heart attack. That confirmed my inability to tell them."[23] If abortions occur to save the feelings of parents – and grand-parents as well – or to avoid painful confrontations, the result may be psychological suffering and family dysfunction.

## Secrecy

Shame and fear are the most frequent motivators for secrecy. These include shame of disappointing parents, fear of the effect pregnancy will have on parents, and/or fear of abandonment. Many decisions to abort are made by young women without the knowledge of their parents. Because there is generally no legal requirement for parental consent or notification, these decisions often include an earlier decision to hide the pregnancy from the family. Secrecy can have a profound effect on the relationship of a daughter to her parents or siblings. Rue summarizes the literature on secrecy in the family the following way: "When an adolescent elects abortion without parental consultation, she must inevitably return to her family context. However, she returns with a secret that shames and emotionally strains her coping abilities. She must employ increased deception to protect her secret and to protect herself from her perceived fears of being found out and condemned by her parents and siblings."[24]

The psychological price of secrecy within the family system is well documented by Webster, Imber-Black, and Ervin.[25] From Ervin's study a woman revealed that: "My sister came and stayed with me...Keeping the secret between us, we never spoke of it for years. My life was a mess...I continued to tell more lies, keep more secrets and deceive those around me to hide the truth within."

**Children in the Aftermath of Abortion**
Much of the discussion in the research literature of the effects of abortion on relationships has been focused on partnership issues. The impact on the family system, however, is seldom addressed. Therapists working with women who have had abortions have noted that some women become numbed by the abortion experience, resulting in a lack of feeling that impedes their ability to relate in a positive, maternal way with their already-born children.

**Relationship Between Aborting Mother and Living Children**
There has been significant evidence in death and dying studies to link failures in parenting to the fact that a parent is grieving the death of a family member. When abortion is considered in the context of bereavement and loss, Raphael argues that "the pattern of grief and mourning is not dissimilar for that for spontaneous abortion, except that suppression and inhibition of grief and mourning are much more likely."[26] Suppression is often accompanied by a lack of emotional affect and an inability to bond with other children. Women often report a feeling of numbness, as described by

one of the women in Ervin's study: "I love my children so much but I didn't want them to touch me. It was like being in a trance."

In a Canadian study, Kent and colleagues used standard self-report questionnaires for post-abortal women and found that fewer than twenty per cent seemed to have suffered serious emotional consequences. However, using their experience as psychiatrists, they looked into the original data and found that "...Alerted by the painfulness of the feeling expressed by women in therapy, we examined the overall emotional picture...absence of affect was the most striking finding from our questionnaire study and in some cases, especially of teenagers, was so marked as to be judged an adverse re-action in itself."[27] Kumar and Robson found that "unresolved feelings of grief, guilt and loss may remain dormant long after an abortion until they are apparently re-awakened by another pregnancy." The authors hypothesize that "the abortion treatment-setting contributes to a suppression of mourning and accentuates ambivalence about motherhood."[28]

**Effect of Abortion upon Living Children**
The effect of an abortion on a family where there are already children is seldom mentioned. What research has been done indicates negative outcomes as a result of two possible mechanisms: the child-rearing approach of the parents and/or the developmental impact on children raised in a family where one child has been eliminated from the family structure. (See also Chapter 12 dealing with the effects of genetic abortion on already-existing children.)

Post-abortal women report that their ability to respond to the remaining or future child(ren) can be manifested in several ways: a feeling of emotional numbness which leads to a lack of bonding, acting out of hostility and anger which can result in child abuse, and considering future children as "replacement children" who become overindulged.

**Emotional Numbing and Lack of Bonding**
Following abortion, some women report an inability to re-spond in caring, appropriate ways to living children or to

children conceived and born later, usually to a different father. This reaction can be the result of ongoing depression or of the fact that children are a constant reminder of the abortion experience and the lost child. Such reminders bring up feelings of guilt and shame. Women in this state of mind have made comments like the following:

"I didn't want [my children] to touch me."

"With my husband's love and support, I am conquering the fear of bonding with my children...."[29]

Mattinson refers to a couple (who had had a previous abortion) whose baby gave them great pleasure for eight months after it was born, but who returned to therapy when the wife turned against the child and had a nervous break-down. Brown and colleagues analyzed letters from women who felt they had experienced negative post-abortion reactions, and in 13.3 per cent of the cases, they reported what the authors call "phobic responses to infants".[30]

**Abuse or Neglect**
Child abuse and neglect may occur if post-abortion trauma is unresolved and the woman goes on to deliver a baby. Ney and Peeters state, "Our research has shown that people who have had an abortion are more likely to abuse their children and people who have been abused are more likely to have an abortion...Abortion results in more post-partum depression and therefore less bonding, less touching and less breast feeding."[31]

Similar findings emerge from a recent study headed by Priscilla Coleman. Drawing from the National Longitudinal Survey of Youth funded by the U.S. Deparment of Labor, her study shows that "children of aborting women had higher rates of behavior problems" than the children of non-aborting mothers.[32]

For many researchers, this finding would be counterintuitive. In 1971, Silverman and Silverman wrote a popular book extolling the virtues of childlessness and denouncing large

families. They contended that large families were the cause
of child abuse because in "certain large families...yet another
unwanted pregnancy may be the final pressure leading to a
battered child." They also said, "Mothers and fathers who
limit the numbers of their children tend to be more
emotionally stable and experience fewer marital problems."[33]
To the extent that legitimate methods of limitation included
induced abortion, an emphasis on small family size as a way
to reduce child abuse contributed to the pressure toward
abortion for "unwanted children". Indeed, the small family
became synonymous with marital stability and the cessation
of child abuse. As Ney and Peeters point out, however,
"...one of the earliest arguments [in support of legalizing
abortion] was that aborting unwanted children would diminish the incidence of child abuse. Statistics show precisely the
opposite, that is, with more frequent abortions all kinds of
child abuse have increased."[34]

The reality is that traumatic, unresolved events connected
to pregnancy and childbirth, including induced abortion,
probably contribute to later child abuse. Benedict, White,
and Cornely studied abusive mothers and found that
"reproductive history (stillbirth/abortion/prior child death)
and the circumstances surrounding past pregnancies may
provide important clues in eliciting more precisely what
family dynamics may be related to subsequent maltreatment." In this study, the level of abuse was found to rise
with the number of previous stillbirths or abortions.[35]

**The Replacement Child**
After abortion, "replacement" children may find themselves
the object of obsessive parenting styles of post-abortal
parents who focus inordinate time, affection, or material
goods on them. In a confused action of compensation for
the abortion, parents may attempt to replace the lost child
with a "wanted" child soon after the abortion. For example,
one woman in Ervin's 1985 study said: "I wanted my baby
back...Nine months later I gave birth to a healthy baby
boy...."

According to Ney and Peeters, "When one infant is aborted the parents may seek to absolve their guilt by pouring their love into the survivor, the child of a subsequent pregnancy. This displaced compensation only makes the survivor's life more difficult. Being a chosen or wanted child is its own hell."[36]

Such indulgence can create in the wanted child a mixed message. To the extent that society accepts that parents will tell their children the truth about the abortion of an unwanted sibling, a growing number of children must cognitively accommodate two important ideas: I am special because I am wanted and, for that reason, I am alive; my sibling was not wanted, so he or she was aborted.

But how is a young child to accept that "wantedness" is a quality that cannot be withdrawn? How can she or he know that tomorrow he or she may not be wanted? Actually, a young child cannot make these distinctions. Knowledge that a sibling has been aborted can lead to behavior disturbances, emotional insecurity, and delayed grief which may surface years later. Rue reports that, clinically, "For the preschool child...comprehending the necessary and intentional death of one's younger sibling in abortion is impossible, prompting considerable confusion and anxiety. Children at this stage attempt mastery of...basic trust and a sense of autonomy. Abortion impedes these development tasks and promotes a sense of mistrust, fear, doubt and latent or manifest hostility...For children of school age or older, Death is seen as irreversible, and they are likely to experience the death of a sibling as personification and attribute external motives for the death...as 'murder' committed by either the doctor or the parents. They may also experience considerable survivor guilt."[37]

One wonders about the impact on the daughter described by Inmate 52 in Pierce's study of women in prison: "[The woman] was still messed up after the abortion. She kept telling her daughter, 'I killed your little brother or sister'."[38]

The negative effects of knowing that a sibling has been aborted can also occur when the surviving child finds out as an adolescent. A client came to Torre Bueno with the following history:

> When I was eighteen my mother told me about her abortion...I was aghast, and said something cruel to her like, "How could you do something so terrible?" We let it drop and I forgot about it. But I had not *really* forgotten. I didn't think about it *consciously* for years...Suddenly I found myself thinking about my little brother!...I became disoriented and lost control of the car for a moment as I burst into tears having lost him. I was astounded by my reaction, but I couldn't shake the sadness and longing to have known him.[39]

If the sibling was aborted for medical or genetic reasons, then the concept of the sibling's disease as a reason for abortion may make the surviving child frightened by illness. In the concrete thinking of children, illness or disease may be incompatible with their continued existence. How will parents react if they become ill? Will they be abandoned by their parents as their baby brother or sister was abandoned? The research literature suggests that children can engage in these thought processes after learning of the death-by-abortion of a genetically-defective sibling.

**Conclusion**
The medical research community has put little effort into investigating the psychological effect abortion has on a woman's life, let alone its effects on her interpersonal and family relationships. It seems, however, from sources investigating breakdowns in marital or partnership or family relations, that the relationships of women who abort are at high risk of either dysfunction or dissolution.

**Key Points Chapter 15**

• Women's marital or partner or family relationships can be significantly affected by abortion.

• After abortion, many relationships come to an end, and if the woman stays with her partner or husband, sexual dysfunction often results as does difficulty bonding with children born later on.

• When a woman or adolescent girl has been coerced into having an abortion, typical reactions include feelings of betrayal (by partners or family members), anger, depression, sadness, and breakdown of trust and intimacy in relationships.

• Some men are negatively affected and sense a loss of control and pride, especially when their partner has had an abortion without their being consulted

• "Suppressed mourning" has very negative outcomes, often leading to feelings of numbness and/or hostility and anger, and to difficulties in forming future relationships and in bonding with later-born children; in some instances, post-abortion trauma can lead to actual abuse of later children.

• Already-born children are affected by the abortion of a sibling, often demonstrating feelings of sadness, fear, confusion, and anxiety; parent-child trust is damaged.

## Notes

1  Sen, A. More than 100 Million Women are Missing. New York Review of Books (20 Dec. 1990): 61-66.

2  Rue V. *Postabortion Trauma*. Lewisville, Texas: Life Dynamics, 1994a; p. 28.

3  Sherman DH, Mandelman N, Kerenyi TD, Scher J. The abortion experience in private practice. In: Finn W, Tallmer M, Seeland I, Kutscher AH, Clark E, editors. *Women and Loss: Psychobiological Perspectives.* New York; Praeger, 1985: 98-107.

4  Barnett W, Freudenberg N, Wille R. Partnership after induced abortion: a prospective controlled study. Archives of Sexual Behavior 1992 October;21(5):443-55.

5  Teichman Y, Shenhar S, Segal S. Emotional distress in Israeli women before and after abortion. American Journal of Orthopsychiatry 1993 April;63(2):277-88.

6  Torre-Bueno A. *Peace After Abortion*. San Diego, California: Pimpernel Press, 1997; p. 45, p. 44.

7  Firestein SK. Special features of grief reactions with reproductive catastrophe. Loss, Grief & Care. 1989 3(3-4);37-45; p. 37.

8  Reisser T. The effects of abortion on marriage and other committed relationships. Newsletter of the Association for Interdisciplinary Research in Values and Social Change 1994 May-June;6(4):1-8; p. 2.

9  Shostak AB, Mclouth G, Seng L. *Men and Abortion: Lessons, Losses, and Love*. New York: Praeger, 1984; p. 152.

10  Baker M. Men and abortion. Esquire. 1990 March:116-26.

11  Franco KN, Tamburrino MB, Campbell NB, Pentz JE, Jurs SG. Psychological profile of dysphoric women postabortion. Journal of the American Medical Women's Association 1989 July-August;44(4):113-5.

12  Morabito S. Abortion and the compromise of fatherhood. Human Life Review. 1991 Fall;17(4):83-100; p. 124.

13  Shostak 1984. See n. 9.

14  Reisser 1994. See n. 8, p. 6.

15  Strahan, T. Portraits of post-abortive fathers devastated by the abortion experience. Newsletter of the Association for Interdisciplinary Research in Values and Social Change. 1994 Nov-Dec;7(3):1-8; pp. 4-5.

16  Reisser 1994. See n. 8, p. 3.

17  Franco 1989. See n.11, p. 113.

18  Rue 1994. See n. 2.

19  Ervin P. *Women Exploited: the other victims of abortion*. Huntington, Indiana: Our Sunday Visitor, 1985; pp. 31, 33.

20  Ervin 1985. See n. 19; pp. 145, 147.

21  Crawford D, Mannion M. *Psycho-Spiritual Healing After Abortion*. Kansas City: Sheed and Ward, 1989; p. 12.

22  Franz W. Post abortion trauma and the adolescent. In: Mannion M, ed. *Post-Abortion Aftermath*. Kansas City: Sheed and Ward, 1994: 119-30; p. 125.

23  Ervin 1985. See n. 19, p. 37.

24  Rue 1994. See n. 2, p. 66.

25  Webster H. *Family Secrets: how telling and not telling affect our children, our relationships, and our lives*. Reading, Mass.: Addison-Wesley, 1991.

Imber-Black E. *Secrets in Families and Family Therapy*. New York: Norton, 1993.

Ervin 1985. See n. 19.

26  Raphael B. *The Anatomy of Bereavement*. New York: Basic Books, 1983.

27  Kent I, Greenwood RC, Loeken J, Nicholls W. Emotional sequelae of elective abortion. BC Medical Journal 1978 April;20(4):118-9; p. 118.

28  Kumar R, Robson K. Previous induced abortion and ante-natal depression in primiparae: preliminary report of a survey of mental health in pregnancy. Psychological Medicine 1978 November;8(4):711-5; p. 714.

29  Ervin 1985. See n. 19.

Mannion M. Abortion and healing: A pastoral church responds in word and sacrament. In: Mannion M, ed. *Post-Abortion Aftermath: A Comprehensive Consideration: Writings Generated by Various Experts at a 'Post-Abortion Summit Conference'*. Kansas City: Sheed and Ward, 1994: 106-18.

30  Mattinson J. The effects of abortion on a marriage. Ciba Foundation Symposium 1985;115:165-77.

Brown D, Elkins TE, Larson DB. Prolonged grieving after abortion: a descriptive study. Journal of Clinical Ethics 1993 Summer;4(2):118-23; p. 120.

31  Ney P, Peeters A. *Hope Alive: Post Abortion and Abuse Treatment. A Training Manual for Therapists.* Victoria, B.C.: Pioneer Publishing, 1993, p. 28.

32  Coleman PK. Reardon DC, Cougle JR. Child developmental outcomes associated with maternal history of abortion using the NLSY data. Archives of Women's Mental Health 2001;3(4)Supp.2:104.

33  Silverman A, Silverman A. *The Case Against Having Children.* New York: David McKay Company, 1971.

34  Ney and Peeters 1993. See n. 31, p. 28.

35  Benedict MI, RB. White RB, Cornely DA. Maternal perinatal risk factors and child abuse. Child Abuse and Neglect 1985;9(2): 217-24.

36  Ney and Peeters 1993. See n. 31, p. 27.

37  Rue, V. The psychological realities of induced abortion. In *Post-Abortion Aftermath*, ed. M Mannion. Kansas City: Sheed and Ward, 1994b, pp. 27-28.

38  Pierce L. Abortion attitudes and experiences in a group of male prisoners. Newsletter of the Association for Interdisciplinary Research in Values and Social Change 1994 January/February;6(2):1-8; p. 8.

39  Torre-Bueno 1997. See n. 6, pp. 70-71.

# Chapter 16

# Abortion: Its Effect on Men

There have been very few studies done on the effects of abortion on men, and what few there are seem to disagree as to whether men are affected or not. A number of studies, however, point to the fact that men often experience depression, guilt, anger, grief, and shame after their partner has an abortion, feelings commonly experienced by the woman herself. In the aftermath of abortion, particularly where the feelings around the decision to abort are ambivalent, men often feel depressed and when they have not been consulted about the decision, they often feel angry about being legally disenfranchised.

As with women, men whose partners abort may demonstrate self-destructive behavior by abusing drugs, alcohol, and sex. On the other hand, men often push women to have an abortion, and in these cases, their initial reaction is relief; in later therapy, however, some of these men demonstrate symptoms of distress, guilt, and grief. It is well documented that a large percentage of unmarried relationships dissolve after an abortion, sometimes because the woman feels that she and her baby have been abandoned and sometimes because the man has not been consulted and feels powerless. There are few counseling programs for men, and some researchers are now calling for further studies of the effect of abortion on men and follow-up therapy for them.

# Abortion: Its Effect on Men

In the recently emerging literature on post-abortion healing, a key area of disagreement is whether abortion affects men. Do men walk away unscathed from the experience, or do they suffer as women do following the abortion decision?

### Male Reactions to Abortion

On one side of the question of whether or not men are affected by abortion are therapists such as Candace De Puy and Dana Dovitch. Their book, *The Healing Choice*, cursorily mentions that, "Some of the men we interviewed were distressed about the practical implications of the pregnancy...Other men who were already fathers did experience a connection to the fetus. For them, the decision to abort was more difficult." However, the authors then cite researcher Benvenuti who reports that even if men express deep "emotional concern," it is over the unwanted pregnancy, not the abortion, and that they do not show depression. The authors state that women are "baffled by the apparent lack of distress some men display during a pregnancy or after it has been resolved."[1]

De Puy and Dovitch, who describe the male partner of the aborting woman as the "man who impregnated her", focus on the loss of relationship and a numbness felt by the male. But they do not speculate on the question of whether the abortion and its aftermath ended the relationship, or whether it played a role in the emotional numbness displayed by the male partner. In the exercises that accompany their discussion, they do ask: "If it [the relationship] ended, how did it end? Did it relate to the abortion?"[2]

On the other side of the question, there is Kim Kluger-Bell who reports, "In my practice I have known a number of women (and men, as well) for whom the psychological consequences of abortion were surprisingly long-term."[3] The men she is referring to, however, are usually involved in abortion for genetic reasons and do not appear in her discussion of early elective abortion.

**Depression, Guilt, and Shame**

Ava Torre-Bueno devotes a chapter of her book *Peace after Abortion* to the effects of abortion on men. She cites the lack of control men feel – their anger at their own legal disenfranchisement from the decision, their guilt about contraceptive failure, and their empathy with their partner. In some cases, "men are confused when their partners are OK with having had an abortion, but they themselves are depressed, guilty, grieving or shame-filled."[4]

Following a common practice of writers in this area, Torre-Bueno uses case studies to illustrate the points she wishes to make. According to her research, just as women who are ambivalent about abortion suffer negative effects, so do men. She discusses the relationship between ambivalence and depression and addresses men directly in this way: "If...you are sleeping too little, or too much; if you have difficulty concentrating, are eating more or less than usual, feel hopeless, helpless, tearful or suicidal, please read Chapter Six of this book, "Depression and Anger", and if you recognize that you are depressed seek help immediately." In her discussion of guilt, Torre-Bueno recognizes the variable nature of this emotion in men. It can arise from feelings of personal failure for not helping raise the child, for forcing the abortion, or for causing their partner to have a general feeling of "having harmed someone."[5]

The precise nature of male grief she professes not to understand: "He knew rationally that it hadn't been a baby at all but an embryo too tiny to see with the naked eye – so why was he so sad?"[6] That the underlying reason for a man's feelings may be an understanding that he has lost a child does not seem to occur to her. Her question suggests in addition that she is unaware that the vast majority of abortions kill easily visible fetuses that are at least one cm in length.

Shame, she argues, arises in one of two possible ways: the man's sense of being "flawed" or "incompetent" and thus not helping his partner to have the baby or "fear of exposure of their irresponsible behavior."[7] Shame is something expressed as negative acting-out: "Some men find that they are acting out in ways that are self-destructive and counter-productive after a partner's abortion. They will find themselves compelled to test fate by having unprotected intercourse and being involved in several more abortions. Or they will have trouble being sexual at all and may become impotent."[8] It would seem that many of the behaviors of men following an abortion mirror those of women who become self-destructive (see Chapter 15), and that these behaviors lead in the end to "more guilt, anger, shame and grief."

A team of Canadian researchers headed by Lauzon recently found that 56.9 per cent of women and 39.6 per cent of men involved in first-trimester abortions were much more distressed than the control groups who were not involved in abortions. The abortion brought emotional relief to only a small fraction of these women and men. Three weeks after the abortion 41.7 per cent of the women and 30.9 per cent of the men were still highly distressed. The researchers conclude that "Being involved in a first-trimester abortion can be highly distressing for both women and men."[9]

**Are Male Grief Reactions New?**
References in the literature from the early 1970s indicate that men suffer following abortion, but there has been little concerted effort to do follow-up research in this area. As Rue notes, "How abortion affects men is even less well documented [than how it affects women]."[10] In 1985, Ervin studied post-abortion disorders and noted, "There is no denying the fact that men too suffer psychological trauma after the abortion of their offspring."[11]

At the very outset of legalized abortion in North America, Wallerstein studied women who aborted at a Planned Parenthood clinic. She mentions that several women noted that their boyfriends/partners "were comparably stressed by the pregnancy and abortion events,"and continues: "It would seem that treatment services should be made equally available to the young men involved."[12] More than 25 years later no such support programs exist for men. Indeed, in the discussion of abortion, men's issues seem to have dropped off the radar screen. They are dealt with only in relation to the women they are in partnership with or if, on their own, they seek out a one-on-one therapeutic relationship,

An exhaustive search between 1995 and 1997 of Medline, the database for all articles in medical, psychiatric, and psychological journals, found a large number of articles and reviews related to abortion but none of them focused on men's reactions or needs before, during, or after abortion. Ryan and Dunn point to "the ethical issue of excluding one partner, the male, from participating in a decision that affects a jointly conceived fetus."[13] The authors report that between 1973 and 1981 only three abortion-related studies focused on men. These studies – Milling, Rothstein, and Francke[14] – considered a limited sample of partners. "In each case, the reports dealt with the male waiting in the abortion clinic." By definition, such men are not representative of all men whose partners choose abortion. Missing from such a sample are those who did not know about the decision as well as those whose moral beliefs about abortion did not allow them to participate.

**Unsupportive Fathers**
In addition to the exclusion from post-abortion research of men who grieve, are men who do not care about the woman or her abortion. It is unknown what percentage of these men later realize the import of the decision and its effect on their lives. Ervin studied women who reported distress following abortion. She reports, "Although some of the men stuck by the women...about 75 per cent of the men fled after paying part or all the costs of the abortion. Some of them just fled – paying nothing...."[15]

Lack of male support does not appear to be limited to a woman's decision to abort. Men leaving women who continue a pregnancy was also reported by Ajzenstat and colleagues in her study of single parents in Canada, *Going It Alone: Unplanned Single Motherhood in Canada*. "Only thirteen per cent of the fathers were emotionally supportive after the baby's birth and during the child's first two years."[16]

*Going it Alone* also looked at the role of the father in the decision-making process. Fifty-six per cent of the social service agencies felt that the father influenced the decision, but only 25 per cent of the mothers themselves felt that the father had influenced their decision. The mothers ranked their male partners behind parents, friends, and other family members. Essentially, the mothers overwhelmingly felt that the input of fathers was not supportive, and indeed was negative, toward their decision to parent. "The least likely person of all to express positive views about the woman's decision to parent is the baby's father," they report. "Close to half the women report that the baby's father expressed disapproval. Only 28 per cent found the father supportive."[17]

Miller surveyed 82 women about who had had input into their abortion decisions. To the question, "Was one of you more motivated to have the abortion than the other?" 23 per cent responded that the boyfriend or husband was more motivated.[18] It is interesting that two quite different studies found that 23 per cent of fathers were the prime movers in the decision to abort. When women acted independently and chose to continue the pregnancy, a similar percentage of fathers gave negative, non-supportive input.

**Negative Post-Abortion Sequelae for Men**
As with women, the problems men have following abortion are most often identified only in a clinical setting. This means, among other things, that only those motivated enough to seek professional help will form the basis for study. The abortion experience may trigger symptoms that can only be plumbed in the context of psychodynamic therapy. In a report of clinical case histories of men, McAll and McAll reported a man of 41 who had first been diagnosed as having anorexia nervosa at age 22: "At the time of examination he was not only anorexic but severely depressed. On close questioning he admitted to having precipitated the abortion of his wife's first child. Within a week of this admission and after following through a process of mourning for and committal of the child he was no longer depressed and was eating normally."[19]

Raphael discussed the reactions of men in his study of bereavement and found that in relation to abortion: "Some fathers will feel angry and cheated by the woman's decision...Many men involved in the termination of the pregnancy they have fathered will experience grief too and may need recognition of their mourning for the lost child."[20]

**Legal Status of Males in the Decision to Abort**
Men in North America currently have no legal rights in abortion decision-making. The only way they can sway a woman's decision is by persuasion. In our legal system, a woman makes the decision to abort or to carry her pregnancy to term and the biological father has only three options: Support of the aborting woman, support of the child until adulthood if the woman chooses not to abort, or to become a socially disapproved, perhaps legally hunted, deadbeat dad. The father's personal views on abortion, however strongly believed, carry no weight. As Rue puts it, "For most men abortion is a private exercise in powerlessness."[21] Perhaps this is one reason so many men vote with their feet.

Indeed, the law has placed fathers in a difficult situation. Redmond studied the role of Canadian men in the abortion/parenting decision. She found that the majority, whether in casual partnerships or involved in a serious relationship, expressed the wish that the woman carry the pregnancy to term. But, as Redmond notes, in the end, few of the men felt that they could "exert any real control in the decision-making process."[22]

**Long-Term Effects of Abortion on Men**
However immaturely men may act at the time of a partner's abortion, is there a later impact when they realize what they have participated in? Shostak contends that, given the problems men have, "the abortion experience of many American males may cast a long and troubled shadow over their future fatherhood experiences."[23]

Milling's study is not representative of all male partners because it focused only on males who waited in the abortion clinic, and it provided only short-term follow up of the 400 men studied. Nonetheless, it is interesting that, although none of them felt that they would later come to regret the decision, within one month of the abortion, 70 per cent of the unmarried relationships had broken up.[24]

Shostak identified 50 young men who were involved with abortion for the first time. His results on decision-making mirrored Milling's and Rothstein's, but he also found that 40 per cent of these men "thought about the child that might-have-been." This "sizable minority reported the persistence of day and night dreams about the child that never was, and some represented these moments as times of guilt, remorse, and sadness." In addition, while 82 per cent felt that men should be offered counseling and/or education about abortion and family planning, Shostak found that abortion clinic staff were indifferent to the possibility of educating these males. Clearly, while the male partners denied experiencing any serious emotional consequences, "many relationships between unmarried partners appeared unable to survive the strains inherent in the abortion experience."[25]

Reardon and Sutton approach abortion from the perspective of clinical psychology. Sutton sees the denial of fatherhood as a powerful factor in pathological guilt and shame which also leads to a type of self-alienation that affects the psychology of decision-making.[26]

Rue reports that abortion is an unrecognized trauma for men, which many suffer without any help. Most men feel isolated, angry at themselves and their partners, and fearful of the emotional damage to their partners. Furthermore, most men feel helpless – while women may choose motherhood, men are not permitted to choose fatherhood. The law in both the U.S. and Canada forbids them any role in the abortion decision. For most men, therefore, "abortion is a private exercise in powerlessness."[27]

**Cultural or Ethnic Factors**
There appears to be a cultural basis to some male reactions. Buchanan and Robbins found that among adolescent males in Texas those whose girlfriends had abortions were more

distressed than those who went on to be fathers. Of those whose partners aborted, Hispanic males were more distressed than males from other ethnic backgrounds.[28] In 1987, the research wing of Planned Parenthood reported that more white women said that they were influenced by their partners' desire for them to have an abortion. This research suggests that among men there is a cultural or ethnic aspect to their response to abortion.

In another American study, Strahan found that "black males are less involved in pregnancy decision-making than males of other races."[29]

**Abuse after Abortion**
Does previous abortion affect relationships that continue? Amarro and colleagues reviewed 1243 obstetrical cases from a Boston hospital. Seven per cent reported physical or sexual violence during their pregnancy. Victims were more likely to have had a previous elective abortion than non-victims.[30] As Bittman and Zalk put it: "A man may have guilt feelings or anger during his wife's pregnancy which may occur if his wife has had a previous miscarriage or abortion. The male may feel somehow responsible and if so, he will resent the baby and his wife that much more."[31]

**In-depth Interviews: Inmates in State Reformatory**
Perhaps one of the most stirring pieces of research comes from Pierce's non-quantitative, interview-based study of male prisoners whose wives/partners had had an abortion. Inmates from a state reformatory were randomly chosen by staff to participate in the interviews. No statistical data were generated from the results. Instead, Pierce chose to recount their stories, recording nothing more than the men's ages and marital status. In all, 57 interviews are reported and the author notes, "Perhaps some of the most touching interviews were lost due to grief. More than once, after a brief introduction...some looked down or away and said they just couldn't talk about it."[32] (In Chapter 17 there is a discussion of the high rate at which women who have aborted are lost to long-term follow up. The consensus is that these are women who find the topic too painful to discuss.

Similarly, it would seem that those men most disturbed by a previous abortion experience may also be lost to follow up. This makes it difficult to determine the full extent of the effect of abortion on the men involved.)

Among the men whose wives had abortions, three expressed neutral or positive reactions. Although they said that abortion did not bother them, these men contextualized the decision in light of major financial, emotional and health problems affecting their lives:

Four married men expressed negative reactions as follows:

> Inmate 1: "I'm hurting just as bad as she."
> Inmate 2: "It's not the child's fault. It was wrong."
> Inmate 3: "I resent her for doing that. It drew a piece from me."
> Inmate 6: "My wife's abortion about killed me. It was rough. There's always room for one more."

Only Inmate 1 indicated acquiescence in the decision saying, "It was also my decision." The others noted their disagreement with the decision and/or their attempts to stop it. Inmate 6 indicated that his wife had had the abortion without his knowledge: "She did it behind my back. I wouldn't have let her do it."[33]

The remaining 49 inmates who were interviewed fell into three other categories: 27 whose girlfriends aborted, nine whose family members aborted, and thirteen whose friends aborted.

In the group whose girlfriends aborted, seven of the 27 blamed the abortion for the breakdown of the relationship. Of particular note is the interview with Inmate 27 who stated, "Abortion didn't change the relationship. Everything fell back into normal. But there always was the thought about it. She talked about it when we had sex." This couple are no longer together. Twenty of the men reported not feeling that the decision was right and wanting the mother to have the child. Only one inmate expressed an unreservedly positive view of the outcome while two reported an objective, impersonal sentiment: "It should be outlawed except for rape or incest" and "I didn't feel it was right, to do it just for freedom, just because she just didn't feel like it."

Inmate 32 whose girlfriend did not tell him of the decision displays the ambivalence present in so many abortion situations: "I was relieved and thought it was a good decision, although I wish she would have told me...I am not affected in any way except that I'm glad she did it. I'm kind of glad that she didn't tell me."

The 22 men who have been touched by abortion because of family members or friends offer a more dispassionate view of the effects of abortion on others and themselves. One man reported stress as a result of supporting his sister during an abortion. Four men point to abortion as the main cause of marriage breakup in their families. Their accounts of the abortions include family pressure to abort in four cases, fathers not wanting the abortion in four cases, and four cases where the inmates themselves tried to talk their friends out of aborting. These men also describe the significant suffering of six of their women friends following their abortions. As Inmate 52 described it, "She was still messed up after the abortion. She kept telling her daughter, I killed your little brother or sister."

Inmate 48, who described himself as a church pastor, described the young women who had had abortions and who came to his church: "They had a lot of guilt. They wondered if they could be forgiven." Likewise, the men described the pain their male family members and friends suffered:

Inmate 39: "He quit school and then lost his job because of major depression."

Inmate 49: "He [my friend] turned to alcohol. He's always talking about the baby. He is miserable about the whole thing...."

Inmate 45: "My friend went through a lot of
          pain...Through the years it caused problems.
          He talked about it several times. Women
          don't take the man into consideration."[34]

## Male Emotional Reactions

It is quite possible that men experience the same range of
emotions following abortion as do women, but because of
differences in the psychology of the sexes, they have difficulty putting their emotions into words. Ney suggests that
they seem to have "fewer words to describe their feelings."
Or, possibly, they have just as many words, but are less
practiced in expressing their feelings. Men tend to use
activity as a defense or escape. Activities may include thrill
seeking, risk taking, or impulsive action which become the
mechanisms by which they can repress or avoid facing their
consequences of abandoning their partners and their children. Internal repression is often accompanied by external
anger. Ney says, "They tend to funnel many of their feelings
into anger. This is often self-destructive or self-defeating."[35]

In an effort to support men who are suffering following an
abortion, clinicians such as Ava Torre-Bueno and Philip Ney
recommend that they enter into the healing process in the
same way as women. For these men, however, the underlying psychodynamics must be recognized and addressed.
There is an underlying male feeling of failure or impotence
either due to allowing the abortion or forcing the abortion.
As Torre-Bueno puts it, "Men don't get much recognition in
our culture for having feelings."[36]

Those men who learn of the abortion only later or by accidental disclosure display significant ambivalence. This is
clearly the case for Inmate 32 in the Pierce study. On the
one hand, there is a feeling of relief; on the other, a fatalistic
sense that nothing could be done. Yet, there is also a feeling
of guilt.

For men who know about the abortion decision, surprisingly
few protest, though in their lack of protest there is often a
sense of resignation and dejection.[37] Such was the case of

Phil McCombs who, in his *Washington Post* article in 1995 says, "Whatever physical, emotional and spiritual agony the woman suffered, I was not by her side to support her. I turned my face away. My behavior was in all respects craven, immoral...my feelings of responsibility and guilt are undiminished by the fact that the woman had full legal authority to make the decision on her own...I could have made a strong case for having the child. Instead, I urged her along the path of death."[38]

**Conclusion**

From the studies cited above, it is clear that men do suffer after abortion: Men who pressure their partners to abort often suffer a sense of guilt and sorrow later on, and men who are not allowed to participate in the decision or who oppose their partner's decision to abort experience anger and frustration, often leading to the breakup of the relationship. Little research has been carried out, however, to fully document the problem and few programs have been set up to help men resolve the issues that haunt them.

**Key Points Chapter 16**

• There is not much literature on the effects of abortion on men, but what there is clearly demonstrates that many men suffer after an abortion.

• Symptoms include depression, guilt, anger, grief, and feelings of powerlessness.

• In Canada and the United States, men have no legal rights in the decision to abort a child they helped to conceive, which often leads to frustration at their legal disenfranchisement.

• Post-abortion, self-defeating behavior patterns emerge in some men, including abuse of alcohol, drugs, and sex.

• Unmarried relationships often do not remain intact after an abortion.

• Future relationships and fatherhood can be adversely affected by past abortion(s).

• There are few programs for men in which they can express their feelings of ambivalence, grief, or anger after a partner has had an abortion. Many researchers are calling for more studies on the effects of abortion on men and therapeutic counseling for them.

## Notes

1   De Puy C, Dovitch D. *The Healing Choice: Your Guide to Emotional Recovery After an Abortion.* N.Y.: Fireside, 1997.p. 35.

2   De Puy and Dovitch 1997. See n. 1, p. 168.

3   Kluger-Bell K. *Unspeakable Losses: Understanding the Experience of Pregnancy Loss, Miscarriage, and Abortion.* N.Y.: W.W. Norton, 1998; p. 70.

4   Torre-Bueno A. *Peace After Abortion.* San Diego, California: Pimpernel Press, 1997; p. 116.

5   Torre-Bueno 1997. See n. 4, pp. 119-20.

6   Torre-Bueno 1997. See n. 4, p. 126.

7   Torre-Bueno 1997. See n. 4, p. 127.

8   Torre-Bueno 1997. See n. 4, p. 131.

9   Lauzon P, Roger-Achim D, Achim A, Boyer R. Emotional distress among couples involved in first-trimester induced abortions. Canadian Family Physician 2000;46:2033-2040; p. 2033.

10  Rue V. The psychological realities of induced abortion. In: Mannion M, editor. *Post-Abortion Aftermath.* Kansas City: Sheed and Ward, 1994a, p. 24.

11  Ervin P. *Women Exploited: The Other Victims of Abortion.* Huntington, Indiana: Our Sunday Visitor, 1985.

12  Wallerstein JS, Kurtz P, Bar-Din M. Psychosocial sequelae of therapeutic abortion in young unmarried women. Archives of General Psychiatry 1972 December;27(6):828-32; p. 832.

13  Ryan IJ, Dunn PC. College students' attitudes toward shared responsibility in decisions about abortion: implications for counseling. Journal of American College Health 1983 June;31(6):231-5; p. 235.

14  Milling E. The men who wait. Woman's Life 1975 April:48-9,69-71.

Rothstein AA. Men's reactions to their partners' elective abortions. American Journal of Obstetrics and Gynecology 1977 August 15;128(8):831-7.

(a) Francke LB. Abortion and Men. Esquire 1978 September:58-60.
(b) Francke LB. *The Ambivalence of Abortion.* New York: Dell, 1982.

15 Ervin 1984. See n. 11, p. 140.

16 Ajzenstat J, Cassidy E, Carter E, Bierling G. *Going It Alone: Unplanned Single Motherhood in Canada.* Toronto: The de Veber Institute, 1994; p. 65.

17 Ajzenstat et al. 1994. See n. 16, pp. 46-7.

18 Miller WB. An empirical study of the psychological antecedents and consequences of induced abortion. Journal of Social Issues 1992 Fall;48(3):67-93; p. 76.

19 McAll RK, McAll FM. Ritual mourning in anorexia nervosa. The Lancet. 1980 Aug 16;2(8190):368; p. 368.

20 Raphael B. *The Anatomy of Bereavement.* New York: Basic Books, 1983; p. 240.

21 Rue 1994 a. See n. 10.

22 Redmond MA. Attitudes of adolescent males toward adolescent pregnancy and fatherhood. Family Relations: Journal of Applied Family & Child Studies. 1985 July;34(3):337-42.

23 Shostak AB, Mclouth G, Seng L. *Men and Abortion: Lessons, Losses, and Love.* New York: Praeger, 1984; p. 574.

24 Milling 1975. See n. 14.

25 Shostak, Arthur B. Abortion as fatherhood lost: problems and reforms. The Family Coordinator 1979 October:569-74; p. 574.

26 Reardon D. *Aborted Women, Silent No More.* Chicago: Loyola University Press, 1987.

Sutton PM. Fathers, Become Who You Are!: Confronting the Cultures of Fatherlessness and Restoring a Culture of Fatherhood. 11 October 1997. First Presented at the Annual Meeting of the Society of Catholic Social Scientists, October 1996.

27 Rue 1994 a. See n. 10, p. 26.

28 Buchanan M, Robbins C. Early adult psychological consequences for males of adolescent pregnancy and its resolution. Journal of Youth and Adolescence 1990;19(4):413-24.

29 Strahan T. African-Americans and induced abortion. Newsletter of the Association for Interdisciplinary Research in Values and Social Change Nov/Dec 1993;6(1):1-8; p. 4.

30  Amaro H, Fried LE, Cabral H, Zuckerman B. Violence during pregnancy and substance use. American Journal of Public Health 1990 May;80(5):575-9.

31  Bittman S, Zalk Rosenberg S. *Expectant Fathers* (1978). Reprinted. New York: Hawthorn Books, 1980.

32  Pierce L. Abortion attitudes and experiences in a group of male prisoners. Newsletter of the Association for Interdisciplinary Research in Values and Social Change January/February 1994;6(2):1-8; pp. 1-2.

33  Pierce 1994. See n. 32, pp. 2-3.

34  Pierce 1994. See n. 32, pp. 5-7.

35  Ney P, Peeters A. *Hope Alive: Post Abortion and Abuse Treatment. A Training Manual for Therapists*. Victoria, B.C.: Pioneer Publishing, 1993, p. 171.

36  Torre-Bueno 1997. See n. 4.

37  Ney 1993. See n. 35.

38  McCombs P. Remembering Thomas. Washington Post 1995 February 3.

# Chapter 17

# Methodology and Bias:
## Problems with the Way Post-Abortion Research is Done

17

Research on the effects of abortion on women's health, especially in North America, is highly prone to the problem of selective citation: Some researchers refer only to previous studies with which they agree and do not consult, or mention, those studies whose conclusions differ from their own.

Other methodological problems exist: short-term follow up which results in many post-abortion complications not being noted because they present themselves after the woman has left the abortion clinic; bias against any negative news about abortion on the part of many researchers whose vested interest is to make abortion appear safe and trouble-free; coding irregularities that do not connect diseases such as uterine perforations, PID, or ectopic pregnancies (sometimes leading to the patient's death), with previous abortions; and infertility attributed to PID and ectopic pregnancy which are actually consequences of previous abortion(s).

Correctives to these biases are epidemiological studies of the reproductive history of patients which may reveal previous abortions as conditions leading to reproductive difficulties.

# Methodology and Bias:
## Problems with the Way Post-Abortion Research is Done

## A. Problems with the Medical Research

When a literature review is done at the beginning of any new research study, the previous works cited are most often those that support the findings of the author or in which the author has participated as a primary or secondary author (i.e., the author appears in the list of authors but as the third name or later). A database search of the whole field will uncover many more studies. But most of these will be treated as secondary or unimportant, while others will be cited over and over until it appears that they are the seminal works in the field, regardless of the extent to which they obey fundamental rules of research or are regarded as seminal by researchers other than the authors of the study that cites them.

Post-abortion research is plagued, to an especially high degree, by this problem of selective citation. It is subject to a number of other methodological weaknesses as well, including the following:

### 1. Lack of Long-term Follow Up
Most post-abortion research is short-term. This may have a particular impact where late second- trimester abortions are concerned because these women are often lost to follow up altogether.

For example, a Canadian study by Jacot and colleagues shows the difficulty of achieving accurate follow up on women who abort later in pregnancy, even where an effort is made to do so. Researchers were able to contact 90 per cent of women who aborted at five to fourteen weeks gestation, but only 82 per cent of those who aborted at fifteen to twenty weeks. Among women who aborted at seventeen to twenty weeks the researchers were able to contact only 77 per cent, *of whom the vast majority could not or would not be seen in person.*[1]

Claims that there are no complications need to be
considered in light of the unwillingness of many subjects to
participate in studies.

## 2. Bias Against Negative Findings

Many post-abortion problems that have been identified by
researchers in Europe have not become widely accepted in
the North-American literature because on this continent there
is a bias against reporting any kind of negative findings
about induced abortion.

## 3. Underreporting

In addition to the overall bias against negative findings,
there is underreporting in the literature of several specific
problems, as follows:

### a. Uterine Perforations and Adhesions

The literature indicates that there is a high likelihood of
underreporting of uterine perforations which do not cause
excessive bleeding or infection. As a result, conditions such
as Asherman's Syndrome – which produces adhesions that
are not immediately detectable – are only discovered much
later when a patient seeks treatment for infertility. Pelvic
examinations fail to reveal abnormalities.[2] Thus only when a
full work-up is done on those women who attend fertility
clinics is the syndrome detected. This means that three
groups of women will not be identified: 1) Those who
would like to conceive but cannot afford fertility treatment;
2) those who believe that the contraceptive devices they
continue to use are preventing conception when they are in
fact unable to conceive; and 3) those who never later
attempt to conceive children. This inability to identify the
whole population of affected women confounds the
statistical analysis.

### b. Pelvic Inflammatory Disease

Pelvic Inflammatory Disease (PID) may develop one or more
weeks following the abortion but may or may not be linked
to the procedure. How the disease will be coded depends
upon the physician treating the patient, the questions asked,
and the coding provided by the doctor's staff or the hospital

clerks. If the patient has a history of sexually transmitted diseases (STDs), then that fact would be considered as sufficient explanation for the development of PID and the actual trigger event of the abortion may never be recorded.

The European literature is very clear about the significant impact of abortion on women with previous STDs: that they are at high risk for developing PID. But in North America, pre-abortion screening for PID is not mandatory. Indeed, while the North-American literature discusses antibiotic regimes for such cases, it is not certain that most abortion clinics even discuss this risk as part of their intake procedure.

### c. Failed "Medical" Abortion

When a "medical" or drug-induced abortion fails, the woman will most likely be referred for a second attempt – a surgical one. Her body will have sustained two abortion procedures within a few weeks. For the purpose of establishing *epidemiological* risks, does this equal one or two abortions? The subject is not discussed in the literature but, given the growing promotion of drug-induced abortion procedures, it merits more attention than it has been given.

### d. Repeat Abortions

Repeat abortions now make up a significant percentage of all abortions (see Chapter 7). The ways in which these multiple events impact on later health requires further investigation. If women are aborting because they believe that abortion is safe, simple, and without impact on future fertility, they believe too that multiple abortion is also without serious consequences. The recent literature suggests otherwise, but few studies actually consider the long-term epidemiological implications of repeat abortion.

### e. Ectopic Pregnancies

Within fifteen years of the legalization of abortion ectopic pregnancy became epidemic in North America as the title of an article in *Obstetrics & Gynecology* indicates.[3] However, if a woman is admitted to hospital for this condition, the coding may not reflect the fact that she had recently attended for an induced abortion. In fact, the American Centers for Disease Control use the International Classification of Disease (called the revised version of ICD 10) for all death records. The reporting codes available for complications specific to abortion omit Code 633 which designates an ectopic pregnancy. Thus hospitals must enter a code which cannot be cross-referenced to induced abortion.[4]

Indeed, recent case reports in the *Journal of Emergency Medicine* and the *Journal of Pathology* note that ectopic pregnancies were not suspected or identified before the women left the facility. Of such a case, Nugent records that the patient "had an uncomplicated intrauterine abortive procedure two weeks earlier."[6]

In a Canadian study, Jacot and colleagues reported that an ectopic pregnancy "discovered after an unsuccessful uterine aspiration...resulted in a hysterectomy, performed in part for voluntary sterilization."[7] When, upon the discovery of an ectopic pregnancy, hysterectomy is performed "in part" for voluntary sterilization, the abortion connection can easily be missed in the coding.

When ectopic pregnancy follows an induced abortion, the literature usually identifies the cause in some earlier reproductive event such as pelvic inflammatory disease, without ever identifying the PID as a consequence of the abortion.

### 4. Epidemiology

Epidemiology is the discipline that studies the incidence and prevalence of diseases within and across populations. Working at arm's length from the procedure or disease they are investigating, epidemiologists try to identify public health issues and to provide practitioners and regulatory bodies with the information that will assist them in counseling patients, treating disease, or developing public policy.

Because of the limitations inherent in the direct study of abortion, it is becoming evident that the epidemiological approach may be the most fruitful in determining the long-term effects of abortion. When obstetrical or gynecological conditions are considered from an epidemiological perspective, there is some hope that abortion, as it affects later medical problems, may be included as part of the reproductive history of the individual patient.

This area of research, however, is fraught with problems. Presently in North America induced abortion is all too likely to be conflated with spontaneous abortion (miscarriages) or, in some cases, included in a study but never discussed in the body of the text of a given research study. As a result, researchers looking at these papers must extrapolate information from raw data – and be prepared to discover that the raw data presented in the results section of a paper may not support the conclusions as stated in the discussion or abstract section of the same paper. Below are some examples of the discrepancies often found between the hard data and the interpretive conclusions:

### Lipworth

In the Results Section of this study, it was observed that there was a 100 per cent increased risk of breast cancer for women whose first pregnancy ended in abortion, and a 60 per cent increased risk for women who had an induced abortion after first pregnancy.

In the Discussion Section, the author observes, "...perhaps all that can be definitely stated is that any increase associated with induced abortion is at most statistically marginal."[8]

The question arises, however, would most women consider a 60 to 100 per cent increased risk of a serious medical problem to be "statistically marginal"?

### Ewertz and Duffy

In the Results Section of this study, the authors noted that among women who underwent an early terminated first pregnancy and did not experience a subsequent full-term pregnancy, "Induced abortions were associated with a R[elative]R[isk] of 3.85"[9] (or the women who had had an induced abortion were at an almost *fourfold increased* risk of breast cancer).

In the Discussion Section, the authors simply observed that "[our findings] gave further evidence that pregnancies must go to term to exert a protective effect against breast cancer."[10] There is no mention here of the connection of induced abortion to a higher risk of breast cancer.

The authors also lump spontaneous and induced abortion together. In the Abstract (the summary at the beginning of the article) they report the risk effects of spontaneous and induced abortion *together* (our italics) as "...an early terminated first pregnancy RR of 1.43."[11]

### Daling and Colleagues

In the Results Section of their study, these researchers note a RR of 1.2 for breast cancer in nulliparous women whose abortions occurred before age eighteen, and refer to an earlier study in 1994 which came up with a relative risk of 2.5.

Yet they concluded that the "...results of the present study give only slight support to the hypothesis that there is an increase in breast cancer incidence...among women of reproductive age."[12]

How many women would consider a twenty to 150 per cent increase in the risk of breast cancer only "slight"?

In general, the reporting of abortion in national surveys may be approximately 30 per cent less than the actual abortion rate. National reporting is therefore not a reliable method of connecting abortion to future medical conditions, unless a corrective calculation is performed. Exactly what form such a calculation would take is at present unknown.

## B. Problems with the Psychological Research

### Analytic Shortcomings

To look more closely at the literature in the field of psychological outcomes, Rogers and colleagues published a detailed analysis of all 280 research studies which dealt specifically with abortion sequelae. These authors found that of these

280 journal articles, 204 had to be excluded "...because they did not report original empirical data." In other words, only 27 per cent (76 studies) were what would be considered real research with actual subjects. The remaining 73 per cent were reviews that rehashed the findings of the 27 per cent. Indeed, of these 76 studies, only 34 were done after the full legalization in 1973 of abortion in the United States.[13]

Through this analytic approach, Rogers and his colleagues identified twenty different methodological limitations that occurred in the abortion literature. They then calculated the occurrence of each of these flaws within the original research articles. The authors found an average of 6.5 methodological weaknesses in each article. They identified the following problems:

- sample inadequacies because of too few subjects
- often no control group for participants who had had multiple abortions
- samples unrepresentative because of selection bias
- information incomplete: data, methods, follow-up interval, or outcome not reported
- no separation of sample for pre-existing psychiatric history
- no before and after measurements for baseline comparisons
- no control for the potential biases of the experimenter or interviewer
- a significant loss (more than fifteen per cent) of subjects to follow up
- when the decision to abort was for psychiatric reasons, the symptoms might be exaggerated in order to obtain permission for the abortion
- the reliability or validity of the assessment instrument low or unknown

Canadian psychiatrist Philip Ney also considered method-ological difficulties in the psychiatric literature. His classifica-tions bear a striking resemblance to the weaknesses in the psychological articles identified by Rogers and colleagues.

Ney concluded that the main failings were:

* a lack of control or comparison groups (For example, only ten per cent of the 250 studies used by Doane and Quigley used control or comparison groups.[14])
* no analysis of pre-pregnant state to determine the comparative health of the woman after an abortion
* no long-term follow up
* no attempt to relate psychiatric to medical sequelae[15]

Another difficulty has plagued the psychological research: the delegitimation of the finds of researchers known to have a pro-life philosophy.

When David Reardon, a researcher who is pro-life, published a large study using 7500 women who were experiencing post-abortion distress, he was criticized for his retrospective approach and sample inadequacy, even though the majority of post-abortion studies are flawed by small samples and significant sample drop-outs. Similarly, the work of Speckhard and Rue has been ignored or criticized because they have suggested the possibility of *Post-traumatic Stress Disorder (PTSD)* following abortion. In his review, Wilmoth stresses that Reardon, Speckhard and Rue, Barnard, and Vaughan are pro-life researchers, whereas pro-abortion researchers are not designated as pro-abortion. A case in point is a review of Adler's research in Wilmoth: Adler, who is pro-abortion and reports no negative outcomes after abortion, is simply identified as a member of the American Psychological Association's "panel of scientists", thus legitimating her results.[16]

**Political Constraints**

Any technically complex issue lends itself to political manipulation, most notably to attempts to debunk a finding whose key "flaw" may be that it is politically unpopular.

A significant example of defective epidemiological research in North America is the possible link between induced abortion and breast cancer. It has proven difficult to research the subject in North America because of the political issues that surround abortion (see Chapter 2).

The epidemiological impact of factors in the environment and diet on later breast cancer rates is still in the experimental stage. Controversies arise over the effects of certain chemicals and pollutants but the information from breast cancer centers acknowledges both the possible impact as well as the controversial nature of such factors. Unlike diet and environment, induced abortion is seldom mentioned in the patient information material (see Chapter 2).

**Conclusion**

As we have seen, the present state of research misleadingly minimizes the effects of induced abortion in a number of ways. In addition, an undetermined number of post-abortion women who are infertile may be unaware of their infertility because they are (quite unnecessarily) using contraceptives. Another undetermined number may know that they are infertile, but be unable to afford treatment or unwilling to venture into the high-technology fertility area because of ethical concerns. None of these groups will be identified as infertile, even though they are.

It would be prudent to assume that there are more health problems after induced abortion than are being reported under the present system. Women deserve a more careful and accurate system of risk assessment, one that captures more of the data reflecting the actual risk of abortion to their health.

**Key Points Chapter 17**

• Post-abortion research in North America is often
hindered by methodological problems which make it
difficult to ascertain accurately the actual effects of abortion
on women's future health and fertility.

• Post-abortion follow up tends to be short-term, to
suffer from inadequate sample size, no control group, or
incomplete information; consequently, many complications
are not attributed to the procedure.

• Vested interests in North America do not want the public
to hear any bad news about abortion; hence, there is a great
deal of underreporting in the literature about the negative
sequelae of abortion and their possible connection to a
number of medical problems, including low fertility,
prematurity, and breast cancer.

• Irregular coding in hospitals and by the Centers for
Disease Control does not connect many reproductive
problems, such as infertility, pelvic inflammatory disease,
Asherman's Syndrome, complications of failed drug-induced
and repeat abortions, and ectopic pregnancies to previous
abortion(s) when, in fact, abortion is often the trigger cause.
Deaths are inaccurately attributed.

• Women deserve a more accountable system of risk
assessment where research data accurately reflect the true
risks of abortion to their future health and fertility.

## Notes

1  Jacot FR, Poulin C, Bilodeau AP, Morin M, Moreau S, Gendron F, et al. A five-year experience with second- trimester induced abortions: no increase in complication rate as compared to the first trimester. American Journal of Obstetrics and Gynecology 1993 February;168(2):633-7.

2  Heisterberg L. Factors influencing spontaneous abortion, dyspareunia, dysmenorrhea, and pelvic pain. Obstetrics & Gynecology 1993 April;81(4):594-7.

3  Weinstein L, Morris MB, Dotters D, Christian CD. Ectopic pregnancy--a new surgical epidemic. Obstetrics & Gynecology 1983 June;61(6):698-701.

4  World Health Organization. International Classification of Diseases (ICD-10) International Statistical Classification of Diseases and Related Health Problems (ICD-10) Tenth Revision 1992. Geneva.

Crutcher M. *Lime 5: Exploited by Choice*. Denton, Texas: Life Dynamics, 1996:136.

5  Li L, Smialek JE. Sudden death due to rupture of ectopic pregnancy concurrent with theraputic abortion. Archives of Pathology and Laboratory Medicine 1993 July;117(7):698-700.

6  Nugent PJ. Ruptured ectopic pregnancy in a patient with a recent intrauterine abortion. Annals of Emergency Medicine 1992 January;21(1):97-9, p. 97.

7  Jacot et al. 1993. See n. 1, p. 635.

8  Lipworth L, Katsouyanni K, Ekbom A, Michels KB, Trichopoulos D. Abortion and the risk of breast cancer: a case-control study in Greece. International Journal of Cancer 1995 April;61(2):181-4, p. 184.

9  Ewertz M, Duffy SW. Risk of breast cancer in relation to reproductive factors in Denmark. British Journal of Cancer 1988 July;58(1):99-104, p. 102.

10  Ewertz and Duffy, 1988. See n. 9, p. 103.

11  Ewertz and Duffy, 1988. See n. 9, p. 99.

12  Daling JR, Brinton LA, Voigt LF, Weiss NS, Coates RJ, Malone KE, and colleagues. Risk of breast cancer among white women following induced abortion. American Journal of Epidemiology 1996 August;144(4):373-80, p. 379.

13   Rogers JL, Stoms GB, Phifer JL. Psychological impact of abortion: methodological and outcomes summary of empirical research between 1966 and 1988. Health Care for Women International 1989;10(4):347-76.

14   Doane BK, Quigley BG. Psychiatric aspects of therapeutic abortion. Canadian Medical Association Journal 1981 September 1;125(5):427-32.

15   Ney PG, Wickett AR. Mental health and abortion: review and analysis. Psychiatric Journal of the University of Ottawa 1989 November;14(4): 506-16.

16   Reardon D. *Aborted Women, Silent No More*. Chicago: Loyola University Press, 1987.

Wilmoth GH, de Alteriis M, Bussell D. Prevalence of psychological risks following legal abortion in the U.S.: Limits of the evidence. Journal of Social Issues 1992 Fall;48(3):37-66.

Speckhard AC, Rue VM. Postabortion syndrome: an emerging public health concern. Journal of Social Issues 1992 Fall;48:95-119.

Barnard C. The Long Term Psychosocial Effects of Abortion. Portsmouth, N.H.: Institute for Abortion Recovery and Research, 1990.

Vaughan HP. Canonical Variates of Postabortion Syndrome [Doctoral Dissertation]. University of North Carolina at Greensboro, 1990.

Chapter 18

# Informed Consent and Abortion: A Woman's Right to Know

Over the past 30 to 40 years patient autonomy – the principle that patients have the right to know about the nature and the risks of the treatments they are being asked to undergo – has become widely accepted. As a consequence, the idea of informed consent has also developed and become much broader. The courts have established that patients have the right to full information from their doctors about the risks involved in medical treatment, even when the risks are slight. Doctors who fail to provide full information about these risks, and to ensure that their patients have understood the information, are liable to prosecution.

Based on an analysis of nearly 500 medical studies, *Women's Health after Abortion* has documented significant risks associated with induced abortion. They include hemorrhaging, uterine perforation, infection, infertility, subsequent ectopic pregnancy, premature delivery, and death. Doctors have a duty to educate themselves about these risks, and to relay this new knowledge to patients contemplating abortion.

# Informed Consent and Abortion:
# A Woman's Right to Know

The concept of informed consent has evolved considerably over the past century. It began with an early recognition that doctors should not violate the bodily integrity of another person without their permission. From there it progressed to the current concept that informed consent, properly understood, must be considered an essential ingredient of good patient care.

Most medical schools now foster some instruction in law and ethics, exploring the nuances of how truly informed consent is realized when doctors and patients enter into a discussion about proposed treatments or procedures. The concept of informed consent has been clarified and broadened by legal cases before the Supreme Courts of the United States and Canada, and by similar courts in other western countries. A legal precedent is often established when a lawsuit against a physician is advanced on behalf of a patient who has suffered a serious complication of a treatment or procedure about which they feel they were not properly warned. A number of patients have been successful and awarded damages by the courts.

**Informed Consent in Law**
Some of the principles involved in the current legal concepts of informed consent could apply directly to the situation where a woman is considering an induced abortion.[1] The following summary of pertinent health law is drawn from *Canadian Health Law and Policy* and *Legal Liability of Doctors and Hospitals in Canada*.

• The doctor is ultimately liable for information given to a patient, whether or not this has been delegated to a nurse or resident.

• The standard of disclosure has shifted to what a "reasonable or prudent" patient or person might want to know about a procedure, rather than what a "reasonable" doctor might disclose.

- Although the Supreme Court of Canada has allowed that doctors can withhold important information from patients for extenuating or other circumstances, this "therapeutic privilege"[2] should only be exercised in a truly exceptional situation and should not be used to interfere with the patient's right to be informed. Using the information to manipulate a patient's decision, or to protect the health care professional is "ethically inappropriate". The legal role of the information is to allow the patient to exercise choices that accord with his or her wishes.[3]

- Court cases have tended to focus on what the patient was told, but Canadian Chief Justice Bora Laskin has stated that the health care professional must make sure that the patient has understood what he or she was told, particularly if there is a language difference, or extensive technical detail given by the doctor.

- Common but minor risks such as pain after surgery must be disclosed. Rare risks must also be disclosed if they have serious or fatal consequences.

The following are examples of rare risks that were not disclosed to patients, but which resulted in the doctor being found liable:

- A fatal reaction to the dye used in an intravenous pyelogram. The risk ranges between one in 40,000 and one in 100,000.

- Stroke or paralysis from neck manipulation. Here the risk is between one in 100,000 and one in 300,000.

Elective procedures (for example induced abortion) require a greater degree of disclosure than emergency procedures.

Furthermore, the complications from induced abortion, as outlined in this book, carry a risk many times greater than those associated with diagnostic kidney procedures, neck manipulation, etc. It would not be surprising, therefore,

271

to see lawsuits due to failure to obtain proper informed consent to the abortion procedure.

**Informing Consent Prior to Abortion**

Although the practice of abortion has largely broken free of legal restraint in many western countries, intense ongoing social debate about its morality has distracted the medical profession from the type of close scrutiny to which other forms of surgery are subject. The findings of *Women's Health after Abortion* on the breadth of serious potential complications of induced abortion reported throughout the world literature, raise the question of just how informed is the consent obtained from women who presently seek abortion as a solution to an unwanted or troubled pregnancy.

The full realization of patient autonomy in this setting depends on three aspects of medical consent:

1. How *well informed* is the patient?
2. Is the patient fully *competent*, at that moment, to make such a major decision?
3. To what extent is consent given *voluntarily*?

**Uninformed Consent**

In the context of abortion, the likelihood of uninformed consent is very real. Aside from the natural reluctance of abortion doctors to disclose their true immediate surgical complication rate, these practitioners are not in a position to outline medium- or longer-term complications of the procedure, even if they were inclined to do so. Private abortion clinics do not provide after-hours care, or any form of higher-level care for complications such as excessive bleeding, uterine perforation, or systemic infection. Moreover, abortion doctors are unlikely ever to learn of later sequelae such as infertility, life-threatening ectopic pregnancy, subsequent birth prematurity (with its high rate of cerebral palsy), or the late complications of any needed blood transfusions. Nor are they trained to weigh the risks of non-gynecological complications such as breast cancer or depression. As this book documents, the potential complications of abortion are complex, and continue to be uncovered by new research, as the first generation of women to whom abortion was widely available now reaches middle age.

U.S. courts have ruled that it is a doctor's "continuing duty" to inform patients, with up-to-date information, of potential risks. In a similar vein, the Canadian Supreme Court has ruled that manufacturers have a "continuing duty"[5] to inform customers of developing risks. Finally, the marked political polarization of the morality of abortion raises the question of whether individual or establishment bias may prevent these complications from being revealed, in the literature and in consent discussions, thus subverting a woman's access to full disclosure.

**Competent and Voluntary**
The competence of a woman seeking abortion is often assumed because of her young age and otherwise good health. However, competence is relative, and the highly charged atmosphere of an abortion decision may not be conducive to a woman who is emotionally vulnerable, and may be in the midst of a frank clinical depression. True respect for the woman's ability to make a potentially life-altering decision to abort her pregnancy recognizes that depression and other emotional issues may need to be addressed first, especially for a procedure that is almost always elective.

Finally, the voluntary nature of the abortion consent must be considered in context. Many women are referred by a family physician or clinic to a private abortion clinic or hospital gynecologist without an in-depth exploration of the potential risks and complications, on the assumption that "the specialist will deal with it". In fact, the procedure is often then "booked", and, at times, the first and only opportunity for a woman to enter into a discussion to inform her "consent" is on the surgical stretcher as a pre-operative patient, a highly coercive setting in which all of the individuals around her have an expectation of acquiescence.

**A Woman's Right to Know**
A British inquiry into the physical and psycho-social aspects of abortion found it difficult to establish how much informa-

tion is actually given to women prior to abortion. Medical practitioners in Australia and New Zealand have reported concerns over the dearth of information about risks given to women considering abortion. As well, the inadequacy of the current voluntary system of reporting by Statistics Canada and the World Health Organization has led some to call for mandatory reporting of abortion complications.

In order to regulate the timely disclosure of pertinent information to women by abortion providers, fourteen American states have enacted "women's right to know" statutes.[6] At time of writing at least ten other states are considering similar statutes. The Virginia statute mandates a 24-hour wait for women seeking abortion, requiring the facility to give women an explanation of abortion risks, dangers and alternatives, and then wait at least a day before performing the abortion.

The Louisiana Department of Health and Hospitals Act requires a physician to present a document outlining the risks of medical and psychological complications both of pregnancy and abortion, as well as showing various states of fetal development. Pennsylvania includes information about assistance available should the woman decide to carry her pregnancy to full term.

The American Supreme Court has upheld the constitutionality of laws that protect the right of informed consent prior to abortion. In its 1992 ruling upholding the Pennsylvania law the court declared, "In attempting to ensure that a woman apprehend the full consequences of her decision, the State furthers the legitimate purpose of reducing the risk that a woman may elect an abortion, only to discover later, with devastating psychological consequences, that her decision was not fully informed."[7]

**Conclusion**
The unique medical, psychological and political issues surrounding induced abortion pose a challenge to the often frail practice of informed consent. Since the only true choice is an informed choice, women who are considering an

abortion, and the doctors and other health workers who provide them, bear a particular responsibility to ensure that any consent is obtained with full and comprehensive disclosure of the potential risks, that it is fully understood, and that it is presented in a non-coercive setting.

**Key Points Chapter 18**

• The concept of informed consent has been clarified and broadened by the Supreme Courts of the United States and Canada, as well as by courts in other western countries.

• The courts have ruled that doctors have a "continuing duty" to be familiar with up-to-date information about potential and developing risks of treatments or procedures in order to inform patients properly.

• The standard of disclosure has shifted to what a "reasonable or prudent" patient might want to know about a procedure, rather than what a "reasonable" doctor might disclose.

• Common but minor risks must be disclosed, while rare risks must be disclosed if the consequences are potentially serious or fatal.

• The doctor must also ensure that the patient has understood what he or she has been told.

• Doctors who fail to inform their patients about the documented risks associated with induced abortion may be liable to prosecution in the courts.

## Notes

1  Picard EI and Robertson GB. *Legal Liability of Doctors and Hospitals in Canada.* Toronto: Carswell, 1996; Chapter 3. 110-157.

Dickens BM. "Informed Consent: The Doctor's Duty of Disclosure" Chapter 5 in Downie J. and Caulfield T. *Canadian Health Law and Policy.* Toronto: Butterworths, 1999; pp. 117-141.

2  Dickens 1999. See n. 1, p. 137.

3  Dickens 1999. See n. 1, p. 118.

4  Picard and Robertson 1996. See n. 1, p. .127.

6  Picard and Robertson 1996 . See n. 1, p. 153.

5  Arkansas, Kansas, Louisiana, Michigan, Mississippi, Nebraska, North Dakota, Ohio, Pennsylvania, South Carolina, South Dakota, Utah, Virginia, and Wisconsin.

7  Planned Parenthood of Southeastern Pennsylvania v. Casey, 112 S. Ct. 2791, 2823-24 (1992).

# Conclusion

In this book we have seen that the consequences of induced abortion for women and for the health of their future children is much graver than used to be thought. Of the 25 to 30 million women in North America who have undergone an induced abortion over the past 33-34 years, at least eleven per cent, at a conservative estimate, have experienced physical or psychological complications.

Some of these complications are short term and manageable. They range from pain, bleeding and fevers to perforation of the uterus, retained fetal or placental tissue, and sepsis. Other consequences are longer term and profoundly serious in their implications. They include a higher rate of pelvic inflammatory disease (PID) and sexually-transmitted diseases (STDs), placenta previa, and damage to the uterus and cervix which impair a woman's ability to conceive and bear children. There is also a higher rate of ectopic pregnancy.

Not only does abortion drastically increase a woman's risk of having a premature delivery the next time she becomes pregnant, prematurity itself is associated with a huge increase in cerebral palsy among newborns. Abortion leads to an 86 to 267 per cent increase in the risk of prematurity. Prematurity in turn leads to a more than 3700 per cent increase in cerebral palsy. Induced abortion is therefore directly responsible for a medical tragedy of serious proportions.

Many studies downplay the impact of abortion on women's future fertility. But a British study done under the auspices of the Royal College of Physicians and Surgeons found that women who had abortions experienced six per cent lower fertility than those who did not. Infertility is such a significant consequence of abortion that it needs to be studied more intensively and over a much longer period of time. At present many women do not even know that they are at risk or should be seeking treatment for infertility.

The abortion pill misopristone (RU-486) has been hailed in some quarters as a simple, safe, effective alternative to surgical abortion. According to one glowing testimonial this pill enables physicians now to do abortions in their offices, thereby making the procedure available to many more women. The reality is more sobering:

1. The failure rate is higher than with surgical abortion;
2. The complication rate is higher;
3. Women have to wait an average of 24 days to find out if their abortion has actually worked. The emotional effect of this long period of uncertainty can easily be imagined.

Although its incidence is low, maternal death is one of the real risks of abortion. Abortion's defenders have long asserted that it is safer than childbirth. Recent massive studies in Scandinavia, Britain and the U.S. have now relegated this claim to the realm of fiction. The death rate among women, one to four years after their abortions, is many times greater than among women who deliver their babies. These recent studies, based on record-linkage, serve to underline the limitations of conventional methods of examining abortion mortality. The conventional methods have long been bedeviled by coding problems and by deliberate obfuscation of the problem.

This book has also shown that a history of previous induced abortion is associated with a higher risk of cervical, ovarian and colorectal cancer. More disturbingly, 27 studies worldwide have documented an average 30 per cent increased risk of breast cancer among women who have abortions. The chilling reality is that a young woman who opts to abort her first pregnancy rather than carry the pregnancy through to delivery nearly doubles her lifetime risk of breast cancer. Until recently the North-American research community has been loath to recognize the validity of these findings. Only in the past two years has the pioneering work of Joel Brind in this field begun to win grudging acceptance.

The difficulties of measuring the physical consequences of abortion are legion. These difficulties are compounded when it comes to the emotional and psychological aftermath of abortion. To begin with, a significant proportion of women simply refuse to be interviewed about their experience. Much more work needs to be done, but already we know that women who have an abortion are much likelier to commit suicide than women who deliver their babies. We also know that women often feel ambivalent about their decision to abort. When offered supportive counseling, as they are in Sweden, they are more likely not to abort. In many instances, abortion, far from being a woman's free choice, is the product of coercive pressure from her male partner or family. It is also known that abortion is often not a good solution for women who have a psychiatric history, live in abusive relationships, believe abortion is morally wrong, or are adolescents. Abortion deepens the tribulation of these women. Our findings lead us to pose the question: Should those who counsel women contemplating an abortion not be more alert to these negative psychological sequelae? Should they not consider, in some cases at least, steering depressed, guilty, angry, anxious, or young women *away* from abortion?

Women who have abortions experience greater rates of substance abuse (including tobacco, alcohol and non-medical drugs). There is some evidence that they are also susceptible to eating disorders such as anorexia, to sexual dysfunction, and to psychic numbing or absence of affect. Abortion is also associated with higher rates of marital breakups and relationship dissolution. A mother's relationship with her other children may also be adversely affected.

This survey of the medical and psychological literature has led us to conclude that the consequences we have outlined are more numerous and far reaching than most specialists in the field have suspected. Much more research is needed, particularly to determine abortion's long-term impact on women physical and mental health.

For the present, those professionals who deal with women considering abortion have a duty to acquaint themselves with the evidence that has been accumulated so far. Women have a right to know about the evidence of abortion's consequences. Without this knowledge they are in no position to give their informed consent to the procedure.

# References

1 Adam S, Wiggins S, Whyte P, Bloch M, Shokeir MH, Soltan H, et al. "Five Year Study of Prenatal Testing for Huntington's Disease: Demand, Attitudes, and Psychological Assessment." *Journal of Medical Genetics* 30, no. 7 (July 1993): 549-56.

2. Adami HO, Bergstrom R, Lund E and Meirik O. "Absence of Association between Reproductive Variables and the Risk of Breast Cancer in Young Women in Sweden and Norway." *British Journal of Cancer* 62, no. 1 (July 1990): 122-6.

3. Adler NE, David HP, Major BN, Roth SH, Russo NF and Wyatt GE. "Psychological Responses after Abortion." *Science* 248, no. 4951 (6 April 1990): 41-4.

4. Adler, Nancy E. "Abortion: A Social-Psychological Perspective." *The Journal of Social Issues* 35, no. 1 (1979): 100-19.

5. Ajzenstat, J, E. Cassidy, E. Carter and G Bierling. *Going It Alone: Unplanned Single Motherhood in Canada.* Toronto: The deVeber Institute, 1994.

6. Albrektsen, G, I Heuch, S Tretli and G Kvale. "Is the Risk of Cancer of the Corpus Uteri Reduced by a Recent Pregnancy? A Prospective Study of 765,756 Norwegian Women." *International Journal of Cancer* 61, no. 4 (16 May 1995): 485-90.

7. Alexander PC. "Application of Attachment Theory to the Study of Sexual Abuse." *Journal of Consulting and Clinical Psychology* 60, no. 2 (April 1992): 185-95.

8. Allanson S and Astbury J. "The Abortion Decision: Reasons and Ambivalence." *Journal of Psychosomatic Obstetrics and Gynecology* 16, no. 3 (September 1995): 123-36.

9. Amaro H, Fried LE, Cabral H and Zuckerman B. "Violence During Pregnancy and Substance Use." *American Journal of Public Health* 80, no. 5 (May 1990): 575-9.

10. Ancel PY, Saurel-Cubizolles MJ, Di Renzo GC, Papiernik E and Breart G. "Very and Moderate Preterm Births: Are the Risk Factors Different?" *British Journal of Obstetrics and Gynaecology* 106, no. 11 (November 1999): 1162-70.

11. Andrieu N, Clavel F, Gairard B, Piana LBremond A, Lansac J, Flamant R and Renaud R. "Familial Risk of Breast Cancer and Abortion." *Cancer Detection and Prevention* 18, no. 1 (1994): 51-5.

281

12. Andrieu N, Duffy SW, Rohan TE, Le MG, Luporsi E, Gerber M, et al. "Familial Risk, Abortion and Their Interactive Effect on the Risk of Breast Cancer–a Combined Analysis of Six Case-Control Studies." *British Journal of Cancer* 72, no. 3 (September 1995.): 744-51.

13. Appleby L. "Suicide During Pregnancy and in the First Postnatal Year." *British Medical Journal* 302, no. 6769 (19 January 1991): 137-40.

14. Armstrong K, Eisen A and Weber B. "Assessing the Risk of Breast Cancer." *New England Journal of Medicine* 342, no. 8 (24 February 2000): 564-71.

15. Atrash HK, Cheek TG and Hogue CJ. "Legal Abortion Mortality and General Anesthesia." *American Journal of Obstetrics and Gynecology* 158, no. 2 (February 1988): 420-4.

16. Atrash HK, Koonin LM, Lawson HW, Franks AL and Smith JC. "Maternal Mortality in the United States, 1979-1986." *Obstetrics & Gynecology* 76, no. 6 (December 1990): 1055-60.

17. Atrash HK, MacKay HT and Hogue CJ. "Ectopic Pregnancy Concurrent with Induced Abortion: Incidence and Mortality." *American Journal of Obstetrics and Gynecology* 162, no. 3 (March 1990): 726-30.

18. Bacelar AC, Wilcock D, Powell M and Worthington BS. "The Value of MRI in the Assessment of Traumatic Intra-Uterine Adhesions (Asherman's Syndrome)." *Clinical Radiology* 50, no. 2 (February 1995): 80-3.

19. Bader, Eleanor J. "Stranger In A Strange Land: Attending A Right To Life Conference." *On The Issues: The Journal of Substance For Progressive Women* 13 (1989): 10-3.

20. Baker A. "Helping Clients Manage Pain and Fear of Pain." In *Abortion and Options Counseling: A Comprehensive Reference.* Granite City, Illinois: Hope Clinic For Women, 1995.

21. Baker, M. "Men and Abortion." *Esquire,* March 1990, 116-26.

22. Barbacci MB, Spence MR, Kappus EW, Burkman RC, Rao L and Quinn TC. "Postabortal Endometritis and Isolation of Chlamydia Trachomatis." *Obstetrics & Gynecology* 68, no. 5 (November 1986): 686-90.

23. Barnard C. *The Long Term Psychosocial Effects of Abortion.* Portsmouth, N.H.: Institute for Abortion Recovery and Research, 1990.

24. Barnett W, Freudenberg N and Wille R. "Partnership after Induced Abortion: A Prospective Controlled Study." *Archives of Sexual Behavior* 21, no. 5 (October 1992): 443-55.

25. Barrett JM, Boehm FH and Killam AP. "Induced Abortion: A Risk Factor for Placenta Previa." *American Journal of Obstetrics Gynecology* 141, no. 7 (1 December 1981): 769-72.

26. Beckwith FJ. "Absolute Autonomy and Physician-Assisted Suicide: Putting A Bad Idea Out Of Its Misery." In *Life and Learning VII: Proceedings of Seventh University Faculty for Life Conference in Loyola College, Baltimore 1997*, ed. Joseph Koterski, S.J. Washington, D.C.: University Faculty for Life, 1998.

27. Bégin, I. "Mortality and Morbidity Coding in Canada and the World – Pitfalls and Shortcomings", 1999 [Unpublished Paper].

28. Belanger E, Melzack R and Lauzon P. "Pain of the First Trimester Abortion: A Study of Psychosocial and Medical Predictors." *Pain* 36, no. 3 (March 1989): 339-50.

29. Bellingham FR. "Endometrial Bone Formation." *Australian and New Zealand Journal of Obstetrics and Gynecology* 36, no. 1 (February 1996): 109-10.

30. Belsey EM, Greer HS, Lal S, Lewis SC and Beard RW. "Predictive Factors in Emotional Response to Abortion: King's Termination Study–IV." *Social Science and Medicine* 11, no. 2 (January 1977): 71-82.

31. Benedict, MI, White, RB, and Cornely DA. "Maternal Perinatal Risk Factors and Child Abuse." *Child Abuse and Neglect* 9, no. 2 (1985): 217-24.

32. Berg CJ, Atrash HK, Koonin LM and Tucker M. "Pregnancy-Related Mortality in the United States, 1987-1990." *Obstetrics & Gynecology* 88, no. 2 (August 1996): 161-7.

33. Berger C, Gold D, Andres D, Gillett P and Kinch R. "Repeat Abortion: Is It a Problem?" *Family Planning Perspectives* 16, no. 2 (March-April 1984): 70-5.

34. Berkowitz GS. "An Epidemiologic Study of Preterm Delivery." *American Journal of Epidemiology* 113, no. 1 (January 1981): 81-92.

35. Berkowitz RL, Lynch L, Stone J and Alvarez M. "The Current Status of Multifetal Pregnancy Reduction." *American Journal of Obstetrics and Gynecology* 174, no. 4 (April 1996): 1265-72.

36. Bernal A, Mendez-Moran L, Fajardo-Gutierrez A, Gonzalez-Lira G, Escudero P and Ortiz H. "Univariate and Multivariate Analysis of Risk Factors for Ovarian Cancer: Case-Control Study, Mexico City." *Archives of Medical Research* 26, no. 3 (1995, Autumn): 245-9.

37. Bierling, G, E Cassidy, and E Carter. "Agency and Maternal Perceptions of the Decision to Parent." In *Life and Learning IV: Proceedings of Fourth University Faculty for Life Conference in Fordham University*, ed. Joseph Koterski, S.J. Washington, D.C.: University Faculty for Life, 1995.

38. Bittman, Sam and Sue Zalk Rosenberg. *Expectant Fathers*. 1978; reprint, New York: Hawthorn Books, 1980.

39. Black RB. "A 1 and 6 Month Follow-Up of Prenatal Diagnosis Patients Who Lost Pregnancies." Prenatal Diagnosis 9, no. 11 (November 1989): 795-804.

40. Blackwell AL, Thomas PD, Wareham K and Emery SJ. "Health Gains from Screening for Infection of the Lower Genital Tract in Women Attending for Termination of Pregnancy." *The Lancet* 342, no. 8865 (24 July 1993): 206-10.

41. Blomain, Karen. "Customer Review of An Empty Lap : One Couple's Journey to Parenthood, by Jill Smolowe." [http://www.amazon.com/exec/obidos/tg/stores/detail/-/books/0671004379/customer-reviews/107-9690183-1333303]. 31 October 1997.

42. Bluestein D and Rutledge CM. "Family Relationships and Depressive Symptoms Preceding Induced Abortion." *The Family Practice Research Journal* 13, no. 2 (June 1993): 149-56.

43. Blumberg BD, Golbus MS and Hanson KH. "The Psychological Sequelae of Abortion Performed for a Genetic Indication." American Journal of Obstetrics and Gynecology 122, no. 7 (1 August 1975): 799-808

44. Bognar Z and Czeizel A. "Mortality and Morbidity Associated with Legal Abortions in Hungary, 1960-1973." *American Journal of Public Health* 66, no. 6 (June 1976): 568-75.

45. Boivin J, Andersson L, Skoog-Svanberg A, Hjelmstedt A, Collins A, Bergh T. "Psychological Reactions During In-Vitro Fertilization: Similar Response Pattern in Husbands and Wives." *Human Reproduction* 13, no. 11 (Nov. 1998): 3262-7.

46. Bollen N, Camus M, Tournaye H, Wisanto A, Van Steirteghem A, Devroey P. "Embryo Reduction in Triplet Pregnancies after Assisted Procreation: A Comparative Study." *Fertility and Sterility* 60, no. 3 (September 1993): 504-9.

47. Borgatta L and Nickinovich D. "Pain During Early Abortion." *Journal of Reproductive Medicine* 42, no. 5 (May 1997): 287-93.

48. Boss JA. "First Trimester Prenatal Diagnosis: Earlier Is Not Necessarily Better." *Journal of Medical Ethics* 20, no. 3 (September 1994): 146-51.

49. Boulot P, Hedon B, Pelliccia G, et al. "Effects of Selective Reduction in Triplet Gestation: A Comparative Study of 80 Cases Managed with or without This Procedure." *Fertility and Sterility* 60, no. 3 (September 1993): 497-503.

50. Bracken MB, Klerman LV and Bracken M. "Coping with Pregnancy Resolution Among Never-Married Women." *American Journal of Orthopsychiatry* 48, no. 2 (April 1978): 320-4.

51. Brende, Joel Osler. "Fragmentation of the Personality Associated with Post-Abortion Trauma." *Newsletter of the Association for Interdisciplinary Research in Values and Social Change* 8, no. 3 (July/August 1995): 1-8.

52. Brewer C. "Prevention of Post-Abortion Infection." *The Lancet* 342, no. 8874 (25 September 1993): 802.

53. Brind J, Chinchilli VM, Severs WB and Summy Long J. "Induced Abortion and Risk for Breast Cancer: Reporting (Recall) Bias in a Dutch Case-Control Study [Letter and Comment]." *Journal of the National Cancer Institute* 89, no. 8 (15 April 1997): 588-90.

54. _____. "Induced Abortion as an Independent Risk Factor for Breast Cancer: A Comprehensive Review and Meta-Analysis." *Journal of Epidemiology and Community Health* 50, no. 5 (October 1996): 481-96.

55. Brind J. "Abortion, Breast Cancer, and Ideology." In *Life And Learning VII: Proceedings of University Faculty For Life in Loyola College, Baltimore, Maryland June 1997*, ed. Joseph W. Koterski, S.J., 139-44.

56. Brind, J and VM Chinchilli. "Induced Abortion and Risk of Breast Cancer." *Epidemiology* 11 (2000): 234-5.

57. Brinton LA, Daling JR, Liff JM, Schoenberg JB, Malone KE and Stanford JL. "Oral Contraceptives and Breast Cancer Risk Among Younger Women." *Journal of the National Cancer Institute* 87, no. 11 (7 June 1995): 827-35.

58. Brinton L, Hoover R, Fraumeni JF Jr. "Reproductive Factors in the Aetiology of Breast Cancer." *British Journal of Cancer* 47, no. 6 (June 1983): 757-62.

59. Brock KE, Berry G, Brinton LA, Kerr C, et al. "Sexual, Reproductive and Contraceptive Risk Factors for Carcinoma-in-Situ of the Uterine Cervix in Sydney." *Medical Journal of Australia* 150, no. 3 (6 February 1989): 125-30.

60. Brown D, Elkins T, Larson D. "Prolonged Grieving after Abortion: A Descriptive Study." *Journal of Clinical Ethics* 4, no. 2 (1993 Summer): 118-23.

61. Brown, Judy (pseudonym). "A Piece of My Mind. The Choice." *Journal of the American Medical Association* 262, no. 19 (17 November 1989): 2735.

62. Buchanan, Mary and Cynthia Robbins. "Early Adult Psychological Consequences for Males of Adolescent Pregnancy and Its Resolution." *Journal of Youth and Adolescence* 19, no. 4 (1990): 413-24.

63. Bugalho A, Bique C, Almeida L and Faundes A. "The Effectiveness of Intravaginal Misoprostol (Cytotec) in Inducing Abortion after Eleven Weeks of Pregnancy." *Studies in Family Planning* 24, no. 5 (September-October 1993): 319-23.

64. Bugalho A, Bique C, Almeida L, Bergstrom S. "Pregnancy Interruption by Vaginal Misoprostol." *Gynecologic and Obstetric Investigation* 36, no. 4 (1993): 226-9.

65. Burany B. "[Gestational Characteristics in Women with Breast Cancer].[Article in Serbo-Croatian (Roman)." *Jugosl Ginekol Opstet* 19, no. 5-6 (September-December 1979): 237-47.

66. Busetti MC, Miller AB, To T and Rohan TE. "Risk Factors for Breast Cancer Mortality Among the National Breast Screening Study of Canada Participants." *Cancer Detection and Prevention* 20, no. 2 (1996): 122-9.

67. Calle EE, Mervis CA, Wingo PA, Thun MJ, Rodriguez C and Heath CW Jr. "Spontaneous Abortion and Risk of Fatal Breast Cancer in a Prospective Cohort of United States Women." *Cancer Causes and Control* 6, no. 5 (September 1995): 460-8.

68. Campbell, NB, K Franco and S Jurs. "Abortion in Adolescence." *Adolescence* 23, no. 92 (Winter 1988): 813-23.

69. Campion, Bridget. "An Argument for Continuing a Pregnancy Where the Fetus Is Discovered to Be Anencephalic." In *Life and Learning IX: Proceedings of University Faculty for Life in Trinity International University 1999*, ed. Koterski, JW. Washington, D.C.: University Faculty for Life, 2000.

70. Canadian PID (Pelvic Inflammatory Disease) Society. *Submission to the Royal Commission on Health Care and Costs*, October 1990.

71. Canty, L. "Breast Cancer Risk: Protective Effect of an Early First Full-Term Pregnancy Versus Increased Risk of Induced Abortion [Review]." *Oncological Nurses Forum* 24, no. 6 (July 1997): 1025-31.

72. Capella-Allouc S, Morsad F, Rongieres-Bertrand C, Taylor S and Fernandez H. "Hysteroscopic Treatment of Severe Asherman's Syndrome and Subsequent Fertility." *Human Reproduction* 14, no. 5 (May 1999): 1230-3.

73. Cassidy, Elizabeth. "Multifetal Pregnancy Reduction (MFPR): The Psychology of Desperation and the Ethics of Justification." In *Life and Learning IX: Proceedings of Ninth Annual Meeting, University Faculty for Life in Deerfield, Illinois 1999*, ed. Koterski, Joseph, S.J., 331-46. Washington, D.C.: University Faculty for Life, 2000.

74. _____. "Psychological Decision Making Models: An Extension of Miller's Abortion Decision Models to Miscarriage and Genetic Abortion in Light of the Human Genome Project", June 1997 [Unpublished Conference Paper]. University Faculty for Life.

75. Castadot RG. "Pregnancy Termination: Techniques, Risks, and Complications and Their Management." *Fertility and Sterility* 45, no. 1 (January 1986): 5-17.

76. Chan NS. "Intrauterine Retention of Fetal Bone." *Australian and New Zealand Journal of Obstetrics and Gynecology* 36, no. 3 (August 1996): 368-71.

77. Chen MT, Cook LS, Daling JR and Weiss NS. "Incomplete Pregnancies and Risk of Ovarian Cancer (Washington, United States)." *Cancer Causes and Control* 7, no. 4 (7 July 1996): 415-20.

78. Chervenak FA, McCullough LB and Wapner R. "Three Ethically Justified Indications for Selective Termination in Multifetal Pregnancy: A Practical and Comprehensive Management Strategy." *Journal of Assisted Reproduction and Genetics* 12, no. 8 (September 1995): 531-6.

79. Chipman, John. "Study Claims Abortion Cuts Crime." *The National Post*, 17 May 2001, A, 1.

80. Christin-Maitre S, Bouchard P and Spitz IM. "Medical Termination of Pregnancy." *New England Journal of Medicine* 342, no. 13 (March 2000): 946-56.

81. Chung CS, Smith RG, Steinhoff PG and Mi MP. "Induced Abortion and Ectopic Pregnancy in Subsequent Pregnancies." *American Journal of Epidemiology* 115, no. 6 (June 1982): 879-87.

82. Clare, Anthony and Janette Tyrrell. "Psychiatric Aspects of Abortion." *Irish Journal of Psychological Medicine* 11, no. 2 (June 1994): 92-8.

83. Coccia ME, Becattini C, Bracco GL and Scarselli G. "Ultrasound-Guided Hysteroscopic Management of Endometrial Osseous Metaplasia." *Ultrasound Obstetrics and Gynecology* 8, no. 2 (August 1996): 134-6.

84. Cohen J. "How to Avoid Multiple Pregnancies in Assisted Reproduction." *Human Reproduction* 13, no. Supplement 3 (June 1998): 197-214; discussion 215-8.

85. Cole, P. M. and C. Woolger. "Incest Survivors: The Relation of Their Perceptions of Their Parents and Their Own Parenting Attitudes." *Child Abuse and Neglect* 13, no. 3 (1989): 409-16.

86. Coleman PK, Reardon DC and Cougle JR. "Child Developmental Outcomes Associated with Maternal History of Abortion Using the NLSY Data." *Archives of Women's Mental Health* 3, no. 4 Supp.2 (2001): 104.

87. Coleman, P.K., W. Franz and D. Reardon. "The Salience of Pressure to Obtain an Abortion as a Predictor of Post-Abortion Adjustment in Adolescents and Adult Women", 1998 [Unpublished Manuscript].

88. Collett TS. "Abortion Malpractice: Exploring the Safety of Legal Abortion." In *Proceedings of Fifth University Faculty for Life Conference in Marquette University June 1995*, vol. V, ed. Koterski, JW, S.J., 243-72, Life and Learning.

89. Collins FS and Mahoney MJ. "Hydrocephalus and Abnormal Digits after Failed First-Trimester Prostaglandin Abortion Attempt." *Journal of Pediatrics* 102, no. 4 (April 1983): 620-1.

90. The Commonwealth Fund. *National Survey of Women's Health*, 14 July 1993.

91. Congleton GK and Calhoun LG. "Post-Abortion Perceptions: A Comparison of Self-Identified Distressed and Nondistressed Populations." *International Journal of Social Psychiatry* 39, no. 4 (Winter 1993): 255-65.

92. Coste J, Job-Spira N and Fernandez H. "Risk Factors for Spontaneous Abortion: A Case-Control Study in France." *Human Reproduction* 6, no. 9 (October 1991): 1332-7.

93. Cougle JR, Reardon DC, Rue VM, Shuping MW, Coleman PK and Ney PG. "Psychiatric Admissions Following Abortion and Childbirth: A Record-Based Study of Low-Income Women." *Archives of Women's Mental Health* 3, no. (4) Suppl 2 (2001): 47.

94. Council on Scientific Affairs, American Medical Association. "Induced Termination of Pregnancy Before and After Roe V Wade. Trends in the Mortality and Morbidity of Women." *Journal of the American Medical Association* 268, no. 22 (9 December 1992): 3231-9.

95. Cozzarelli C. "Personality and Self-Efficacy as Predictors of Coping with Abortion." *Journal of Personality and Social Psychology* 65, no. 6 (December 1993): 1224-36.

96. Crawford D and Mannion M. *Psychospiritual Healing After Abortion.* Kansas City: Sheed and Ward, 1989.

97. Creinin MD. "Methotrexate and Misoprostol for Abortion At 57-63 Days Gestation." *Contraception* 50, no. 6 (December 1994): 511-5.

98. _____. "Methotrexate for Abortion at <42 Days." *Contraception* 48, no. 6 (December 1993): 519-25.

99. Creinin MD and Darney PD. "Methotrexate and Misoprostol for Early Abortion." *Contraception* 48, no. 4 (October 1993): 339-48.

100. Creinin MD and Vittinghoff E. "Methotrexate and Misoprostol vs. Misoprostol Alone for Early Abortion: A Randomized Controlled Trial." *Journal of the American Medical Association* 272, no. 15 (19 October 1994): 1190-5.

101. Crutcher M. *Lime 5: Exploited by Choice*. Denton, Texas: Life Dynamics, 1996.

102. Curry MA, Perrin N and Wall E. "Effects of Abuse on Maternal Complications and Birth Weight in Adult and Adolescent Women." *Obstetrics & Gynecology* 92, no. 4 Pt 1 (October 1998): 530-4.

103. Curtis, Melanie and Lionel Standing. "The Decision to Abort: No Sex-Role Bias, and Little Enthusiasm." *Social Behavior & Personality* 20, no. 4 (1992): 237-42.

104. Dagg PK. "The Psychological Sequelae of Therapeutic Abortion–Denied and Completed." *American Journal of Psychiatry* 148, no. 5 (May 1991): 578-85.

105. Daling JR, Brinton LA, Voigt LF, Weiss NS, Coates RJ, Malone KE, et al. "Risk of Breast Cancer Among White Women Following Induced Abortion." *American Journal of Epidemiology* 144, no. 4 (August 1996): 373-80.

106. Daling JR, Chow WH, Weiss NS, Metch BJ and Soderstrom R. "Ectopic Pregnancy in Relation to Previous Induced Abortion." *Journal of the American Medical Association* 253, no. 7 (February 1985): 1005-8.

107. Daling JR, Malone KE, Voigt LF, White E and Weiss NS. "Risk of Breast Cancer Among Young Women: Relationship to Induced Abortion." *Journal of The National Cancer Institute* 86, no. 21 (2 November 1994): 1584-92.

108. David HP. "Post-Abortion and Post-Partum Psychiatric Hospitalization." *Ciba Foundation Symposium* 115 (1985): 150-64.

109. DePuy, C and D Dovitch. *The Healing Choice: Your Guide to Emotional Recovery After an Abortion*. Fireside, 1997.

110. Deutsch, Marjorie B. "Personality Factors, Self Concept, and Family Variables Related to First Time and Repeat Abortion-Seeking Behavior in Adolescent Women." Doctoral Dissertation, The American University, 1982.

111. deVeber, LL, J Ajzenstat and D Chisholm. "Postabortion Grief: Psychological Sequelae of Medical Abortion." *Humane Medicine* (1991): 203-9.

112. Dickens, Bernard M. "Informed Consent." In *Canadian Health Law and Policy*, eds. Jocelyn Downie, J. Caulfield and Timothy Caulfield, 117-41. Toronto and Vancouver: Butterworths, 1999.

113. Dirks, Marth Jean. "Psychological Outcomes of Abortion: An Exploration of Knowledge, Conflict, and Expectancies." Doctoral Dissertation, University of Cincinnati, 1979.

114. Doane BK, Quigley B. "Psychiatric Aspects of Therapeutic Abortion." *Canadian Medical Association Journal* 125, no. 5 (1 Sept. 1981): 427-32.

115. Donati S, Medda E, Proietti S, Rizzo L, Spinelli A, Subrizi D, et al. "Reducing Pain of First Trimester Abortion Under Local Anaesthesia." *European Journal of Obstetrics & Gynecology and Reproductive Biology* 70, no. 2 (27 December 1996): 145-9.

116. Donohue, John J. and Steven Levitt. "The Impact of Legalized Abortion on Crime." *The Quarterly Journal of Economics* CXVI, no. 2 (May 2001): 379-420.

117. Donnai P, Charles N and Harris R. "Attitudes of Patients After "Genetic" Termination of Pregnancy." British Medical Journal 282, no. 6264 (21 February 1981): 621-2.

118. Drake H, Reid M and Marteau T. "Attitudes Towards Termination for Fetal Abnormality: Comparisons in Three European Countries." *Clinical Genetics* 49, no. 3 (March 1996): 134-40.

119. Drower, SJ and ES Nash. "Therapeutic Abortion on Psychiatric Grounds: Part I. A Local Study." *South African Medical Journal* (7 October 1978): 604-8.

120. Dunlop JL. "Counselling of Patients Requesting an Abortion." *Practitioner* 220 (June 1978): 847-52.

121 Duthie SJ, Hobson D, Tait IA, BC Pratt, N Lowe, PJL Sequeira and C Hargreaves. "Morbidity after Termination of Pregnancy in First Trimester." *Genitourinary Medicine* 63 (1987): 183-7.

122. Dvoirin, VV and Medvedev AB. "Role of Women's Reproductive Status in the Development of Breast Cancer." In *Methods and Progress in Breast Cancer Epidemiology Research*, Tallin, 1978, 53-63. Moscow: Oncology Science Centre of the USSR Academy of Sciences, 1978.

123. Egeland, B, D Jacobvitz and LA. Sroufe. "Breaking the Cycle of Abuse." *Child Development* 59 (1988): 1080-8.

124. el-Refaey H, Rajasekar D, Abdalla M, Calder L and Templeton A. "Induction of Abortion with Mifepristone (RU 486) and Oral or Vaginal Misoprostol." *New England Journal of Medicine* 332, no. 15 (April 1995): 983-7.

125. el-Refaey H and Templeton A. "Induction of Abortion in the Second Trimester by a Combination of Misoprostol and Mifepristone: A Randomized Comparison Between Two Misoprostol Regimens." *Human Reproduction* 10, no. 2 (February 1995): 475-8

126. el-Refaey H, Templeton A. "Early Induction of Abortion by a Combination of Oral Mifepristone and Misoprostol Administered by the Vaginal Route." *Contraception* 49, no. 2 (February 1994): 111-4.

127. Elder SH and Laurence KM. "The Impact of Supportive Intervention after Second Trimester Termination of Pregnancy for Fetal Abnormality." *Prenatal Diagnosis* 11, no. 1 (January 1991): 47-54.

128 Elliott JP. "Multifetal Reduction of Triplets to Twins Improves Perinatal Outcome." *American Journal of Obstetrics and Gynecology* 171, no. 1 (July 1994): 278.

129. Ervin, Paula. *Women Exploited: The Other Victims of Abortion.* Huntington, Indiana: Our Sunday Visitor, 1985.

130. Escobar GJ, Littenberg B and Petitti DB. "Outcome Among Surviving Very Low Birthweight Infants: A Meta-Analysis." *Archives of Disease in Childhood* 66, no. 2 (February 1991): 204-11.

131. Evans M, Dommergues M, Wapner RJ, Lynch L, Dumez Y, Goldberg JD, et al. "Efficacy of Transabdominal Multifetal Pregnancy Reduction: Collaborative Experience Among the World's Largest Centers." *Obstetrics & Gynecology* 82, no. 1 (July 1993): 61-6.

132. Evans MI, Dommergues M, Wapner RJ, Goldberg JD, Lynch L, Zador IECarpenter RJ Jr., et al. "International, Collaborative Experience of 1789 Patients Having Multifetalpregnancy Reduction: A Plateauing of Risks and Outcomes." *Journal of the Society for Gynecologic Investigation* 3, no. 1 (January-February 1996): 23-6.

133. Evans MI, Goldberg JD, Horenstein J, Wapner RJ, Ayoub MA, Stone J, et al. "Selective Termination for Structural, Chromosomal, and Mendelian Anomalies: International Experience." *American Journal of Obstetrics and Gynecology* 181, no. 4 (October 1999): 893-7.

134. Evans MI, Henry GP, Miller WA, Bui TH, Snidjers RJ, Wapner RJ, Miny P, Johnson MP and Johnson A Peakman D, Nicolaides K, Holzgreve W, Ebrahim SA, Babu R, Jackson L. "International, Collaborative Assessment of 146,000 Prenatal Karyotypes: Expected Limitations If Only Chromosome-Specific Probes and Fluorescent in-Situ Hybridization Are Used." *Human Reproduction* 14, no. 5 (May 1999): 1213-6.

135. Evans MI, Johnson MP, Quintero RA, Fletcher JC. "Ethical Issues Surrounding Multifetal Pregnancy Reduction and Selective Termination." *Clinical Perinatology* 23, no. 3 (September 1996): 437-51.

136. Ewertz M and Duffy SW. "Risk of Breast Cancer in Relation to Reproductive Factors in Denmark." *British Journal of Cancer* 58, no. 1 (July 1988): 99-104.

137. Feitshans IL. "Legislating to Preserve Women's Autonomy During Pregnancy." *Medical Law (South Africa)* 14, no. 5-6 (1995): 397-412.

138. Ferguson JE 2d, Burkett BJ, Pinkerton JV, Thiagarajah S, Flather MM, Martel MM and Hogge WA. "Intraamniotic 15(s)-15-Methyl Prostaglandin F2 Alpha and Termination of Middle and Late Second-Trimester Pregnancy for Genetic Indications: A Contemporary Approach." *American Journal of Obstetrics and Gynecology* 169, no. (2 Pt 1) (August 1993): 332-9; discussion 339-40.

139. Ferris LE and Basinski AS. "Medical Abortion: What Does the Research Tell Us?" *Canadian Medical Association Journal* 154, no. 2 (15 January 1996): 185-7.

140. Ferris LE, McMain-Klein M, Colodny N, Fellows GF and Lamont J. "Factors Associated with Immediate Abortion Complications." *Canadian Medical Association Journal* 154, no. 11 (1 June 1996): 1677-85.

141 Ferris LE, McMain-Klein M and Iron K. "Factors Influencing the Delivery of Abortion Services in Ontario: A Descriptive Study." *Family Planning Perspectives* 30, no. 3 (May-June 1998): 134-8.

142. Fielding WL, Lee SY and Friedman EA. "Continued Pregnancy after Failed First-Trimester Abortion." *Obstetrics & Gynecology* 52, no. 2 (July 1978): 56-8.

143. Firestein, Stephen K. "Special Features of Grief Reactions with Reproductive Catastrophe." *Loss, Grief & Care* 3, no. 3-4 (1989): 37-45.

144. Fisher, Susan. "Reflections on Repeated Abortions: The Meanings and Motivations." *Journal of Social Work Practice* 2, no. 2 (May 1986): 70-87.

145. Fonseca W, Alencar AJ, Pereira RM and Misago C. "Congenital Malformation of the Scalp and Cranium After Failed First Trimester Abortion Attempt with Misoprostol." *Clinical Dysmorphology* 2, no. 1 (January 1993): 76-80.

146. Francke L.B. "Abortion and Men." *Esquire*, September 1978, 58-60.

147. Francke, L.B. *The Ambivalence of Abortion.* New York: Random House, 1978; reprint, New York: Dell, 1982.

148. Franco KN, Tamburrino MB, Campbell NB, Pentz JE and Jurs SG. "Psychological Profile of Dysphoric Women Postabortion." *Journal of the American Medical Women's Association* 44, no. 4 (July-August 1989): 113-5.

149. Frank DA, Zuckerman BS, Amaro H, Aboagye K, Bauchner H, Cabral H, et al. "Cocaine Use During Pregnancy: Prevalence and Correlates." *Pediatrics* 82, no. 6 (December 1988): 888-95.

150. Frank P, McNamee R, Hannaford PC, Kay CR and Hirsch S. "The Effect of Induced Abortion on Subsequent Fertility." *British Journal of Obstetrics and Gynaecology* 100, no. 6 (June 1993): 575-80.

151. Frank PI, Kay CR, Lewis TL and Parish S. "Outcome of Pregnancy Following Induced Abortion. Report From the Joint Study of the Royal College of General Practitioners and the Royal College of Obstetricians and Gynaecologists." *British Journal of Obstetrics and Gynaecology* 92, no. 4 (April 1985): 308-16.

152. Frank PI, Kay CR, Scott LM, Hannaford PC and Haran D. "Pregnancy Following Induced Abortion: Maternal Morbidity, Congenital Abnormalities and Neonataldeath. Royal College of General Practitioners/Royal College of Obstetricians and Gynaecologists Joint Study." *British Journal of Obstetrics and Gynaecology* 94, no. 9 (September 1987): 836-42.

153. Franz W and Reardon D. "Differential Impact of Abortion on Adolescents and Adults." *Adolescence* 27, no. 105 (Spring 1992): 161-72.

154. Franz, W. "Post Abortion Trauma and the Adolescent." In *Post Abortion Aftermath*, ed. Mannion M, 119-30. Kansas City: Sheed and Ward, 1994.

155. Freeman EW, Rickels K, Huggins GR, Garcia CR and Polin J. "Emotional Distress Patterns Among Women Having First or Repeat Abortions." *Obstetrics & Gynecology* 55, no. 5 (May 1980): 630-6.

156. Furlong RM and Black RB. "Pregnancy Termination for Genetic Indications: The Impact on Families." *Social Work in Health Care* 10, no. 1 (Fall 1984): 17-34.

157. Garel M, Stark C, Blondel B, Lefebvre G, Vauthier-Brouzes D and Zorn JR. "Psychological Reactions After Multifetal Pregnancy Reduction: A 2-Year Follow-Up Study." *Human Reproduction* 12, no. 3 (March 1997): 617-22.

158. Garfinkel, B. D., H. Hoberman, J. Parsons and J. Walker. "Stress, Depression and Suicide: A Study of Adolescents in Minnesota", 1986 [Proceedings from: Responding to High Risk Youth]. Minnesota Extension Service, University of Minnesota.

159. Garton, J. "The Cultural Impact of Abortion and Its Implications for a Future Society." In *Post-Abortion Aftermath*, ed. M. Mannion, 88-99. Kansas City: Sheed and Ward, 1994.

160. "Genetic Testing for Cystic Fibrosis. National Institutes of Health Consensus Development Conference Statement on Genetic Testing for Cystic Fibrosis." *Archives of Internal Medicine* 159, no. 14 (26 July 1999): 1529-39.

161. Gentles, I and E Cassidy. *Evaluating the Evaluators: Child Sexual Abuse Prevention - Do We Know It Works?* Toronto: Human Life Research Institute, 1988.

162. Giertz G, Kallings I, Nordenvall M and Fuchs T. "A Prospective Study of Chlamydia Trachomatis Infection Following Legal Abortion." *Acta Obstetricia et Gynecologica Scandanavica* 66, no. 2 (1987): 107-9.

163. Gilchrist AC, Hannaford PC, Frank P and Kay CR. "Termination of Pregnancy and Psychiatric Morbidity." *British Journal of Psychiatry* 167, no. 2 (August 1995): 243-8.

164. Gissler M, Kauppila R, Merilainen J, Toukomaa H and Hemminki E. "Pregnancy-Associated Deaths in Finland 1987 - 1994 -- Definition Problems and Benefits of Record Linkage." *Acta Obstetricia et Gynecologica Scandanavica* 76, no. 7 (August 1997): 651-7.

165. Gissler M, Hemminki E and Lonnqvist J. "Suicides After Pregnancy in Finland, 1987-94: Register Linkage Study." *British Medical Journal* 313, no. 7070 (7 December 1996): 1431-4.

166. Gissler, M., E. Hemminki and J. Lonnqvist. "Letters: Suicides After Pregnancy - Author's Reply." *British Medical Journal* 314, no. 7084 (22 March 1997): 902-3.

167. Glander SS, Moore ML, Michielutte R and Parsons LH. "The Prevalence of Domestic Violence Among Women Seeking Abortion." *Obstetrics & Gynecology* 91, no. 6 (June 1998): 1002-6.

168. Gleicher N, Campbell DP, Chan CL, Karande V, Rao R, Balin M and Pratt D. "The Desire for Multiple Births in Couples with Infertility Problems Contradicts Present Practice Patterns." *Human Reproduction* 10, no. 5 (May 1995): 1079-84.

169. Goldner TE, Lawson HW, Xia Z and Atrash HK. "Surveillance for Ectopic Pregnancy--United States, 1970-1989." *Morbidity and Mortality Weekly Report, Center for Disease Control, Surveillance Summary* 42, no. (SS-6) (December 1993): 73-85.

170. Gonzalez CH, Vargas FR, Perez AB, Kim CA, Brunoni D, Marques-Dias MJ, et al. "Limb Deficiency with or Without Mobius Sequence in Seven Brazilian Children Associated with Misoprostol Use in the First Trimester of Pregnancy." *American Journal of Medical Genetics* 47, no. 1 (1 August 1993): 59-64.

171. Green JM. "Obstetricians' Views on Prenatal Diagnosis and Termination of Pregnancy: 1980 Compared with 1993." *British Journal of Obstetrics and Gynaecology* 102, no. 3 (March 1995): 228-132.

172. Greer HS, Lal S, Lewis SC, Belsey EM and Beard RW. "Psychosocial Consequences of Therapeutic Abortion King's Termination Study III." *British Journal of Psychiatry* 128 (January 1976): 74-9.

173. Grimes D, Schultz K and Cates WJ. "Prevention of Perforation During Cutterage Abortion." *Journal of the American Medical Association* 251, no. 16 (27 April 1984): 2108-11.

174. Grimes D. "Medical Abortion In Early Pregnancy: A Review Of The Evidence [Review]." *Obstetrics & Gynecology* 89, no. (5 Pt 1) (May 1997): 790-6.

175. Grimes DA and Cates W Jr. "Complications From Legally-Induced Abortion: A Review." *Obstetrical and Gynecological Survey* 34, no. 3 (March 1979): 177-91.

176. Groutz A, Yovel I, Amit A, Yaron Y, Azem F and Lessing JB. "Pregnancy Outcome After Multifetal Pregnancy Reduction to Twins Compared with Spontaneously Conceived Twins." *Human Reproduction* 11, no. 6 (June 1996): 1334-6.

177. Guidozzi F, van der Griendt M and Israelstam D. "Major Complications Associated with Extra-Amniotic Prostaglandin F2 Alpha Termination of the Mid-Trimester Pregnancy." *South African Medical Journal* 82, no. 2 (August 1992): 102-4.

178. Hadjimichael OC, Boyle CA and Meigs JW. "Abortion Before First Livebirth and Risk of Breast Cancer." *British Journal of Cancer* 53, no. 2 (February 1986): 281-4.

179. Hakim-Elahi E, Tovell HM and Burnhill MS. "Complications of First-Trimester Abortion; A Report of 170,000 Cases." *Obstetrics & Gynecology* 76, no. 1 (July 1990): 129-35.

180. Hall JG. "Arthrogryposis Associated with Unsuccessful Attempts at Termination of Pregnancy." *American Journal of Medical Genetics* 63, no. 1 (3 May 1996): 293-300.

181. Hamark B, Uddenberg N and Forssman L. "The Influence of Social Class on Parity and Psychological Reactions in Women Coming for Induced Abortion." *Acta Obstetricia et Gynecologica Scandanavica* 74, no. 4 (April 1995): 302-6.

182. Hamilton Regional Cancer Centre. "Early Stage Breast Cancer." *Cancer Centre Update* 5, no. 1 (1997): 1-8.

183. Harris BM, Eklund G, Meirik O, Rutqvist LE and Wiklund K. "Risk of Cancer of the Breast after Legal Abortion during First Trimester: A Swedish Register Study." *British Medical Journal* 299, no. (6713) (9 December 1989): 1430-2.

184. Harris JR, Lippman ME, Veronesi U and Willett W. "Breast Cancer (1)." *New England Journal of Medicine* 327, no. 5 (30 July 1992): 319-28.

185. _____. "Breast Cancer (2)." *New England Journal of Medicine* 327, no. 6 (6 August 1992): 390-8.

186. _____. "Breast Cancer (3)." *New England Journal of Medicine* 327, no. 7 (13 August 1992): 473-80.

187. Hartoov J, Geva E, Wolman I, Lerner-Geva L, Lessing JB, Amster R, Amit A and Jaffa A. "A 3 Year, Prospectively-Designed Study of Late Selective Multifetal Pregnancy Reduction." *Human Reproduction* 13, no. 7 (July 1998): 1996-8.

188. Hausknecht RU. "Methetrexate And Misoprostol To Terminate Early Pregnancy." *New England Journal of Medicine* 333, no. 9 (31 August 1995): 537-40.

189. Heisterberg L. "Factors Influencing Spontaneous Abortion, Dyspareunia, Dysmenorrhea, and Pelvic Pain." *Obstetrics & Gynecology* 81, no. 4 (April 1993): 594-7.

190. Heisterberg L, Hebjorn S, Andersen LF and Petersen H. "Sequelae of Induced First-Trimester Abortion. A Prospective Study Assessing the Role of Postabortal Pelvic Inflammatory Disease and Prophylactic Antibiotics." *American Journal of Obstetrics and Gynecology* 155, no. 1 (July 1986): 76-80.

191. Heisterberg L and Kringelbach M. "Early Complications After Induced First-Trimester Abortion." *Acta Obstetricia et Gynecologica Scandanavica* 66, no. 3 (1987): 201-4.

192. Henshaw RC, Naji SA, Russell IT and Templeton AA. "A Comparison of Medical Abortion (Using Mifepristone and Gemeprost) with Surgical Vacuum Aspiration: Efficacy and Early Medical Sequelae." *Human Reproduction* 9, no. 11 (November 1994): 2167-72.

193. Henshaw RC, Naji SA, Russell IT and Templeton AA. "Comparison of Medical Abortion with Surgical Vacuum Aspiration: Women's Preferences and Acceptability of Treatment." *British Medical Journal* 307, no. (6906) (18 September 1993): 714-7

194. Henshaw SK, Forrest JD and Van Vort J. "Abortion Services in the United States, 1984 and 1985." *Family Planning Perspectives* 19, no. 2 (March-April 1987): 63-70.

195. Henshaw SK and Van Vort J. "Abortion Services in the United States, 1991 and 1992." *Family Planning Perspectives* 26, no. 3 (May-June 1994): 100-6, 112.

196. Herman JL, Perry JC and van der Kolk BA. "Childhood Trauma in Borderline Personality Disorder." *American Journal of Psychiatry* 146, no. 4 (April 1989): 490-5.

197. Hirohata T, Shigematsu T, Nomura AM, Nomura Y, Horie A and Hirohata I. "Occurrence of Breast Cancer in Relation to Diet and Reproductive History: A Case-Control Study in Fukuoka, Japan." *National Cancer Institute Monograph* (December 1985): 187-90.

198. Holmes-Siedle M, Ryynanen M and Lindenbaum RH. "Parental Decisions Regarding Termination of Pregnancy Following Prenatal Detection of Sex Chromosome Abnormality." *Prenatal Diagnosis* 7, no. 4 (May 1987): 239-44.

199. Holmes LB. "Possible Fetal Effects of Cervical Dilation and Uterine Curettage During the First Trimester of Pregnancy." *Journal of Pediatrics* 126, no. 1 (January 1995): 131-4.

200. Holmgren K and Uddenberg N. "Abortion Ethics--Women's Post Abortion Assessments." *Acta Obstetricia et Gynecologica Scandanavica* 73, no. 6 (July 1994): 492-6.

201. _____. "Ambivalence During Early Pregnancy Among Expectant Mothers." *Gynecologic and Obstetric Investigation* 36, no. 1 (1993): 15-20.

202. Holmgren K. "Women's Evaluation of Three Early Abortion Methods." *Acta Obstetricia et Gynecologica Scandanavica* 71, no. 8 (December 1992): 616-23.

203. Holt VL, Daling JR, Voigt LF, McKnight B, Stergachis A, Chu J, et al. "Induced Abortion and the Risk of Subsequent Ectopic Pregnancy." *American Journal of Public Health* 79, no. 9 (September 1989): 1234-8.

204. "Hospital Pays $8.7M Settlement: Premature Baby Was Abandoned with Dead Foetuses." *The National Post*, 31 July 1999, A, 1.

205. Howe HL, Senie RT, Bzduch H and Herzfeld P. "Early Abortion And Breast Cancer Risk Among Women Under Age 40." *International Journal Of Epidemiology* 18, no. 2 (June 1989): 300-4.

206. Huggins GR and Cullins VE. "Fertility after Contraception or Abortion." *Fertility and Sterility* 54, no. 4 (October 1990): 559-73.

207. Hunfeld JA, Wladimiroff JW and Passchier J. "Pregnancy Termination, Perceived Control, and Perinatal Grief." *Psychological Reports* 74, no. 1 (February 1994): 217-8.

208. Hunfeld JA, Wladimiroff JW, Passchier J, Venema-Van Uden MU, Frets PG, Verhage F. "Emotional Reactions in Women in Late Pregnancy (24 Weeks or Longer) Following the Ultrasound Diagnosis of a Severe or Lethal Fetal Malformation." *Prenatal Diagnosis* 13, no. 7 (July 1993): 603-12.

209. Husfeldt C, Hansen SK, Lyngberg A, Noddebo M and Petersson B. "Ambivalence Among Women Applying for Abortion." *Acta Obstetricia et Gynecologica Scandanavica* 74, no. 10 (November 1995): 813-7.

210. Iles S and Gath D. "Psychiatric Outcome of Termination of Pregnancy for Foetal Abnormality." *Psychological Medicine* 232 (May 1993): 407-13.

211. Imber-Black, Evan. *Secrets in Families and Family Therapy.* New York: Norton, 1993.

212. Jacob S, Bloebaum L, Shah G and Varner MW. "Maternal Mortality in Utah." *Obstetrics & Gynecology* 91, no. 2 (February 1998): 187-91.

213. Jacot FR, Poulin C, Bilodeau AP, Morin M, Moreau S, Gendron F, et al. "A Five-Year Experience with Second-Trimester Induced Abortions: No Increase in Complication Rate As Compared to the First Trimester." *American Journal of Obstetrics and Gynecology* 168, no. 2 (February 1993): 633-7.

214. Jones EF and Forrest JD. "Underreporting of Abortion in Surveys of U.S. Women: 1976 to 1988." *Demography* 29, no. 1 (February 1992): 113-26.

215. Jones OW, Penn NE, Shuchter S, Stafford CA, Richards T, Kernahan C, Gutierrez J, Cherkin P, Reinsch S and Dixson B. "Parental Response to Mid-Trimester Therapeutic Abortion Following Amniocentesis." Prenatal Diagnosis 4, no. 4 (July-August 1984): 249-56.

216. Jonsson M, Karlsson R, Persson K, et al. "The Influence of Sexual and Social Factors on the Risk of Chlamydia Trachomatis Infections: A Population-Based Serologic Study." *Sexually Transmitted Diseases* 22, no. 6 (November-December 1995): 355-63.

217. Kaali SG, Szigetvari IA and Bartfai GS. "The Frequency and Management of Uterine Perforations During First-Trimester Abortions." *American Journal of Obstetrics and Gynecology* 161, no. 2 (Aug. 1989): 406-8.

218. Kanhai HH, de Haan M, van Zanten LA, et al. "Follow-Up of Pregnancies, Infants, and Families after Multifetal Pregnancy Reduction." *Fertility and Sterility* 62, no. 5 (November 1994): 955-9.

219. Kelsey JL. "A Review of the Epidemiology of Human Breast Cancer." *Epidemiologic Reviews* 1 (1979): 74-109.

220. Kelsey JL, Fischer DB, Holford TR, LiVoisi VA, Mostow ED, Goldenberg IS, et al. "Exogenous Estrogens and Other Factors in the Epidemiology of Breast Cancer." *Journal of the National Cancer Institute* 67, no. 2 (August 1981): 237-233.

221. Kelsey JL, Gammon MD and John EM. "Reproductive Factors and Breast Cancer." *Epidemiologic Reviews* 15, no. 1 (1993): 36-47.

222. Kent, I, R.C. Greenwood, J Loeken, W Nicholls. "Emotional Sequelae of Elective Abortion." *BC Medical Journal* 20, no. 4 (April 1978): 118-9.

223. Kiel FW. "The Medical Value of Examining Tissue from Therapeutic Abortions: An Analysis of 13,477 Cases." *British Journal of Obstetrics and Gynaecology* 93, no. 6 (June 1986): 594-5.

224. Klassen AD and Wilsnack SC. "Sexual Experience and Drinking Among Women in a U.S. National Survey." *Archives of Sexual Behavior* 15, no. 5 (October 1986): 363-92.

225. Kluger-Bell, Kim. *Unspeakable Losse : Understanding the Experience of Pregnancy Loss, Miscarriage, and Abortion.* W.W. Norton, 1998.

226. Kolker A and Burke BM. "Grieving the Wanted Child: Ramifications of Abortion after Prenatal Diagnosis of Abnormality." *Health Care for Women International* 14, no. 6 (November-December 1993): 513-26.

227. Koller O and Eikhom SN. "Late Sequelae of Induced Abortion in Primigravidae. The Outcome of the Subsequent Pregnancies." *Acta Obstetricia et Gynecologica Scandanavica* 56, no. 4 (1977): 311-7.

228. Koonin LM, Atrash HK, Lawson HW and Smith JC. "Maternal Mortality Surveillance, United States, 1979-1986." *Morbidity and Mortality Weekly Report, Centers for Disease Control* 40, no. 2 (July 1991): 1-13.

229. Koonin LM, Smith JC and Ramick M. "Abortion Surveillance - United States 1991 [Published Erratum Appears in MMWR Morb Mortal Wkly Rep 1995 Jun 30;44(25):479]." *Morbidity and Mortality Weekly Report, Centers for Disease Control, Surveillance Summaries* 44, no. 2 (5 May 1995): 22-53.

230. Koonin LM, Smith JC, Ramick M, Green CA. "Abortion Surveillance-United States, 1992." *Morbidity and Mortality Weekly Report, Centers for Disease Control, Surveillance Summaries* 45, no. 3 (3 May 1996): 1-36.

231. Koonin LM, Smith JC, Ramick M, Lawson HW. "Abortion Surveillance- -United States, 1989." *Morbidity and Mortality Weekly Report, Centers for Disease Control, Surveillance Summaries* 41, no. 5 (4 Sept. 1992): 1-33

232. Koonin LM, Smith JC, Ramick M, Strauss LT. "Abortion Surveillance- United States, 1995." *Morbidity and Mortality Weekly Report, Centers for Disease Control, Surveillance Summaries* 47, no. 2 (3 July 1998): 31-40.

233. Koonin LM, Smith JC, Ramick M, Strauss LT and Hopkins FW. "Abortion Surveillance--United States, 1993 and 1994." *Morbidity and Mortality Weekly Report, Centers for Disease Control, Surveillance Summaries* 46, no. 4 (8 August 1997): 37-98.

234. Koonin LM, Strauss LT, Chrisman C, Parker W. "Abortion Surveillance- -United States, 1997." *Morbidity and Mortality Weekly Report, Centers for Disease Control, Surveillance Summaries* 49, no. 11 (8 Dec. 2000): 1-43.

235. Koonin LM, Strauss LT, Chrisman CE, Montalbano MA, LA Bartlett LA, Smith JG. "Abortion Surveillance-United States, 1996." *Morbidity and Mortality Weekly Report, Centers for Disease Control, Surveillance Summaries* 48, no. 4 (30 July 1999): 1-42.

236. Krieger N. "Exposure, Susceptibility, and Breast Cancer Risk: A Hypothesis Regarding Exogenous Carcinogens, Breast Tissue Development, and Social Gradients, Including Black/White Differences, in Breast Cancer Incidence." *Breast Cancer Research and Treatment* 13, no. 3 (July 1989): 205-23.

237. Kumar R and Robson K. "Previous Induced Abortion and Ante-Natal Depression in Primiparae: Preliminary Report of a Survey of Mental Health in Pregnancy." *Psychological Medicine* 8, no. 4 (November 1978): 711-5.

238. Kunz J and Keller PJ. "HCG, HPL, Oestradiol, Progesterone and AFP in Serum in Patients with Threatened Abortion." *British Journal of Obstetrics and Gynaecology* 83, no. 8 (August 1976): 640-6.

239. Kvale G and Heuch I. "Is the Incidence of Colorectal Cancer Related to Reproduction? A Prospective Study of 63,000 Women." *International Journal of Cancer* 47, no. 3 (1 February 1991): 390-5.

240. Kvale G. "Reproductive Factors In Breast Cancer Epidemiology." *Acta Oncologica* 31, no. 2 (1992): 187-94.

241. Laffont I and Edelmann RJ. "Psychological Aspects of In Vitro Fertilization: A Gender Comparison." *Journal of Psychosomatic Obstetrics and Gynecology* 15, no. 2 (June 1994): 85-92.

242. Laing, AE, Bonney GE Adams-Campbell L, et al. "Reproductive and Lifestyle Risk Factors for Breast Cancer in African-American Women." *Genetic Epidemiology* 11 (1994): 285-310.

243. Laing AE, Demenais FM, Williams R, Kissling G, Chen VW and Bonney GE. "Breast Cancer Risk Factors in African-American Women: The Howard University Tumor Registry Experience." *Journal of the National Medical Association* 85, no. 12 (December 1993): 931-9.

244. Lambe M, Hsieh CC, Chan HW, Ekbom A, Trichopoulos D and Adami HO. "Parity, Age at First And Last Birth and Risk of Breast Cancer: A Population Based Study in Sweden." *Breast Cancer Research And Treatment* 38, no. 3 (1996): 305-11.

245. Lang JM, Lieberman E and Cohen A. "A Comparison of Risk Factors for Preterm Labor and Term Small-for-Gestational-Age Birth." *Epidemiology* 7, no. 4 (July 1996): 369-76.

246. Lauzon P, Roger-Achim D, Achim A and Boyer R. "Emotional Distress Among Couples Involved in First-Trimester Induced Abortions." *Canadian Family Physician* 46 (October 200): 2033-40.

247. LaVecchia C, Negri E, Franceschi S and D'Avanzo B. "Reproductive Factors and the Risk of Hepatocellular Carcinoma in Women." *International Journal of Cancer* 52, no. 3 (30 September 1992): 351-4.

248. LaVecchia C, Negri E, Franceschi S and Parazzini F. "Long-Term Impact of Reproductive Factors on Cancer Risk." *International Journal of Cancer* 53, no. 2 (21 January 1993): 215-9.

249. Lazovich, D, JA Thompson, PJ Mink, TA Sellars and KE Anderson. "Induced Abortion and Breast Cancer Risk." *Epidemiology* 11 (2000): 76-80.

250. Le, M-G, A Bachelot, F Doyon, A Kramar and Hill C. "Oral Contraceptive Use and Breast or Cervical Cancer: Preliminary Results of a French Case-Control Study." In *Hormones and Sexual Factors in Human Cancer Aetiology*, eds. Wolff J-P and Scott JS, 139-47. Amsterdam: Elsevier, 1984.

251. Leach J. "The Repeat Abortion Patient." *Family Planning Perspectives* 9, no. 1 (January-February 1977): 37-9.

252. Leibner EC. "Delayed Presentation of Uterine Perforation." *Annals of Emergency Medicine* 26, no. 5 (November 1995): 643-6.

253. Lekea-Karanika V, Tzoumaka-Bakoula C and Golding J. "Previous Obstetric History and Subsequent Preterm Delivery in Greece." *European Journal of Obstetrics & Gynecology and Reproductive Biology* 37, no. 2 (November 1990): 99-109.

254. Lemkau JP. "Post-Abortion Adjustment of Health Care Professionals in Training." *American Journal of Orthopsychiatry* 61, no. 1 (January 1991): 92-102.

255. Lemkau, Jeanne P. "Emotional Sequelae of Abortion: Implications for Clinical Practice." *Psychology of Women Quarterly. Special Issue: Women's health: Our minds, our bodies.*

256. Levallois P and Rioux JE. "Prophylactic Antibiotics for Suction Curettage Abortion: Results of a Clinical Controlled Trial." *American Journal of Obstetrics and Gynecology* 158, no. 1 (January 1988): 100-5.

257. Levin AA, Schoenbaum SC, Monson RR, Stubblefield PG and Ryan KJ. "Association of Induced Abortion with Subsequent Pregnancy Loss." *Journal of the American Medical Association* 243, no. 24 (27 June 1980): 2495-9.

258. Levin AA, Schoenbaum SC, Stubblefield PG, Zimicki S, Monson RR and Ryan KJ. "Ectopic Pregnancy and Prior Induced Abortion." *American Journal of Public Health* 72, no. 3 (March 1982): 253-6.

259. Li L and Smialek JE. "Sudden Death Due to Rupture of Ectopic Pregnancy Concurrent with Theraputic Abortion." *Archives of Pathology and Laboratory Medicine* 117, no. 7 (July 1993): 698-700.

260. Lieberman E, Ryan KJ, Monson RR and Schoenbaum SC. "Risk Factors Accounting for Racial Differences in the Rate of Premature Birth." *New England Journal of Medicine* 317, no. 12 (September 1987): 743-8.

261. Linares L, Leadbeater B, Jaffe L, et al. "Predictors of Repeat Pregnancy Outcome Among Black and Puerto Rican Adolescent Mothers." *Journal of Developmental and Behavioral Pediatrics* 13, no. 2 (April 1992): 89-94.

262. Lindefors-Harris BM, Eklund G, Adami HO and Meirik O. "Response Bias in a Case-Control Study: Analysis Utilizing Comparative Data Concerning Legal Abortions from Two Independent Swedish Studies." *American Journal of Epidemiology* 134, no. 9 (1 November 1991): 1003-8.

263. Lipworth L, Katsouyanni K, Ekbom A, Michels KB and Trichopoulos D. "Abortion and the Risk of Breast Cancer: A Case-Control Study in Greece." *International Journal of Cancer* 61, no. 2 (April 1995): 181-4.

264. Lloyd J and Laurence KM. "Sequelae and Support After Termination of Pregnancy for Fetal Malformation." British Medical Journal 290, no. 6472 (23 March 1985): 907-9.

265. Lorenzen J and Holzgreve W. "Helping Parents to Grieve after Second Trimester Termination of Pregnancy for Fetopathic Reasons." *Fetal Diagnosis and Therapy* 10, no. 3 (May-June 1995): 147-56.

266. Lott, John, John Whitley. "Abortion and Crime: Unwanted Children and Out-of-Wedlock Births", 15 May 2001 [Working Paper #254]. Yale Law School, Program for Studies in Law, Economics, and Public Policy.

267. Luke, Barbara [forward by Emile Papiernik]. *Every Pregnant Woman's Guide to Preventing Premature Birth: A Program for Reducing the Sixty Proven Risks That Can Lead to Prematurity.* New York: Times Books, 1995.

268. Lukse MP and Vacc NA. "Grief, Depression, and Coping in Women Undergoing Infertility Treatment." *Obstetrics & Gynecology* 93, no. 2 (February 1999): 245-51.

269. Lumley, J. "The Association Between Prior Spontaneous Abortion, Prior Induced Abortion and Preterm Birth in First Singleton Births." *Prenatal and Neonatal Medicine* 3, no. 1998: 21-4

270. _____. "Very Low Birth-Weight (Less Than 1,500 G) and Previous Induced Abortion: Victoria 1982-1983." *Australian and New Zealand Journal of Obstetrics and Gynecology* 26, no. 4 (November 1986): 268-72.

271. Lurie S. and Shoham Z. "Induced Midtrimester Abortion and Future Fertility-Where Are We Today?" *International Journal of Fertility and Menopausal Studies* 40, no. 6 (November-December 1995): 311-5.

272. Lydon J, Dunkel-Schetter C, Cohan CL and Pierce T. "Pregnancy Decision Making as a Significant Life Event: A Commitment Approach." *Journal of Personality and Social Psychology* 71, no. 1 (July 1996): 141-51.

273. MacLean, NE. "Complications of Legal Abortion [Letter]." *New Zealand Medical Journal* 106, no. 955 (12 May 1993): 186.

274. MacMahon, Brian and Dimitrios. Trichopoulos. *Epidemiology: Principles and Methods.* Boston: Little, Brown, 1996.

275. Macones GA, Schemmer G, Pritts E, Weinblatt V and Wapner RJ. "Multifetal Reduction of Triplets to Twins Improves Perinatal Outcome." *American Journal of Obstetrics and Gynecology* 169, no. 4 (October 1993): 982-6.

276. Main, M and R. Goldwyn. "Predicting Rejection of Her Infant from Mother's Representation of Her Own Experience: Implications for the Abused-Abusing Intergenerational Cycle." *Child Abuse and Neglect* 8, no. 2 (1984): 203-17.

277. Major B, Cozzarelli C, Cooper ML, Zubek J, Richards C, Wilhite M and Gramzow RH. "Psychological Responses of Women After First-Trimester Abortion." *Archives of General Psychiatry* 57, no. 8 (August 2000): 777-84.

278. Major B, Cozzarelli C, Sciacchitano AM, Cooper ML, Testa M and Mueller PM. "Perceived Social Support, Self-Efficacy, and Adjustment to Abortion." *Journal of Personality and Social Psychology* 59, no. 3 (September 1990): 452-63.

279. Makinen JI. "Increase of Ectopic Pregnancy in Finland--Combination of Time and Cohort Effects." *Obstetrics & Gynecology* 73, no. 1 (January 1989): 21-4.

280. Makinen JI, Erkkola RU and Laippala PJ. "Causes of the Increase in the Incidence of Ectopic Pregnancy. A Study on 1017 Patients From 1966 to 1985 in Turku, Finland." *American Journal of Obstetrics and Gynecology* 160, no. 3 (March 1989): 642-6.

281. Mander, Rosemary. *Loss and Bereavement in Childbearing.* Oxford: Blackwell Scientific Publications, 1994.

282. Mannion, M. "Abortion and Healing: A Pastoral Church Responds in Word and Sacrament." In *Post-Abortion Aftermath: A Comprehensive Consideration: Writings Generated by Various Experts at a 'Post-Abortion Summit Conference'*, ed. Michael Mannion, 106-18. Kansas City: Sheed and Ward, 1994.

283. Marcus SF, Bhattacharya J, Williams G, Brinsden P and Hamou J. "Endometrial Ossification: A Cause of Secondary Infertility. Report of Two Cases." *American Journal of Obstetrics and Gynecology* 170, no. (5 Pt 1) (May 1994): 1381-3.

284. Martius JA, Steck T, Oehler MK and Wulf KH. "Risk Factors Associated with Preterm (<37+0 Weeks) and Early Preterm Birth  (<32+0 Weeks): Univariate and Multivariate Analysis of 106 345 Singleton Births from the 1994 Statewide Perinatal Survey of Bavaria." *European Journal of Obstetrics & Gynecology and Reproductive Biology* 80, no. 2 (October 1998): 183-9.

285. Marttunen MJ, Aro HM, Henriksson MM, Lonnqvist JK. "Psychosocial Stressors More Common in Adolescent Suicides with Alcohol Abuse Compared with Depressive Adolescent Suicides." *Journal of the American Academy of Child and Adolescent Psychiatry* 33, no. 4 (May 1994): 490-7.

286. Mattinson J. "The Effects of Abortion on a Marriage." *Ciba Foundation Symposium* 115 (1985): 165-77.

287. McAll K and Wilson WP. "Ritual Mourning for Unresolved Grief after Abortion." *Southern Medical Journal* 80, no. 7 (July 1987): 817-21.

288. McAll RK and McAll FM. "Ritual Mourning in Anorexia Nervosa." *The Lancet* 2, no. 8190 (16 August 1980): 368.

289. McCombs, P. "Remembering Thomas." *Washington Post*, 3 Feb. 1995.

290. McGinnis, J. "The Politics of Cancer Research." *The Wall Street Journal*, 28 February 1997.

291. McKinney M, Downey J, Timor-Tritsch I. "The Psychological Effects of Multifetal Pregnancy Reduction." *Fertility and Sterility* 64, no. 1 (July 1995): 51-61

292. McKinney MK, Tuber SB and Downey JI. "Multifetal Pregnancy Reduction: Psychodynamic Implications." *Psychiatry* 59, no. 4 (Winter 1996); 393-407.

293. McPherson CP, Sellers TA, Potter JD, Bostick RM and Folsom AR. "Reproductive Factors and Risk of Endometrical Cancer. The Iowa Women's Health Study." *American Journal of Epidemiology* 143, no. 12 (5 June 1996): 1195-202.

294. Meirik O, Adami HO and Eklund G. Letter on: "Relation Between Induced Abortion and Breast Cancer". *Journal of Epidemiology and Community Health* 52, no. 3 (March 1998): 209-11.

295. Meirik O, Lund E, Adami HO, Bergstrom R, Christoffersen T and Bergsjo P. "Oral Contraceptive Use and Breast Cancer in Young Women. A Joint National Case-Control Study in Sweden and Norway." *The Lancet* 2, no. (8508) (20 September 1986): 650-4.

296. Melbye M, Wohlfahrt J, Olsen JH, Frisch M, Westergaard T, Helweg-Larsen K, et al. "Induced Abortions and the Risk of Breast Cancer." *New England Journal of Medicine* 336, no. 2 (9 January 1997): 81-5.

297. Mensch B and Kandel DB. "Drug Use as a Risk Factor for Premarital Teen Pregnancy and Abortion in a National Sample of Young White Women." *Demography* 29, no. 3 (August 1992): 409-29.

298. Meyer RE and Buescher PA. "Maternal Mortality Related to Induced Abortion in North Carolina: A Historical Study." *Family Planning Perspectives* 26, no. 4 (July-August 1994): 179-80, 191.

299. Michalas S, Minaretzis D, Tsionou C, Maos G, Kioses E and Aravantinos D. "Pelvic Surgery, Reproductive Factors and Risk of Ectopic Pregnancy: A Case Controlled Study." *International Journal of Gynecology and Obstetrics* 38, no. 2 (June 1992): 101-5.

300. Michels KB and Willett WC. "Does Induced or Spontaneous Abortion Affect the Risk of Breast Cancer?" *Epidemiology* 7, no. 5 (September 1996): 521-8.

301. Michels, Nancy. *Helping Women Recover From Abortion*. Minneapolis, MN: Bethany House, 1988.

302. Michielutte R, Ernest JM, Moore ML, Meis PJ, Sharp PC, Wells HB and Buescher PA. "A Comparison of Risk Assessment Models for Term and Preterm Low Birthweight." *Preventive Medicine* 21, no. 1 (January 1992): 98-109.

303. Millar WJ, Wadhera S and Henshaw SK. "Repeat Abortions in Canada, 1975-1993." *Family Planning Perspectives* 29, no. 1 (January-February 1997): 20-4.

304. Miller, Warren B. "An Empirical Study of the Psychological Antecedents and Consequences of Induced Abortion." *Journal of Social Issues* 48, no. 3 (Fall 1992): 67-93.

305. Milling, E. "The Men Who Wait." *Woman's Life*, April 1975, 48-9,69-71.

306. Milner KK, Collins EE, Connors GR and Petty EM. "Attitudes of Young Adults to Prenatal Screening and Genetic Correction for Human Attributes and Psychiatric Conditions." *American Journal of Medical Genetics* 76, no. 2 (March 1998): 111-9.

307. Mittal S and Misra SL. "Uterine Perforation Following Medical Termination of Pregnancy by Vacuum Aspiration." *International Journal of Gynaecology and Obstetrics* 23, no. 1 (February 1985): 45-50.

308. Mogilevkina I, Markote S, Avakyan Y, Mrochek L, Liljestrand J and Hellberg D. "Induced Abortions and Childbirths: Trends in Estonia, Latvia, Lithuania, Russia, Belarussia and the Ukraine During 1970 to 1994." *Acta Obstetricia et Gynecologica Scandanavica* 75, no. 10 (November 1996): 908-11.

309. Molin, A. "Risk of Damage to the Cervix by Dilation for First-Trimester-Induced Abortion by Suction Aspiration." *Gynecologic and Obstetric Investigation* 35, no. 3 (1993): 152-4.

310. Moon HS, Park YH, Kwon HY, Hong SH and Kim SK. "Iatrogenic Secondary Infertility Caused by Residual Intrauterine Fetal Bone After Midtrimester Abortion." *American Journal of Obstetrics and Gynecology* 176, no. 2 (February 1997): 369-70.

311. Moormeier, J. "Breast Cancer In Black Women [Review]." *Annals of Internal Medicine* 124, no. 10 (15 May 1996): 897-905.

312. Morabito, Stella. "Abortion and the Compromise of Fatherhood." *The Human Life Review* 17, no. 4 (Fall, 1991): 83-100.

313. Morgan CL, Evans M and Peters JR. "Suicides After Pregnancy. Mental Health May Deteriorate As a Direct Effect of Induced Abortion." *British Medical Journal* 314, no. 7084 (22 March 1997): 902; discussion 902-3.

314. Moseson M, Koenig KL, Shore RE and Pasternack BS. "The Influence of Medical Conditions Associated with Hormones on the Risk of Breast Cancer." *International Journal of Epidemiology* 22, no. 6 (December 1993): 1000-9.

315. Mueller-Heubach E and Guzick DS. "Evaluation of Risk Scoring in a Preterm Birth Prevention Study of Indigent Patients." *American Journal of Obstetrics and Gynecology* 160, no. 4 (April 1989): 835-7.

316. Myers KA and Farquhar DR. "Improving the Accuracy of Death Certification." *Canadian Medical Association Journal* 158, no. 10 (19 May 1998): 1317-23.

317. Nathanson, Sue. *Soul Crisis : One Woman's Journey Through Abortion to Renewal.* New York: New American Library, 1989.

318. Naziri, D and A Tzavaras. "Mourning and Guilt Among Greek Women Having Repeated Abortions." *Omega: Journal of Death & Dying* 26, no. 2 (1992-1993): 137-44.

319. Neugebauer R, Kline J, Shrout P, Skodol A, O'Connor P, Geller PA, Stein Z and Susser M. "Major Depressive Disorder in the 6 Months After Miscarriage." *Journal of the American Medical Association* 277, no. 5 (February 1997): 383-8.

320. Newcomb PA, Storer BE, Longnecker MP, Mittendorf R, Greenberg ER and Willett WC. "Pregnancy Termination in Relation to Risk of Breast Cancer." *Journal of the American Medical Association* 275, no. 4 (January 1996): 283-7.

321. Ney P. "Relationship Between Abortion and Child Abuse." *Canadian Journal of Psychiatry* 24, no. 7 (November 1979): 610-20.

322. Ney PG. "Post-Abortion Survivors Syndrome." *Canadian Journal of Psychiatry* 38, no. 8 (October 1993): 577-8.

323. Ney PG, Fung T, Wickett AR and Beaman-Dodd C. "The Effects of Pregnancy Loss on Women's Health." *Social Science and Medicine* 38, no. 9 (May 1994): 1193-200.

324. Ney PG and Wickett AR. "Mental Health and Abortion: Review and Analysis." *Psychiatric Journal of the University* of Ottawa 14, no. 4 (November 1989): 506-16.

325. Ney, P. "Abortion and Family  Psychology: A Study in Progress." *Canadian Journal of Diagnosis* (1999): 113-9.

326. Ney, P and A. Peeters. *Hope Alive: Post Abortion and Abuse Treatment. A Training Manual for Therapists.* Victoria, B.C.: Pioneer Publishing, 1993.

327. Nielsen IK, Engdahl E and Larsen T. "[Pelvic Inflammation after Induced Abortion] Danish." *Ugeskr Laeger* 154, no. 40 (28 September 1992): 2743-6.

328. _____. "No Effect of Single Dose Ofloxacin on Postoperative Infection Rate after First-Trimester Abortion. A Clinical, Controlled Trial." *Acta Obstetricia et Gynecologica Scandanavica* 72, no. 7 (October 1993): 556-9.

329. Niemela P, Lehtinen P, Rauramo L, Hermansson R, Karjalainen R, Maki H and Stora CA. "The First Abortion - and the Last? A Study of the Personality Factors Underlying Repeated Failure of Contraception." *International Journal of Gynaecology and Obstetrics* 19, no. 3 (June 1981): 193-200.

330. Nishiyama F. "The Epidemiology of Breast Cancer in Tokushima Prefecture." *Shikou Ichi* 38 (1982): 333-43.

331. Nugent PJ. "Ruptured Ectopic Pregnancy in a Patient with a Recent Intrauterine Abortion." *Annals of Emergency Medicine* 21, no. 1 (January 1992): 97-9.

332. O'Connor, Karen. *No Neutral Ground: Abortion Politics in an Age of Absolutes.* Boulder, Colorado: Westview, 1996.

333. Oakeshott P, Hilton S and Hay P. "Treatment and Causes of Female Infertility." *The Lancet* 344, no. 8918 (30 July 1994): 334.

334. Obel EB. "Pregnancy Complications Following Legally Induced Abortion." *Acta Obstetricia et Gynecologica Scandanavica* 58, no. 5 (1979): 485-90.

335. Oddens BJ, den Tonkelaar I and Nieuwenhuyse H. "Psychosocial Experiences in Women Facing Fertility Problems--a Comparative Survey." *Human Reproduction* 14, no. 1 (January 1999): 255-61.

336. Olsen J. "Options in Making Use of Pregnancy History in Planning and Analysing Studies of Reproductive Failure." *Journal of Epidemiology and Community Health* 48, no. 2 (April 1994): 171-4.

337. Olsson H. "Reproductive Events, Occurring in Adolescence at the Time of Development of Reproductive Organs and at the Time of Tumour Initiation, Have a Bearing on Growth Characteristics and Reproductive Hormone Regulation in Normal and Tumour Tissue Investigated Decades Later--a Hypothesis." *Medical Hypotheses* 28, no. 2 (February 1989): 93-7.

338. Olsson H, Borg A, Ferno M, Ranstam J and Sigurdsson H. "Her-2/Neu and INT2 Proto-Oncogene Amplification in Malignant Breast Tumors in Relation to Reproductive Factors and Exposure to Exogenous Hormones." *Journal of the National Cancer Institute* 83, no. 20 (16 October 1991): 1483-7.

339. Olsson H, Ranstam J, Baldetorp B, Ewers SB, Ferno M, Killander D, et al. "Proliferation and DNA Ploidy in Malignant Breast Tumors in Relation to Early Oral Contraceptive Use and Early Abortions." *Cancer* 67, no. 5 (March 1991): 1285-90.

340. Ortiz CG and Vazquez Nuttall E. "Adolescent Pregnancy: Effects of Family Support, Education, and Religion on the Decision to Carry or Terminate Among Puerto Rican Teenagers." *Adolescence* 22, no. 88 (Winter 1987): 897-917.

341. Osler M, Morgall JM, Jensen B and Osler M. "Repeat Abortion in Denmark." *Danish Medical Bulletin* 39, no. 1 (February 1992): 89-91.

342. Osser S and Persson K. "Postabortal Pelvic Infection Associated with Chlamydia Trachomatis and the Influence of Humoral Immunity." *American Journal of Obstetrics and Gynecology* 150, no. 6 (15 November 1984): 699-703.

343. Ostbye T, Wenghofer EF, Woodward CA, Gold G and Craighead J. "Health Services Utilization after Induced Abortions in Ontario: A Comparison Between Community Clinics and Hospitals." *American Journal of Medical Quality* 16, no. 3 (May 2001): 99-106.

344. Palmer, JR, L Rosenberg, RS Rao, A Zauber, BL Strom, ME Warshauser et al. "Induced and Spontaneous Abortion in Relation to Risk of Breast Cancer (United States)." *Cancer Causes And Control* 8 (1997): 841-9.

345. Pantelakis SN, Papadimitriou GC and Doxiadis SA. "Influence of Induced and Spontaneous Abortions on the Outcome of Subsequent Pregnancies." *American Journal of Obstetrics and Gynecology* 116, no. 6 (July 1973): 799-805.

346. Papaevangelou G, Vrettos AS, Papadatos C and Alexiou D. "The Effect of Spontaneous and Induced Abortion on Prematurity and Birthweight." *Journal of Obstetrics Gynaecology of the British Commonwealth* 80, no. 5 (May 1973): 410-22.

347. Parazzini F, Ferraroni M, Tozzi L, Ricci E, Mezzopane R and LaVecchia C. "Induced Abortions and Risk of Ectopic Pregnancy." *Human Reproduction* 10, no. 7 (July 1995): 1841-4.

348. Parazzini F, LaVecchia C and Negri E. "Spontaneous and Induced Abortion and Risk of Breast Cancer." *International Journal of Cancer* 48, no. 6 (30 July 1991): 816-20.

349. Parker B, McFarlane J and Soeken K. "Abuse During Pregnancy: Effects on Maternal Complications and Birth Weight in Adult and Teenage Women." *Obstetrics & Gynecology* 84, no. 3 (September 1994): 323-8.

350. Parkins, T. "Does Abortion Increase Breast Cancer Risk?" *Journal of the National Cancer Institute* 85, no. 24 (15 December 1993): 1987-88.

351. Parthun M, Kiss A, Morris H and Williams L. *Abortion's Aftermath*. 2nd ed. Toronto: Human Life Research Institute, 1987.

352. Peppers LG. "Grief and Elective Abortion: Breaking the Emotional Bond?" *Omega-Journal of Death and Dying* 18, no. 1 (1987-1988): 1-12.

353. "Personal Stories." In *Post-Abortion Aftermath*, ed. Michael T. Mannion, 164-83. Kansas City, MO: Sheed and Ward, 1994.

354. Pickering R, Deeks J. "Risks of Delivery During the 20th to the 36th Week of Gestation." *International Journal of Epidemiology* 20, no. 2 (June 1991): 456-66.

355. Pickering RM and Forbes JF. "Risks of Preterm Delivery and Small-for-Gestational Age Infants Following Abortion: A Population Study." *British Journal of Obstetrics and Gynaecology* 92, no. 11 (November 1985): 1106-12.

356. Pierce, Lindy. "Abortion Attitudes and Experiences in a Group of Male Prisoners." *Newsletter of the Association for Interdisciplinary Research in Values and Social Change* 6, no. 2 (January/February 1994): 1-8.

357. Pike MC, Henderson BE, Casagrande JT, Rosario I and Gray GE. "Oral Contraceptive Use and Early Abortion As Risk Factors for Breast Cancer in Young Women." *British Journal of Cancer* 43, no. 1 (January 1981): 72-6.

358. Pike MC and Spicer DV. "The Chemoprevention of Breast Cancer by Reducing Sex Steroid Exposure: Perspectives From Epidemiology." *Journal of Cellular Biochemistry Suppl* 17G (1993): 26-36.

359. Pike MC, Spicer DV, Dahmoush L and Press MF. "Estrogens, Progestogens, Normal Breast Cell Proliferation, and Breast Cancer Risk [Review]." *Epidemiologic Reviews* 15, no. 1 (1993): 17-35.

360. Planned Parenthood Federation of America. "The Emotional Effects of Induced Abortion." [http://www.plannedparenthood.org/library/facts/emot-eff_010600.html]. May 2000.

361. Potts M. "Legal Abortion in Eastern Europe." *Eugenics Review* 59, no. 4 (December 1967): 232-50.

362. Qvigstad E, Skaug K, Jerve F, Fylling P and Ulstrup JC. "Pelvic Inflammatory Disease Associated with Chlamydia Trachomatis Infection after Therapeutic Abortion. A Prospective Study." *British Journal of Venereal Disease* 59, no. 3 (June 1983): 189-92.

363. Radestad A, Bui T, Nygren K, et al. "The Utilization Rate and Pregnancy Outcome of Multifetal Pregnancy Reduction in the Nordic Countries." *Acta Obstetricia et Gynecologica Scandanavica* 75, no. 7 (August 1996): 651-3.

364. Raphael, B. *The Anatomy of Bereavement*. New York: Basic Books, 1983.

365. Rayburn WF, Barr M Jr. "The Manformed Fetus: Diagnosis and Pregnancy Management." *Obstetrics and Gynecology Annual* 14 (1985): 112-26.

References

366. Rayburn W, Laferla J. "Mid-Gestational Abortion for Medical or Genetic Indications." *Clinical Obstetrics & Gynecology* 13, no. 1 (March 1986): 71-82.

367. Reardon D. *Aborted Women Silent No More* Chicago: Loyola University Press, 1987.

368. Reardon DC and Ney PG. "Abortion and Subsequent Substance Abuse." *American Journal of Drug and Alcohol Abuse* 26, no. 1 (February 2000): 61-75.

369. Reardon DC, Ney PG, Scheuren FJ, Cougle JR, Coleman PK and Strahan TW. "Suicide Deaths Associated with Pregnancy Outcome A Record Linkage Study of 173,279 Low Income American Women." *Archives of Women's Mental Health* 3, no. (4)Suppl 2 (2001): 104.

370. Reardon, David. "The Abortion/Suicide Connection." *The Post-Abortion Review* 1, no. 2 (Summer 1993): 1-2.

371. _____. "Substance Abuse Subsequent to Abortion", 4 November 1994. Presented to the Society of Catholic Social Scientists, Second Annual Conference.

372. Reardon, David C. "Abortion Risk Factors: An Avenue for New Pro-Life/Pro-Woman Laws." In Life and Learning IX: *Proceedings of Ninth University Faculty for Life Conference in Trinity International University, Deerfield Illinois*, ed. J. Koterski, SJ, 25-40. Washington, D.C.: University Faculty for Life, 2000.

373. Reardon, David C. and Cougle, JR. : "Depression and Unintended Pregnancy in the National Longitudinal Survey of Youth: A Cohort Study." *British Medical Journal* 324, no. 7330 (19 January 2002): 151-2.

374. Redmond, Marcia A. "Attitudes of Adolescent Males Toward Adolescent Pregnancy and Fatherhood." *Family Relations: Journal of Applied Family & Child Studies*. 34, no. 3 (July 1985): 337-42.

375. Reisser, Teri. "The Effects of Abortion on Marriage and Other Committed Relationships." *Newsletter of the Association for Interdisciplinary Research in Values and Social Change* 6, no. 4 (May/June 1994): 1-8.

376. Reist, Melinda Tankard. *Giving Sorrow Words: Women's Stories of Grief After Abortion*. Sydney: Duffy and Snelgrove, 2000.

377. Remennick LI. "Induced Abortion as Cancer Risk Factor: A Review of Epidemiological Evidence." *Journal of Epidemiology And Community Health* 44, no. 4 (December 1990): 259-64.

378. _____. "Reproductive Patterns and Cancer Incidence in Women: A Population-Based Correlation Study in the USSR." *International Journal of Epidemiology* 18, no. 3 (September 1989): 498-510

379. Rich V. "Breast Cancer in Lithuania." *The Lancet* 344 (1994): 947.

380. Richardson JA, Dixon G. "Effects of Legal Termination on Subsequent Pregnancy." *British Medical Journal* 1, no. 6021 (29 May 1976): 1303-4.379.

381 Ries LAG, Kosary CL, Hankey BF, et al. eds. *SEER Cancer Statistics Review*, 1973-1996. Bethesda, Maryland: National Cancer Institute, 1999.

382. Robertson, Gerald B. and Ellen I. Picard. *Legal Liability of Doctors and Hospitals*. 3rd ed. Toronto: Carswell, 1996.

383. Rock JA and Murphy AA. "Anatomic Abnormalities." *Clinical Obstetrics & Gynecology* 29, no. 4 (December 1986): 886-911.

384. Rock J, Parmley T, Murphy A, Jones H Jr. "Malposition of the Ovary Associated with Uterine Anomalies." *Fertility and Sterility* 45, no. 4 (April 1986): 561-3.

385. Rogers JL, Stoms GB and Phifer JL. "Psychological Impact of Abortion: Methodological and Outcomes Summary of Empirical Research Between 1966 and 1988." *Health Care for Women International* 10, no. 4 (1989): 34-776.

386. Rookus MA and van Leeuwen FE. "Induced Abortion and Risk of Breast Cancer: Reporting (Recall) Bias in a Dutch Case-Control Study." *Journal of the National Cancer Institute* 88, no. 23 (4 December 1996): 1759-64.

387. Rooney B. "Elective Surgery Boosts Cerebral Palsy Risk [Letter]." *European Journal of Obstetrics & Gynecology and Reproductive Biology* 96, no. 2 (2001): 739-40.

388. Rose GL and Chapman MG. "Aetiological Factors in Placenta Praevia-- A Case Controlled Study." *British Journal of Obstetrics and Gynaecology* 93, no. 6 (June 1986): 586-8.

389. Rosenberg L, Palmer JR, Kaufman D, Strom BL, Schottenfeld D, Shapiro S. "Breast Cancer in Relation to the Occurrence and Time of Induced and Spontaneous Abortion." *American Journal of Epidemiology* 127, no. 5 (May 1988): 981-9.

390. Rosenberg L. "Induced Abortion and Breast Cancer:More Scientific Data Are Needed." *Journal of the National Cancer Institute* 86, no. 21 (2 November 1994): 1569-70.

391. Rosenfeld JA. "Emotional Responses to Therapeutic Abortion." *American Family Physician* 45, no. 1 (January 1992): 137-40.

392. Rothman, Barbara Katz. *The Tentative Pregnancy: How Amniocentesis Changes the Experience of Motherhood*. Revised ed. New York: W.W. Norton, 1993.

393. Rothstein A. "Abortion: A Dyadic Perspective." *American Journal of Orthopsychiatry* 47, no. 1 (January 1977): 111-8.

394. Rothstein AA. "Men's Reactions to Their Partners' Elective Abortions." *American Journal of Obstetrics and Gynecology* 128, no. 8 (15 Aug 1977): 831-7.

395. Royal College of Obstetricians and Gynaecologists. *Evidence-Based Guideline No. 7: The Care of Women Requesting Induced Abortion.* London, April 2000.

396. Rue V. *Postabortion Trauma.* Life Dynamics, 1994.

397. Rue, V. "The Psychological Realities of Induced Abortion." In *Post-Abortion Aftermath*, ed. M Mannion, 5-43. Kansas City: Sheed and Ward, 1994.

398. Ruiz-Velasco V, Gonzalez Alfani G, Pliego Sanchez L and Alamillo Vera M. "Endometrial Pathology and Infertility." *Fertility and Sterility* 67, no. 4 (April 1997): 687-92.

399. Russo J and Russo IH. "Susceptibility of the Mammary Gland to Carcinogenesis. II. Pregnancy Interruption as a Risk Factor in Tumor Incidence." *American Journal of Pathology* 100, no. 2 (August 1980): 497-512.

400. Ryan IJ and Dunn PC. "College Students' Attitudes Toward Shared Responsibility in Decisions About Abortion: Implications for Counseling." *Journal of American College Health* 31, no. 6 (June 1983): 231-5.

401. Sawaya GF, Grady D, Kerlikowske K and Grimes DA. "Antibiotics at the Time of Induced Abortion: The Case for Universal Prophylaxis Based on a Meta-Analysis." *Obstetrics & Gynecology* 87, no. (5 pt 2) (May 1996): 884-90.

402. Schenker JG. "Etiology of and Therapeutic Approach to Synechia Uteri." *European Journal of Obstetrics & Gynecology and Reproductive Biology* 65, no. 1 (March 1996): 109-13.

403. Schreiner-Engel P, Walther VN, Mindes J, Lynch L and Berkowitz RL. "First-Trimester Multifetal Pregnancy Reduction: Acute and Persistent Psychologic Reactions." *American Journal of Obstetrics and Gynecology* 172, no. (2 Pt 1) (February 1995): 541-7.

404. Schwartz SM, Weiss NS, Daling JR, Newcomb PA, Liff JM, Gammon MD, et al. "Incidence of Histologic Types of Uterine Sarcoma in Relation to Menstrual and Reproductive History." *International Journal of Cancer* 49, no. 3 (30 September 1991): 362-7.

405. Segi M, Fukushima I, Fujisaku S, Kurihara M, Saito S, Asano K, et al. "An Epidemiological Study of Cancer in Japan. *GANN* 48, no. Supplement (April 1957): 1-43.

406. Seller M, Barnes C, Ross S, Barby T and Cowmeadow P. "Grief and Mid-Trimester Fetal Loss." *Prenatal Diagnosis* 13, no. 5 (May 1993): 341-8.

407. Sen, Amartya. "More Than 100 Million Women Are Missing." *New York Review of Books*, 20 December 1990, 61-6.

408. Shaver, Jessica. *Gianna: Aborted ... And Lived to Tell About It.* Colorado Springs, CO: Focus on the Family Publishing, 1995.

409. Sherman, David H., Nathan Mandelman, Thomas D. Kerenyi and Jonathan Scher. "The Abortion Experience in Private Practice." In *Women and Loss: Psychobiological Perspectives*, eds. William Finn, Margot Tallmer, Irene Seeland, Austin H. Kutscher and Elizabeth Clark, 98-107. New York: Praeger, 1985.

410. Shimizu M and Nakayama M. "Endometrial Ossification in a Postmenopausal Woman." *Journal of Clinical Pathology* 50, no. 2 (February 1997): 171-2.

411. Shiono PH and Klebanoff MA. "Ethnic Differences in Preterm and Very Preterm Delivery." *American Journal of Public Health* 76, no. 11 (November 1986): 1317-21.

412. Shostak, Arthur B, Gary. Mclouth and Lynn Seng. *Men and Abortion: Lessons, Losses, and Love.* New York: Praeger, 1984.

413. Shostak, Arthur B. "Abortion as Fatherhood Lost: Problems and Reforms." *The Family Coordinator* (October 1979): 569-74.

414. Shulman, LP. "Pregnancy Termination Procedures." In *Essentials of Prenatal Diagnosis*, eds. Joe Leigh Simpson and Sherman Elias, eds. New York: Churchill Livingston, 1993.

415. Shusterman LR. "Predicting the Psychological Consequences of Abortion." *Social Science and Medicine* 13A, no. 6 (November 1979): 683-9.

416. Sihvo S, Hemminki E, Kosunen E and Koponen P. "Quality of Care in Abortion Services in Finland." *Acta Obstetricia et Gynecologica Scandanavica* 77, no. 2 (February 1998): 210-7.

417. Silber T. "Abortion in Adolescence: The Ethical Dimension." *Adolescence* 15, no. 58 (1980 Summer): 461-74.

418. Silverman, Anna and Arnold Silverman. *The Case Against Having Children.* New York: David McKay Company, 1971.

References

419. Silvestre L, Dubois C, Renault M, Rezvani Y, Baulieu EE and Ulmann A. "Voluntary Interruption of Pregnancy with Mifepristone (RU 486) and a Prostaglandin Analogue. A Large-Scale French Experience." *New England Journal of Medicine* 322, no. 10 (8 March 1990). 645 0.

420. Singer, Eleanor. "Public Attitudes Toward Fetal Diagnosis and the Termination of Life." *Social Indicators Research* 28 (1993): 117-36.

421. Slater PE, Davies AM and Harlap S. "The Effect of Abortion Method on the Outcome of Subsequent Pregnancy." *Journal Of Reproductive Medicine* 26, no. 3 (March 1981): 123-8.

422. Smith GM, Stubblefield PG, Chirchirillo L and McCarthy MJ. "Pain of First-Trimester Abortion: Its Quantification and Relations with Other Variables." *American Journal of Obstetrics and Gynecology* 133, no. 5 (March 1979): 489-98.

423. Soderberg H, Andersson C, Janzon L and Sjoberg NO. "Continued Pregnancy Among Abortion Applications. A Study of Women Having a Change of Mind." *Acta Obstetricia et Gynecologica Scandanavica* 76, no. 10 (November 1997): 942-7.

424. _____. "Selection Bias in a Study on How Women Experienced Induced Abortion." *European Journal of Obstetrics & Gynecology and Reproductive Biology* 77, no. 1 (March 1998): 67-70.

425. Somerville SW. "Does Abortion Increase the Risk of Breast Cancer?" *Journal of the Medical Association of Georgia* 83, no. 4 (April 1994): 209-10.

426. Sorensen JL, Thranov I, Hoff G, Dirach J and Damsgaard MT. "A Double-Blind Randomized Study of the Effect of Erythromycin in Preventing Pelvic Inflammatory Disease after First Trimester Abortion." *British Journal of Obstetrics and Gynaecology* 99, no. 5 (May 1992): 434-8.

427. Sorensen JL, Thranov IR and Hoff GE. "[Genital Chlamydia Trachomatis Infection in Abortion Seekers. Strategy of Examination and Treatment in Order to Reduce the Sequelae of the Infection]. [Article in Danish]." *Ugeskr Laeger* 154, no. 44 (26 October 1992): 3047-53.

428. Sorensen, Jl, I Thranov, G Hoff and Dirach J. "Early and Late-Onset Pelvic Inflammatory Disease Among Women with Cervical Chlamydia Trachomatis Infection at the Time of Induced Abortion - A Follow-Up Study." *Infection* 22, no. 4 (1994): 242-6.

429. Souter I and Goodwin TM. "Decision Making in Multifetal Pregnancy Reduction for Triplets." *American Journal of Perinatology* 15, no. 1 (January 1998): 63-71.

430. Speckhard, Anne C and Vincent M Rue. "Postabortion Syndrome: An Emerging Public Health Concern." *The Journal of Social Issues* 48 (Fall 1992): 95-119.

315

431. Speckhard, Anne. *The Psycho-Social Aspects of Stress Following Abortion.* Kansas City, MO: Sheed & Ward, 1987.

432. Steier A and Bergsjo P. "[Failed Induced Abortion. Pregnancy Continuing After Induced Abortion]." *Tidsskr Nor Laegeforen.* 112, no. 19 (20 August 1992): 2538-40.

433. Stewart DR, Overstreet JW, Nakajima ST and Lasley BL. "Enhanced Ovarian Steroid Secretion Before Implantation in Early Human Pregnancy." *Journal of Clinical Endocrinology and Metabolism* 76, no. 6 (June 1993): 1470-6.

434. Stotland NL. "The Myth of the Abortion Trauma Syndrome." *Journal of the American Medical Association* 268, no. 15 (21 October 1992): 2078-9.

435. Strahan TW. "Induced Abortion as a Contributing Factor in Maternal Mortality or Pregnancy-Related Death in Women." *Association for Research in Values and Social Change, Research Bulletin* 10, no. 3 (Nov/Dec 1996): 1-8.

436. Strahan, T. "African-Americans and Induced Abortion." *Newsletter of the Association for Interdisciplinary Research in Values and Social Change* 6, no. 1 (Nov/Dec 1993): 1-8.

437. _____. "Portraits of Post-Abortive Fathers Devastated by the Abortion Experience." *Newsletter of the Association for Interdisciplinary Research in Values and Social Change* 7, no. 3 (Nov/Dec 1994): 1-8.

438. Stubblefield PG. "Control of Pain for Women Undergoing Abortion." *International Journal of Obstetrics and Gynecology, Supplement 3* (1989): 131-4.

439. Suprapto K and Reed S. "Naproxen Sodium for Pain Relief in First-Trimester Abortion." *American Journal of Obstetrics and Gynecology* 150, no. 8 (15 December 1984): 1000-1.

440. "Survey of Canadian Physicians on Women's Health after Induced Abortion", 1997. The deVeber Institute for Bioethics and Social Research.

441. Sutton, Philip M. "Fathers, Become Who You Are!: Confronting the Cultures of Fatherlessness and Restoring a Culture of Fatherhood", 11 October 1997. First Presented at the Annual Meeting of the Society of Catholic Social Scientists, October, 1996

442. Sykes, P. "Complications of Termination of Pregnancy: A Retrospective Study of Admissions to Christchurch Women's Hospital 1989 and 1990." *New Zealand Medical Journal* 106, no. 951 (10 March 1993): 83-5.

443. Tabsh KM. "A Report of 131 Cases of Multifetal Pregnancy Reduction." *Obstetrics & Gynecology* 82, no. 1 (July 1993): 57-60.

444. Talamani, R, S Franceschi, C LaVecchia, E Negri, L Borsa, M. Montella, et al. "The Role of Reproductive and Menstrual Factors in Cancer of the Breast Before and After Menopause." *European Journal of Cancer* 32A, no. 2 (1996): 303-10.

445. Tamburrino MB, Franco KN, Campbell NB, Pentz JE, Evans CL and Jurs SG. "Postabortion Dysphoria and Religion." *Southern Medical Journal* 83, no. 7 (July 1990): 736-8.

446. Tavani, A, C LaVecchia, Franceschi S, E Negri, B D'Avano, A Decarli, et al. "Abortion and Breast Cancer Risk." *International Journal of Cancer* 65 (1996): 401-5.

447. Taylor VM, Kramer MD, Vaughan TL and Peacock S. "Placental Previa in Relation to Induced and Spontaneous Abortion: A Population-Based Study." *Obstetrics & Gynecology* 82, no. 1 (July 1993): 88-91.

448. Teichman Y, Shenhar S and Segal S. "Emotional Distress in Israeli Women Before and After Abortion." *American Journal of Orthopsychiatry* 63, no. 2 (April 1993): 277-88.

449. Thomas T and Tori CD. "Sequelae of Abortion and Relinquishment of Child Custody Among Women with Major Psychiatric Disorders." *Psychological Reports* 84, no. (3 Pt 1) (June 1999): 773-90.

450. Thorn, Vicki. "Project Rachel: Faith in Action, A Ministry of Compassion and Caring." In *Post-Abortion Aftermath*, ed. M Mannion, 144-63. Kansas City, MO: Sheed and Ward, 1994.

451. Timor-Tritsch IE, Peisner DB, Monteagudo A, Lerner JP and Sharma S. "Multifetal Pregnancy Reduction by Transvaginal Puncture: Evaluation of the Technique Used in 134 Cases." *American Journal of Obstetrics and Gynecology* 168, no. (3 Pt 1) (March 1993): 799-804.

452. Tishler CL. "Adolescent Suicide Attempts Following Elective Abortion: A Special Case of Anniversary Reaction." *Pediatrics* 68, no. 5 (November 1981): 670-1.

453. Tornbom M, Ingelhammar E, Lilja H, Moller A and Svanberg B. "Repeat Abortion: A Comparative Study." *Journal of Psychosomatic Obstetrics and Gynecology* 17, no. 4 (December 1996): 208-14.

454. Tornbom M, Ingelhammar E, Lilja H, Svanberg B and Moller A. "Decision-Making About Unwanted Pregnancy." *Acta Obstetricia et Gynecologica Scandanavica* 78, no. 7 (August 1999): 636-41.

455. Tornbom M and Moller A. "Repeat Abortion: A Qualitative Study." *Journal of Psychosomatic Obstetrics and Gynecology* 20, no. 1 (March 1999): 21-30.

456. Torne A, Jou P, Pagano R, Sanchez I, Ordi J and Vanrell JA. "Endometrial Ossification Successfully Treated by Hysteroscopic Resection." *European Journal of Obstetrics & Gynecology and Reproductive Biology* 66, no. 1 (May 1996): 75-7.

457. Torre-Bueno, Ava. *Peace After Abortion*. San Diego, California: Pimpernel Press, 1997.

458. Trost, JE. "Abortions in Relation to Age, Coital Frequency, and Fecundity." *Archives of Sexual Behavior* 15, no. 6 (December 1986): 505-9.

459. Trott E, Ziegler W and Levey J. "Major Complications Associated with Termination of a Second Trimester Pregnancy: A Case Report." *Delaware Medical Journal* 67, no. 5 (May 1995): 294-6.

460. Tuomivaara L and Kauppila A. "Ectopic Pregnancy: A Case-Control Study of Aetiological Risk Factors." *Archives of Gynecology and Obstetrics* 243, no. 1 (1988): 511.

461. _____. "Radical or Conservative Surgery for Ectopic Pregnancy? A Followup Study of Fertility of 323 Patients." *Fertility and Sterility* 50, no. 4 (October 1988): 5803.

462. Turell Susan C, Armsworth Mary W and Gaa John P. "Emotional Response to Abortion: A Critical Review of the Literature." *Women & Therapy* 9, no. 4 (1990): 49-68.

463. UK Multicentre Trial. "The Efficacy and Tolerance of Mifepristone and Prostaglandin in First Trimester Termination of Pregnancy." *British Journal of Obstetrics and Gynaecology* 97, no. 6 (June 1990): 480-6.

464. van der Slikke JW and Treffers PE. "Influence of Induced Abortion on Gestational Duration in Subsequent Pregnancies." *British Medical Journal* 1, no. 6108 (4 February 1978): 270-2.

465. Vargas FR, Schuler-Faccini L, Brunoni D, Kim C, Meloni VF, Sugayama SM, Albano L, et al. "Prenatal Exposure to Misoprostol and Vascular Disruption Defects: A Case-Control Study." *American Journal of Medical Genetics* 95, no. 4 (11 December 2000): 302-6.

466. Vaughan H. *Canonical Variates of Post Abortion Syndrome*. Portsmouth, N.H.: Institute for Abortion Recovery and Research, 1991.

467. Vaughan, Helen P. "Canonical Variates of Postabortion Syndrome." Doctoral Dissertation, University of North Carolina at Greensboro, 1990.

468. Wadhera S and Millar WJ. "Marital Status and Abortion." *Health Reports* 9, no. 3 (Winter, 1997): 19-26.

469. _____. "Second Trimester Abortions: Trends and Medical Complications." *Health Reports* 6, no. 4 (1994): 441-54.

470. Wadhera, S and WJ Millar. Teenage Pregnancies, 1974 to 1994." *Health Reports* 9, no. 3 (Winter, 1997): 9-17.

471. Walker in JD, Kirby P and Dai Dia M. "Psychosocial Sequelae of Therapeutic Abortion in Young Unmarried Women." *Archives of General Psychiatry* 27, no. 6 (December 1972): 828-32.

472. Washington AE, Johnson RE and Sanders LL Jr. "Chlamydia Trachomatis Infections in the United States. What Are They Costing Us?" *Journal of the American Medical Association* 257, no. 15 (April 1987): 2070-2.

473. Watanabe H and Hirayama T. [Epidemiology and Clinical Aspects of Breast Cancer]." *Nippon Rinsho* 26, no. 8 (August 1968): 1843-9.

474. Webster J, Chandler J and Battistutta D. "Pregnancy Outcomes and Health Care Use: Effects of Abuse." *American Journal of Obstetrics and Gynecology* 174, no. 2 (February 1996): 760-7.

475. Webster, Harriet. *Family Secrets: How Telling and Not Telling Affect Our Children, Our Relationships, and Our Lives.* Reading, Mass.: Addison-Wesley, 1991.

476. Weed DL and Kramer BS. "Induced Abortion, Bias, and Breast Cancer: Why Epidemiology Hasn't Reached Its Limit." *Journal of the National Cancer Institute* 88, no. 23 (4 December 1996): 1698-700.

477. Weiner, Anita H and Eugene C Weiner. "The Aborted Sibling Factor: A Case Study." *Clinical Social Work Journal* 12, no. 3 (Fall 1984): 209-15.

478. Weinstein L, Morris MB, Dotters D and Christian CD. "Ectopic Pregnancy–a New Surgical Epidemic." *Obstetrics & Gynecology* 61, no. 6 (June 1983): 698-701.

479. Wells N. "Management of Pain During Abortion." *Journal of Advanced Nursing* 14, no. 1 (January 1989): 56-62.

480. _____. "Pain and Distress During Abortion." *Health Care for Women International* 12, no. 3 (July/Sept 1991): 293-302.

481. _____. "Reducing Distress During Abortion: A Test of Sensory Information." *Journal of Advanced Nursing* 17, no. 9 (September 1992): 1050-6.

482. Westergaard L, Philipsen T and Scheibel J. "Significance of Cervical Chlamydia Trachomatis Infection in Postabortal Pelvic Inflammatory Disease." *Obstetrics & Gynecology* 60, no. 3 (September 1982): 322-5.

483. Westrom L. "Clinical Manifestations and Diagnosis of Pelvic Inflammatory Disease." *Journal of Reproductive Medicine* 28, no. 10 Supplement (October 1983): 703-8.

484. White-van Mourik MC, Connor JM and Ferguson-Smith MA. "The Psychosocial Sequelae of a Second-Trimester Termination of Pregnancy for Fetal Abnormality." *Prenatal Diagnosis* 12, no. 3 (March 1992): 189-204.

485. White-Van Mourik MC, Connor JM and Ferguson-Smith MA. "The Psychosocial Sequelae of a Second Trimester Termination of Pregnancy for Fetal Abnormality Over a Two Year Period." *Birth Defects Original Article Series* 28, no. 1 (1992): 61-74.

486. White E, Malone KE, Weiss NS and Daling JR. "Breast Cancer Among Young U.S. Women in Relation to Oral Contraceptive Use." *Journal of the National Cancer Institute* 86, no. 7 (6 April 1994): 505-14.

487. Whittemore AS, Harris R and Itnyre J. "Characteristics Relating to Ovarian Cancer Risk: Collaborative Analysis of 12 US Case-Control Studies. II. Invasive Epithelial Ovarian Cancers in White Women. Collaborative Ovarian Cancer Group." *American Journal of Epidemiology* 136, no. 10 (15 November 1992): 1184-203.

488. Wiebe E.R. "Comparing Abortion Induced with Methotrexate and Misoprostol to Methotrexate Alone." *Contraception* 59, no. 1 (January 1999): 7-10.

489. _____. "Oral Methotrexate Compared with Injected Methotrexate When Used with Misoprostol for Abortion." *American Journal of Obstetrics and Gynecology* 181, no. 1 (July 1999): 149-52.

490. Wiebe ER and Rawling M. "Pain Control in Abortion." *International Journal of Gynaecology and Obstetrics* 50, no. 1 (July 1995): 41-6.

491. Wiebe ER, Rawling M and Janssen P. "Comparison of 0.5% and 1.0% Lidocaine for Abortions." *International Journal of Gynaecology and Obstetrics* 55, no. 1 (October 1996): 71-2.

492. Wiebe ER. "Abortion Induced with Methotrexate and Misoprostol." *Canadian Medical Association Journal* 154, no. 2 (15 January 1996): 165-70.

493. Wiebe, ER. "Comparison of the Efficacy of Different Local Anesthetics and Techniques of Local Anesthesia in Therapeutic Abortions." *American Journal of Obstetrics and Gynecology* 167, no. 1 (July 1992): 131-4.

494. Wilmoth Gregory H, Martin de Alteriis and Bussell Danielle. Prevalence of Psychological Risks Following Legal Abortion in the U.S.: Limits of the Evidence." *Journal of Social Issues* 48, no. 3 (Fall 1992): 37-66.

495. Wingo PA, Bolden S, Tong T, Parker SL, Martin LM and Heath CW Jr. "Cancer Statistics for African Americans, 1996." *CA - A Cancer Journal for Clinicians* 46, no. 2 (March-April 1996): 113-25.

496. Wingo PA, Newsome K, Marks JS, Calle EE and Parker SL. "The Risk of Breast Cancer Following Spontaneous or Induced Abortion [Review]." *Cancer Causes and Control* 8, no. 81 (January 1997): 93-108.

497. Wong TW, Lau CC, Yeung A, Lo L and Tai CM. "Efficacy of Transabdominal Ultrasound Examination in the Diagnosis of Early Pregnancy Complications in an Emergency Department." *Journal of Accidental and Emergency Medicine* 15, no. 3 (May 1998): 155-8.

498. World Health Organisation Task Force on Post-ovulatory Methods of Fertility Regulation. "Termination of Pregnancy with Reduced Doses of Mifepristone." *British Medical Journal* 307, no. 6903 (28 August 1993): 532-7.

499. World Health Organization. *International Statistical Classification of Diseases and Related Health Problems, Tenth Revision (ICD-10)*. Geneva, Switzerland: 1992.

500. Wu AH, Ziegler RG, Pike MC, Nomura AMY, West DW, Kolonel LN, et al. "Menstrual and Reproductive Factors and Risk of Breast Cancer in Asian-Americans." *British Journal of Cancer* 73, no. 5 (March 1996): 680-6.

501. Wyatt, Gail E, Donald Guthrie and Cindy M Notgrass. "Differential Effects of Women's Child Sexual Abuse and Subsequent Sexual Revictimization." *Journal of Consulting and Clinical Psychology* 60, no. 2 (April 1992): 167-73.

502. Zeanah CH, Dailey JV, Rosenblatt MJ and Saller DN Jr. "Do Women Grieve after Terminating Pregnancies Because of Fetal Anomalies? A Controlled Investigation." *Obstetrics & Gynecology* 82, no. 2 (August 1993): 270-5.

503. Zhou W, Sorensen HT, Olsen J. "Induced Abortion and Subsequent Pregnancy Duration." *Obstetrics & Gynecology* 94, no. 6 (December 1999): 948-53.

504. Zlatnik FJ, Burmeister LF, Feddersen DA and Brown RC. "Radiological Appearance of the Upper Cervical Canal in Women with a History of Premature Delivery II. Relationship to Clinical Presentation and to Tests of Cervical Compliance." *Journal of Reproductive Medicine* 34, no. 8 (August 1989): 525-30.

505. Zolese G and Blacker CV. "The Psychological Complications of Therapeutic Abortion." *British Journal of Psychiatry*, no. 160 (June 1992): 742-9.

506. Zoricic D, Ambrozic B and Peric D. "[A Fetal Bone As a Foreign Body in the Uterus][Article in Serbo-Croatian (Roman)]." *Lijec Vjesn* 116, no. 11-12 (November-December 1994): 298-300.

# Addendum

Abbott J, Emmans LS, Lowenstein SR. Ectopic Pregnancy: ten common pitfalls in diagnosis. American Journal of Emergency Medicine 1990;8:515-22

Erlandsson G, Montgomery SM, Cnattingius S, Ekbom A. Abortions and breast cancer: a record-based case-control study. *International Journal of Cancer* 2003;103:676-9

"Hungary," 2001, in Demographic Yearbook, 2001 ed., on line, Council of Europe. Available at http://www.coe.int/t/e/social%5fcohesion/population/demographic%5fyear%5Fbook/2001_Edition/Hungary%202001.asp.

Gentles I. In the matter of child care, Canada could learn from Poland. *The Report* 2000 (9 October 2000), p. 46.

Goldacre MJ, Kurina LM, Seagroatt V, Yeates. Abortion and breast cancer: a case-control record linkage study. *Journal of Epidemiology and Community Health* 2001;55:336-7.

Henriet L, Kaminski, M. Impact of induced abortions on subsequent pregnancy outcome: The 1995 French national perinatal survey. *British Journal of Obstetrics and Gynaecology* 2001;108:1036-1042.

Kitchen WH, Richards, A, Ryan, MM, et al. A longitudinal study of the very-low-birth-weight infants. II Results of a controlled trial of intensive care and incidence of handicaps. *Develop Med Child Neurol* 1979;21:582-589

Mahue-Giangreco M, Ursin G, Sullivan-Halley J, Bernstein L. Induced abortion, miscarriage, and breast cancer risk of young women. *Cancer Epidemiology Biomark Prevention* 2003;12:209-14.

Martin JA, Hamilton BE, Ventura SJ, Menacker F, Park MM, Sutton PD. Births: Final Data for 2001. National Vital Statistics Reports 2002 December 18;51(2).

Newcomb PA, Mandelson MT. A record-based evaluation of induced abortion and breast cancer risk (United States). *Cancer Causes Control* 2000;11(9):777-811.

Robertson C, Van Den Donk M, Primic-Zakelj, Macfarlane T, Boyle P. The association between induced and spontaneous abortion and risk of breast cancer in Slovenian women aged 25-54. *Breast* 2001;10:291-8.

Rooney, B, Calhoun, BC. Induced abortion and the risk of later premature births. Journal of American Physicians and Surgeons 2003 (summer); 8 (2): 46-49, p. 47.

Sanderson M, Shu X-O, Jin F, Dai Q, Wen WQ, Hui Y, Gao YT, Zheng W. Abortion history and breast cancer risk: results from the Shanghai breast cancer study. *American Journal of Epidemiology* 2000;151(abstract only).

Tenore J. Ectopic Pregnancy. *American Family Physician* 2000 (Feb. 15): 1080-1088

Thorp JM, Hartmann KE, Shadigian E. Long-term physical and psychological health consequences of induced abortion: review of the evidence. *Obstetrical and Gynecological Survey* 2003;58(1):67-79.

Ye Z, Gao DL, Qin Q, Ray RM, Thomas DB. Breast cancer in relation to induced abortions in a cohort of Chinese women. *British Journal of Cancer* 2002; 87(9):977-81.

# Glossary

**amenorrhea** the absence, temporary or permanent, of menstrual periods.

**amniocentesis** a diagnostic procedure in which a small amount of amniotic fluid is withdrawn from the amniotic sac (the membranous bag that surrounds the fetus in the uterus). This fluid can be used for diagnosis of a fetal genetic abnormality by examination of cells shed by the baby into the fluid.

**Asherman's Syndrome** intra-uterine adhesions (scar tissue connecting the inner walls of the uterus), a complication of surgical curettage, as in a D&C or abortion.

**borderline personality disorder** a condition characterized by impulsive and self-destructive behaviors of the kind potentially magnified by abortion.

**carcinogens** any agent capable of causing cancer such as, chemicals and high-energy radiation, including nuclear radiation and X rays.

**cardiomyopathy** any disease of the heart muscle that causes a reduction in the force of heart contractions and a resultant decrease in the efficiency of circulation of blood through the lungs and the rest of the body.

**cervical incompetence** abnormal weakness of the cervix (the neck of the uterus) that can result in recurrent pregnancy loss.

**cervical os**  entrance to the uterus from the cervix.

**cervical resistance**  a stiffness of the neck of the uterus, making it difficult to expand.

**Chlamydia trachomatis**  a strain of chlamydiae (a group of microorganisms that cause infectious diseases in humans and animals) which causes genital infections, including sexually transmitted diseases.

**chorionic villi sampling**  tissue taken from the edge of the placenta and analyzed in the laboratory to diagnose  possible abnormalities in the fetus; sampling of the chorionic villi is a possible alternative to amniocentesis and can be performed earlier in the pregnancy.

**coding**  the way hospitals report patients' diseases or disorders. On discharge, doctors write the diagnosis and hospital clerks categorize it according to a list or code.

**cognitive dissonance**  a term used in psychology referring to the intellectual difficulty in reconciling seemingly contradictory propositions.

**denial**  a psychological term referring to a refusal to acknowledge.

**dilation and curettage (D&C)**  a gynecological procedure in which the lining of the uterus is scraped away to diagnose and treat disorders of the uterus. It can also be used for a first-trimester abortion.

**dilation and evacuation (D&E)**  abortion, specifically in the second trimester, in which the uterine cervix is dilated by instrumentation or medication, to allow the uterine contents, including the embryo or fetus, to be sucked out with a vacuum aspirator.

**dysmenorrhoea**  pain or discomfort during or just before a menstrual period.

**dysphoria** adverse emotional state.

**dyspareunia** pain during sexual intercourse (generally in reference to the woman).

**ectopic pregnancy** a pregnancy that develops outside the uterus, most commonly in the fallopian tube, but sometimes in the ovary or rarely, in the abdominal cavity or cervix; the condition creates a life-threatening situation that requires emergency treatment.

**embolism** the blockage of an artery or vein by a fragment of material (a blood clot, a bubble of air or other gas, or various other substances) traveling in the bloodstream causing heart problems, strokes, or death.

**endometrial adhesions** fibrous scar tissue connecting the inner walls of the uterus, a complication of surgical curettage, as in abortion; Asherman's Syndrome.

**endometrial ossification** see *osseous metaplasia*.

**endometriosis** a condition in which fragments of the endometrium (lining of the uterus) are located in other parts of the body, usually in the pelvic cavity, sometimes leading to infertility.

**endometritis** inflammation of the endometrium due to infection which can be caused by complications after abortion.

**epidemiological** pertaining to disease as it affects groups of people (as opposed to individuals), dealing mainly with epidemics of infectious and non-infectious diseases.

**estradiol** see **oestradiol** and **(maternal) oestradiol**.

**et al.** Latin abbreviation used in scientific notation meaning *and others*.

**Human Genome Project** a multicenter scientific endeavor to map every gene in the human DNA contained within the 46 chromosomes of every human cell.

**hypomenorrhea**  scanty menstrual periods; a reduction in the amount of menstrual flow.

**hysterectomy**  surgical removal of the uterus which can be a form of late-term abortion in pregnant women.

**hysteroscopy**  diagnostic or therapeutic exploration of the uterine cavity with a fiberoptic tube.

**hysterotomy**  opening the uterus, usually with a surgical incision. The best example of this is a Caesarean section to deliver a baby. Now, with early-gestation fetal surgery, surgeons can open up the uterus with a small incision, operate to correct a fetal problem, close up the womb, and allow the balance of the pregnancy to proceed. This procedure can also be used in hospitals and abortion clinics to extract a late-term fetus, thus terminating a woman's pregnancy.

***in vitro* fertilization (IVF)**  a method of treating infertility in which an egg is surgically removed from the ovary and fertilized outside the body. *In vitro* (in glass) refers to the glass Petri dish that is used in the fertilization process.

**induced abortion**  deliberate termination of pregnancy, resulting in destruction of the embryo or fetus, by means of a surgical procedure, pharmaceutical product, or other means.

**intrapartum hemorrhage**  bleeding from the uterus or other parts of the birth canal during the process of labor and/or birth.

**KCl injection** (abortion related)  injection of potassium chloride into the bloodstream, including the heart, in a high enough concentration to cause instant death.

**Laminaria tents**  small stick-like devices which absorb fluid, gradually increasing in size. They are inserted into the cervical os over one or two days to create the expansion necessary to remove a large fetus in a late-term abortion.

**laparoscopic sterilization** obstructing fallopian tubes to prevent fertilization of ovum using small incisions and a fibre optic telescope to direct the instruments

**legal abortion** an induced abortion by a licensed medical practitioner and allowed by law.

**leiomyosarcoma** a cancerous tumor in the smooth muscle of the uterus.

**(maternal) oestradiol** oestradiol is the most important of the estrogen hormones essential for the healthy functioning of the reproductive system. See also **oestradiol, estradiol**.

**medical abortion** is a term used for an abortion that is drug-induced; for example, contractions are induced by introducing a prostaglandin hormone into the uterus.

**menorrhagia** excessive blood loss during menstruation which is caused by a hormone imbalance, fibroids, polyps, an intra-uterine device (IUD), or a pelvic infection.

**meta-analysis** a statistical method in which data from subjects participating in a number of similar experimental trials are combined and analyzed together, in order to increase statistical power. This is a relatively new epidemiological tool accepted at leading epidemiological centers, including those at McMaster University (Canada) and Oxford University (England), and by the prestigious medical journal, *The Lancet.*

**morbidity** the state or condition of being diseased.

**Mullerian tumor** a very rare cancerous tumor of the uterus.

**multifetal pregnancy reduction (MFPR)** termination of one or more fetuses in a multiple-conception pregnancy, usually the result of in vitro fertilization, and achieved by injecting the fetuses with a needle containing potassium chloride (KCl). The dead fetuses remain with the living ones in utero until delivery.

**neonatal hypotension**  low blood pressure in a newborn infant.

**nulliparous (woman)**  a woman who has never borne a child.

**oestradiol**  the most powerful of three female hormones, produced in the ovaries, with small amounts produced in the adrenal glands and testes. It is responsible for the control of menstrual periods and the development of secondary sex characteristics in women.

**osseous metaplasia of the endometrium (endometrial ossification)**  calcium formation in the lining of the wall of the uterus.

**parous (woman)**  a woman who has been pregnant and borne a child.

**pelvic inflammatory disease (PID)**  an infection of the internal female reproductive organs which may be caused by a sexually transmitted disease, other bacteria, an IUD, or after a miscarriage, abortion, or childbirth.

*placenta previa*  the implantation of the placenta in the lower part of the uterus, near or over the cervix.

**post-abortion survivor syndrome**  the symptom complex of one who has suffered psychic trauma from abortion.

**post-abortion morbidity**  disease after an abortion directly related to the abortion procedure.

**post-traumatic stress disorder (PTSD)**  a specific form of delayed anxiety that comes on after a stressful or frightening event.

**prenatal**  a term meaning before birth.

*primigravid* **(woman)**  a woman who is pregnant for the first time.

**prophylactic antibiotics** administration of antibiotics in advance of an anticipated medical procedure that might cause bacterial infection

**prostaglandins** one of a group of fatty acids that is made naturally in the body and acts in a similar way to hormones; some prostaglandins are prepared synthetically for use as drugs.

**recall bias** a term used in psychology referring to a bias in answering questions because, although people generally intend to be truthful, they have trouble recalling things they do not wish to think about or admit to.

**relative risk (RR)** the proportion by which a given procedure or behavior increases or diminishes the risk of contracting a disease where 1.0 is a normal risk.
Thus a relative risk of 0.8 means that the risk is twenty per cent less than normal; a relative risk of 2.0 means that the risk is 100 per cent higher than normal, etc.

**RU-486** mifepristone; a drug used in medical/drug-induced abortion.

**salpingitis** inflammation of the fallopian tube, commonly caused by infection spreading upward from the vagina, cervix, or uterus.

**secondary infertility** inability to conceive after a previous pregnancy.

**sepsis** infection of a wound or body tissues with bacteria that leads to the formation of pus or to the multiplication of the bacteria in the blood.

**sequelae** a condition that results from or follows a disease, a disorder, or an injury; the term, used in its plural form, refers to the resulting complications.

**seroprevalence rate** the prevalence in a population of the occurrence of a certain infectious marker in the blood (i.e., "serum").

**sexually transmitted disease (STD)**  infection transmitted primarily, but not exclusively, by sexual intercourse and sexual touching; can also be transmitted by blood.

**spontaneous abortion**  a medical term for a miscarriage with the loss of a fetus before the end of the twentieth week (in Canada) of pregnancy.

**sublimation**  a psychological mechanism whereby a person diverts their thoughts and feelings about a negative experience.

**surgical abortion**  the most common form of induced abortion, using surgical instruments such as a curette or suction device (aspirator); the method varies with the stage of pregnancy.

**symptomology**  a collection of symptoms of a disease or condition.

**synechia uteri**  uterine adhesions.

**systemic**  affecting the whole body or system.

# Index

331

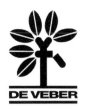

**DE VEBER**

*Need additional copies for business,*
*education, family, or friends?*

**Order NOW as supplies are limited!**
**First Edition sold out FAST!**

# Women's Health after Abortion
## (Second Edition)

*A clear insightful analysis and summary of recent medical evidence*

*Please return completed form with your cheque or money order payable to:*
*The deVeber Institute.*

**Please send me ———— copies**

Name: ————————————————————————

Organization (if applicable): ——————————————————

Street: ————————————————————————

Apartment/Suite: ————————————————————

City/Town: ——————————————————————

Province/State: ————————————————————

Postal Code/Zip Code: ————————————————

Telephone: (    ) ———————— Fax: (    ) ——————————

Email: ————————————————————————

Canadian Orders- $24.95 + $8.00 shipping (Cdn. Funds)
U.S.A. Orders- $19.95 + $8.00 shipping (US Funds)      •Bulk rates on request

*Send to:*
**The deVeber Institute**
**for Bioethics and Social Research**
**3089 Bathurst Street**
**Suite 316**
**Toronto, ON, Canada**
**M6A 2A4**
**Phone: (416) 256-0555    Fax: (416) 256-0611**
**email: bioethics@deveber.org    Web Site: www.deveber.org**

*"Research and Scholarship for an Informed Social Response to Human Life Questions"*

## DATE DUE

| NOV 1 1 2004 | | | |
|---|---|---|---|
| | | | |
| | | | |
| | | | |
| | | | |
| | | | |
| | | | |
| | | | |
| | | | |
| | | | |
| | | | |
| | | | |
| | | | |
| | | | |